Prostaglandins and related substances

a practical approach

TITLES PUBLISHED IN
THE
PRACTICAL APPROACH
SERIES

Affinity chromatography
Animal cell culture
Biochemical toxicology
Biological membranes
Carbohydrate analysis
Centrifugation (2nd Edition)
DNA cloning
Drosophila
Electron microscopy in molecular biology
Gel electrophoresis of nucleic acids
Gel electrophoresis of proteins
H.p.l.c. of small molecules
Human cytogenetics
Human genetic diseases
Immobilised cells and enzymes
Iodinated density-gradient media
Lymphokines and interferons
Microcomputers in biology
Mutagenicity testing
Neurochemistry
Nucleic acid and protein sequence analysis
Nucleic acid hybridisation
Oligonucleotide synthesis
Photosynthesis: energy transduction
Plant cell culture
Plasmids
Spectrophotometry and spectrofluorimetry
Steroid hormones
Teratocarcinomas and embryonic stem cells
Transcription and translation
Virology

Prostaglandins and related substances

a practical approach

Edited by
C Benedetto
Institute of Obstetrics and Gynecology, Università di Torino, Via Ventimiglia 3, Torino 10126, Italy

R G McDonald-Gibson
Department of Biochemistry, Brunel University, Uxbridge, Middlesex UB8 3PH, UK

S Nigam
Department of Gynecological Endocrinology, Prostaglandin Research Laboratories, Klinikum Steglitz, Freie Universität, D-1000 Berlin 45, FRG

T F Slater
Department of Biochemistry, Brunel University, Uxbridge, Middlesex UB8 3PH, UK

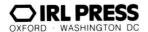
OXFORD · WASHINGTON DC

IRL Press Limited
PO Box 1,
Eynsham,
Oxford OX8 1JJ,
England

British Library Cataloguing in Publication Data

Prostaglandins and related substances : a practical approach.—(Practical
  approach series)
  1. Prostaglandins
  I. Benedetto,C. II. Series
  599.01′927   QP801.P68

ISBN 1-85221-032-X (hardbound)
ISBN 1-85221-031-1 (softbound)

Printed in England by Information Printing, Oxford, England

Preface

The last few years have witnessed an increasing interest in prostaglandins and related substances with respect to many important areas of biology and medicine. The diverse metabolic functions of prostaglandins as second messengers has become firmly established, linking extracellular signals with intracellular events. Moreover, in certain circumstances, some prostaglandins and a number of related substances can exert profound effects in the extracellular milieu and may also influence neighbouring cells; for example, prostacyclin, PGD_2, PGE_2, PAF and lipid hydroperoxides. Indeed the administration of specific prostaglandins is known to be clinically advantageous in certain circumstances, as in obstetrics or in microcirculatory disorders.

Disturbances of prostaglandins and related substances have been identified in many different types of cell injuries and diseases, and these disturbances may be important to the overall metabolic perturbations that occur: for example in inflammation, in hypersensitivity reactions, in asthma, in cancer, etc.

Because of the ever widening interest in prostaglandins and related substances by biological scientists and clinicians we have thought it useful to provide this volume in the Practical Approach series, and cover the main experimental methods used to detect and measure these substances in biological material. In this book, with the help of a considerable number of distinguished experts, we have provided practical outlines on the techniques used to extract prostaglandins, and to measure them using radio-immunoassay, gas-chromatography and mass spectrometry, high pressure liquid chromatography, or bioassay procedures. In addition, there are substantial contributions on lipoxygenases, lipid peroxidation, prostaglandin receptors and platelet activating factor, together with a chapter on prostaglandin metabolism with a critical evaluation of the value of measuring different prostaglandin metabolites.

In assembling this book we have been greatly helped and encouraged by the diligence and enthusiasm of our expert contributors: the book owes its good features to their co-operation. We are also grateful to Miss Jacqueline Boyers and Mrs Eva Gooding of IRL Press who have kept us moving in the right direction, and to Mrs W.Ditschler who has done all of the secretarial work for us from Brunel University.

T.F.Slater
R.McDonald-Gibson
C.Benedetto
S.Nigam

Contributors

S.E.Barrow
Department of Clinical Pharmacology, Royal Postgraduate Medical School, Ducane Road, London W12 0HS, UK

C.Benedetto
Istituto di Ginecologia e Ostetricia, Cattedra A, Università di Torino, Via Ventimiglia 3, 10126 Torino, Italy

J.Benveniste
Inserm U.20, Université Paris-Sud, 32 Rue des Carnets, 92140 Clamart, France

K.H.Cheeseman
Department of Biochemistry, Brunel University, Uxbridge, Middlesex UB8 3PH, UK

R.A.Coleman
Department of Respiratory Pharmacology and Biochemistry, Glaxo Group Research Ltd, Ware, Hertfordshire SG12 0DJ, UK

S.Flatman
Department of Biochemistry, Brunel University, Uxbridge, Middlesex UB8 3PH, UK

E.Granström
Department of Physiological Chemistry, Karolinska Institutet, PO Box 60400, S-10401 Stockholm, Sweden

Y.Hayashi
Department of Biochemistry, Tokushima University School of Medicine, Kuramoto-cho, Tokushima 770, Japan

J.S.Hurst
Department of Biochemistry, Brunel University, Uxbridge, Middlesex UB8 3PH, UK

H.Kindahl
Department of Physiological Chemistry, Karolinska Institutet, PO Box 60400, S-10401 Stockholm, Sweden

H.Kühn
Institut für Physiologische und Biologische Chemie, Bereich Medizin (Charité) der Humboldt-Universität zu Berlin, Hessische Strasse 3 – 4, 104 Berlin, DDR

R.J.Kulmacz
Department of Biological Chemistry, University of Illinois at Chicago, 1853 W.Polk Street, Chicago, IL 60680, USA

M.Kumlin
Department of Physiological Chemistry, Karolinska Institutet, PO Box 60400, S-10401 Stockholm, Sweden

W.E.M.Lands
Department of Biological Chemistry, University of Illinois at Chicago, 1853 W.Polk Street, Chicago, IL 60680, USA

R.G.McDonald-Gibson
Department of Biochemistry, Brunel University, Uxbridge, Middlesex UB8 3PH, UK

S.Nigam
Prostaglandin Research Laboratory, Klinikum Steglitz, Freie Universität Berlin, Hindenburgdamm 30, D-1000 Berlin 45, FRG

P.J.Piper
Department of Pharmacology, Royal College of Surgeons of England, Institute of Basic Medical Sciences, 35 – 43 Lincoln's Inn Fields, London WC2A 3PN, UK

W.S.Powell
Endocrine Laboratory, Royal Victoria Hospital, 687 Pine Avenue West, and Department of Medicine, McGill University, Montreal, Quebec H3A IA1, Canada

S.W.Rapoport
Institut für Physiologische und Biologische Chemie, Bereich Medizin (Charité) der Humboldt-Universität zu Berlin, Hessische Strasse 3 – 4, 104 Berlin, DDR

T.Schewe
Institut für Physiologische und Biologische Chemie, Bereich Medizin (Charité) der Humboldt-Universität zu Berlin, Hessische Strasse 3 – 4, 104 Berlin, DDR

F.Shono
Department of Biochemistry, Tokushima University School of Medicine, Kuramoto-cho, Tokushima 770, Japan

T.F.Slater
Department of Biochemistry, Brunel University, Uxbridge, Middlesex UB8 3PH, UK

G.W.Taylor
Department of Clinical Pharmacology, Royal Postgraduate Medical School, Ducane Road, London W12 0HS, UK

T.Tonai
Department of Biochemistry, Tokushima University School of Medicine, Kuramoto-cho, Tokushima 770, Japan

B.J.R.Whittle
Department of Mediator Pharmacology, Wellcome Research Laboratories, Langley Court, Beckenham, Kent BR3 3BS, UK

S.Yamamoto
Department of Biochemistry, Tokushima University School of Medicine, Kuramoto-cho, Tokushima 770, Japan

K.Yokota
Department of Biochemistry, Tokushima University School of Medicine, Kuramoto-cho, Tokushima 770, Japan

Contents

Abbreviations

13-APA	13-azoprostanoic acid
BDMS	*tert*-butyl-bis-(dimethylsilyl)
BHT	butylated hydroxytoluene
BSA	bovine serum albumin
BSTFA	bis-(trimethylsilyl)trifluoroacetamide
CDI	carbodiimide
c.i.	chemical ionization
CR	concentration ratio
DCC	dextran-coated charcoal
d.c.i.	desorption chemical ionization
DPP	di-4-phloretin phosphate
DEGS	diethylene glycol succinate
d.e.i.	desorption electron impact
DHETE	dihydroxyeicosatetraenoic acid
DMSO	dimethyl sulphoxide
e.i.	electron impact
EIA	enzyme immunoassay
f.a.b.	fast atom bombardment
FID	flame ionization detector
HBSS	Hank's balanced salt sodium
HETE	hydroxyeicosatetraenoic acid
HHT	12-hydroxyheptadecatrienoic acid
HPETE	hydroperoxyeicosatetraenoic acid
KLH	keyhole limpet haemocyanin
LT	leukotriene
LX	lipoxin
MDA	malondialdehyde
n.i.c.i.	negative ion chemical ionization
NSAID	non-steroidal anti-inflammatory drug
ODS	octadecylsilyl
PAF	platelet-activating factor
PEG	polyethylene glycol
PG	prostaglandin
PGI_2	prostacyclin
p.i.c.i.	positive ion chemical ionization
PMNL	polymorphonuclear leukocytes
PPP	platelet-poor plasma
PRP	platelet-rich plasma
PUFAH	polyunsaturated fatty acid
RIA	radioimmunoassay
SRS-A	slow-reacting substance of anaphylaxis
TCA	trichloroacetic acid
TFA	trifluoroacetic acid
THETE	trihydroxyeicosatetraenoic acid
TMPD	N,N,N',N'-tetramethylphenylenediamine
TMS	trimethylsilyl
TX	thromboxane
UFAH	unsaturated fatty acid

CHAPTER 1

Introduction to the eicosanoids

TREVOR F.SLATER and ROBERT G.McDONALD-GIBSON

1. GENERAL BACKGROUND

'Eicosanoids' is the collective name for unsaturated lipids derived from arachidonic acid ($C_{20:4\ n\text{-}6}$), or similar polyunsaturated fatty acid precursors, via the cyclo-oxygenase or lipoxygenase metabolic pathways. This group of compounds includes prostaglandins, thromboxanes, leukotrienes, lipoxins and various hydroxy- and hydro-peroxy-fatty acids.

The term 'prostanoid' relates strictly only to those products of the cyclo-oxygenase pathway that contain the 5-membered cyclopentane ring characteristic of the theoretical parent structure prostanoic acid. As well as the prostaglandins, thromboxanes which contain an oxane ring, are frequently included in the prostanoid group because they are also derived from the cyclo-oxygenase pathway.

The lipoxygenase products, such as leukotrienes, lipoxins and various hydroxy-fatty acids, differ structurally from prostanoids. However, interest in all these compounds centres around their ubiquity, biological activity and the fact that many of them have diverse and potent pharmacological activities that may also be of physiological or pathological significance.

2. NOMENCLATURE, STRUCTURE AND BIOSYNTHESIS

Prostaglandins (PGs) are oxygenated polyunsaturated 20-carbon fatty acids containing a cyclopentane ring, and may be considered chemically as derivatives of the theoretical parent structure prostanoic acid [*Figure 1(1)*]. Each prostaglandin is designated by a letter $A-J$ indicating the nature and position of substituents on the cyclopentane ring and the presence and position of double bonds within the ring [*Figure 1(1)* − *(11)*] and by a numerical subscript (1, 2 or 3) indicating the number of double bonds in the alkyl side chains. Prostaglandins of the 1-series are derived from eicosatrienoic acid ($C_{20:3\ n\text{-}6}$), those of the 2-series from eicosatetraenoic acid (arachidonic acid $C_{20:4\ n\text{-}6}$) and the 3-series from eicosapentaenoic acid ($C_{20:5\ n\text{-}3}$). Subscript (α or β) is added for prostaglandins of the F series to indicate the spatial position of the hydroxyl group at C-9 in the cyclopentane ring. All prostaglandins possess an α-hydroxyl group at C-15 and a C-13,14 *trans* double bond. Series 2 and 3 prostaglandins have additional double bonds in the 5,6 and 17,18 positions, respectively.

PGG_2 and PGH_2 are relatively short-lived biosynthetic endoperoxide intermediates possessing a di-oxygen bridge between C-9 and C-11 on the ring. Prostacyclin (PGI_2) has an oxygen bridge between C-6 and C-9. The stable metabolite of PGI_2 is 6-keto (or oxo)-$PGF_{1\alpha}$.

1

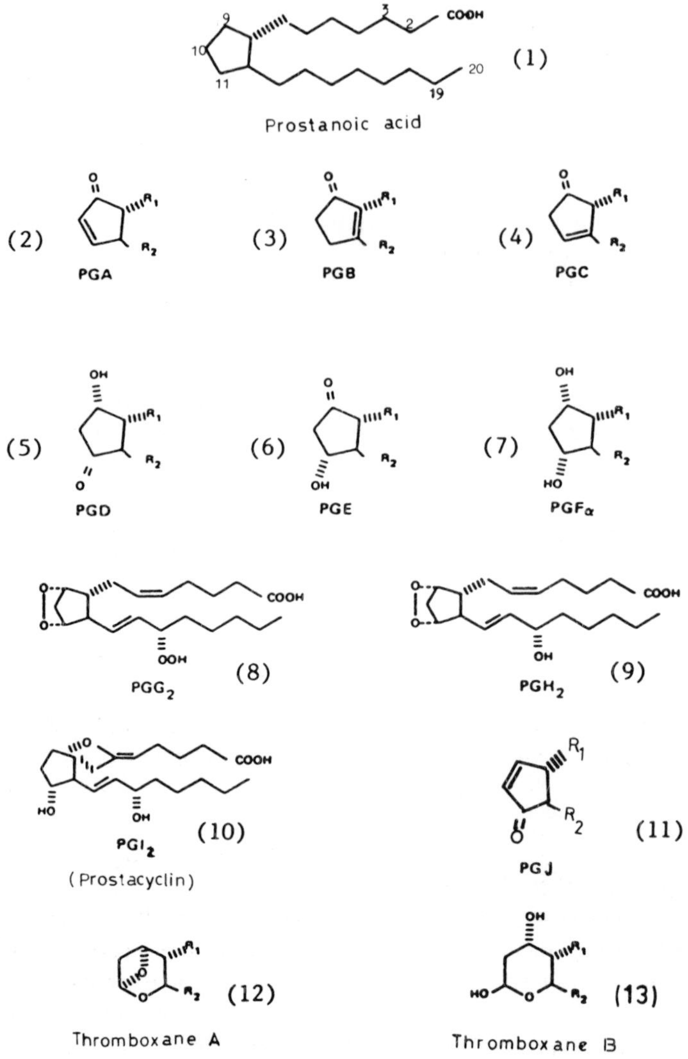

Figure 1. Some prostanoid structures.

Thromboxane A_2 has an unstable bicyclic oxane−oxetane ring structure which rapidly converts to the stable oxane derivative TXB_2.

The first step in all lipoxygenase pathways (*Figure 4*) (5, 12 or 15 lipoxygenases for example) is the formation of the hydroperoxide of the parent straight chain C-20 polyunsaturated fatty acid. Hydroperoxides derived from arachidonic acid are termed hydroperoxyeicosatetraenoic acids (HPETEs) and are subsequently converted to hydroxyeicosatetraenoic acids (HETEs).

Leukotrienes (LT, *Figure 2*) are conjugated trienes produced by the action of 5-lipoxy-

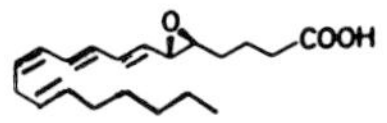

LTA$_4$

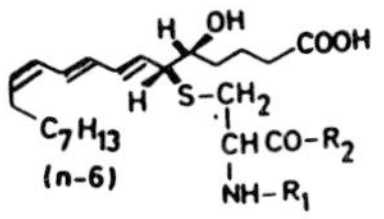

	R_1	R_2
LTC$_4$	Glu	Gly
LTD$_4$	H	Gly
LTE$_4$	H	OH
LTF$_4$	Glu	OH

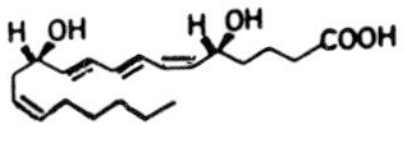

LTB$_4$

Figure. 2. Some leukotriene structures of the 4-series. Note that in the 3-series the conjugated triene system is the same but the 14,15 double bond is absent. In the 5-series an additional double bond is present in the 17,18 position.

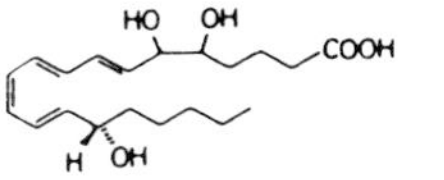

Lipoxin A

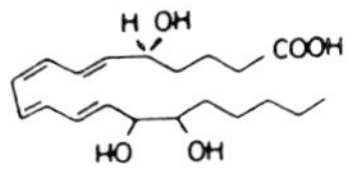

Lipoxin B

Figure 3. Lipoxin structures.

genase. Leukotrienes of the 4-series (LTA_4, LTB_4, etc.) are derived from arachidonic (eicosatetraenoic) acid while the 3-series is derived from eicosatrienoic acid and the 5-series from eicosapentaenoic acid. LTA_4 is an unstable 5,6-epoxy intermediate in the formation of LTB_4. LTC_4 is also formed from LTA_4 by the action of γ-glutamyl-S-transferase; it is a conjugated triene with a γ-glutamyl-cysteinyl-glycine (glutathione) residue coupled to C-6 of the fatty acid chain by a thioether linkage with the cysteine group of glutathione. LTD_4 is formed from LTC_4 by the action of γ-glutamyl transpeptidase which removes glutamic acid, and further removal of glycine by cysteinyl glycinase give rise to LTE_4. LTF_4 can arise from LTE_4 by re-incorporation of glutamic acid.

Lipoxins A and·B (*Figure 3*) are members of a recently discovered group of trihydroxy tetraenes derived from arachidonic acid.

A summary of the general biosynthetic pathways for the formation of eicosanoids is shown in *Figure 4*. Please note that for the biosynthesis of cyclo-oxygenase and lipoxygenase products non-esterified (free) arachidonic acid (or similar polyunsaturated fatty acid) precursor is required. It is generally thought that this is provided from membrane phospholipids by the action of phospholipase A_2 although alternative sources and routes of supply may also exist.

For a more detailed appraisal of the eicosanoids the reader is referred to the many excellent reviews and books on the subject (e.g. 1–5), and the series '*Advances in Prostaglandin, Thromboxane and Leukotriene Research*' published by Raven Press, volumes 1–15.

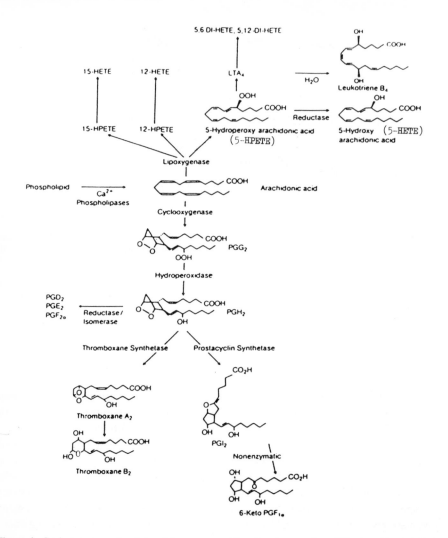

Figure 4. Cyclo-oxygenase (cyclic) and lipoxygenase (linear) pathways of arachidonic acid metabolism.

3. REFERENCES

1. Moore,P.K. (1985) *Prostanoids: Pharmacological, Physiological and Clinical Relevance.* Cambridge University Press, London.
2. Johnson,M., Carey,F. and McMillan,R.M. (1983) In *Essays in Biochemistry.* Campbell,P.N. and Marshall,R.D. (eds), Academic Press Inc., London, Vol. 19, p. 40.
3. Piper,P.J., ed. (1983) *Leukotrienes and Other Lipoxygenase Products.* Research Studies Press (a division of John Wiley and Sons).
4. Moncada,S., ed. (1983) *Br. Med. Bull.,* **39**, 3.
5. Honn,K.V. and Marnett,L.J., eds. (1985) *Prostaglandins, Leukotrienes and Cancer.* Martinus Nijhoff, Dordrecht, Netherlands.

CHAPTER 2

Metabolism of prostaglandins and lipoxygenase products: relevance for eicosanoid assay

ELISABETH GRANSTRÖM and MARIA KUMLIN

1. INTRODUCTION: THE 'WHAT, WHEN, AND WHERE' PROBLEM

In attempts to assay prostaglandins or related compounds in biological material, several serious difficulties are encountered. First, because of their generally very high potencies, the eicosanoids usually occur only in minute amounts in most tissues or body fluids, requiring assay methods of very high sensitivity. Second, the growing complexity of the field, with a multitude of structurally similar compounds being formed from the same precursor, implies that the employed analytical method must be highly specific, if one compound is to be reliably measured (see *Figure 1*, which, despite its complexity, shows only a scanty summary of a few of the more important metabolic pathways in one of several eicosanoid series).

The greatest problem, however, is often the initial decision of *what* compound to measure *when* and *where*. This important decision requires detailed knowledge of metabolic events pertaining to this area: in what forms do these compounds occur in tissues, circulate in blood and appear in urine or other body fluids? Are they present as the primary compounds or as metabolically altered products? Can any of the monitored compounds be formed as an artifact during collection or processing of the sample, thus overshadowing the endogenous levels? Are the assayed prostanoids chemically and metabolically stable in the biological material under study, or would it be better to monitor a stable degradation product? and so on.

Our knowledge is still incomplete for many compounds belonging to this area, particularly the most recently discovered substances, the leukotrienes and the lipoxins. However, also compounds discovered long ago have presented great analytical problems, some of which have been solved only recently, whereas others still await a definitive solution, as with PGE and PGD compounds, for example.

The present chapter will discuss such aspects, and present for each category of compounds the current recommendations for the proper choice of assay target. It is, however, important that these recommendations are not regarded as absolute truths: due to our gradually increasing metabolic knowledge, the opinion of the optimal targets for monitoring has already changed several times and might be expected to change again (*Figure 2*).

Until recently, the general attitude favoured the specific measurement of single prostaglandins or related products, with the aim of pin-pointing the role of a certain

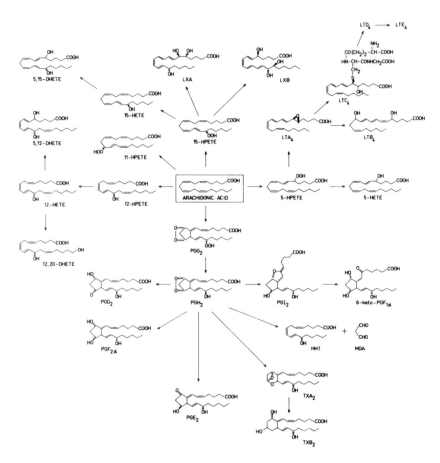

Figure 1. Conversion of arachidonic acid via the cyclo-oxygenase and several lipoxygenase-catalysed pathways.

eicosanoid in some biological process. Since the mid-1960s and to the late 1970s, the methods of choice for this purpose were bioassay, radioimmunoassay (RIA) and gas chromatography−mass spectrometry (g.c.−m.s.), and all these methods are still widely in use. However, with the increasing realization of the complexity of this field, and of how the different metabolic pathways may interfere with one another, this attitude is now gradually being replaced by a quite different approach. A great deal of effort is at present going into the development of profiling assays, based on chromatographic separation of the eicosanoids, where the aim is to obtain as complete a picture of form-ed products as possible. This particular approach has received more attention recently with the growing interest in how the proportion of prostanoids belonging to the 1-, 2- and 3-series (or leukotrienes of the 3-, 4- and 5-series) can be modulated by dietary variations in the content of their respective precursor fatty acids. The minor structural differences between such compounds add further difficulties to the already great analytical problems in this field.

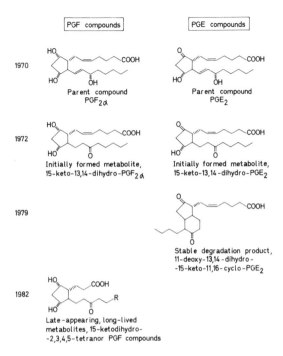

Figure 2. Plasma prostaglandins of the F and E type: preferred targets for measurement have changed with increasing metabolic and chemical knowledge, from the primary compounds to highly degraded circulating metabolites or stable decomposition products thereof.

2. METABOLISM OF PROSTAGLANDINS

2.1 General comments

Early metabolic studies demonstrated a widespread occurrence of prostaglandin metabolizing enzymes in the body, and consequently a rapid inactivation of prostaglandins exposed to a number of different tissues. Furthermore, infusion experiments *in vivo* showed that the metabolic clearance of the compounds from the circulation was extremely rapid. The half-life of a prostaglandin that had reached the blood stream was in fact estimated at less than 1 min (1). It could be calculated that if the primary prostaglandins were circulating at all, their endogenous concentration in peripheral plasma could not exceed about 2 pg/ml. In addition to this, it was also known that several of the prostaglandins were chemically unstable, which might lead to a further reduction of the already low amounts.

Nonetheless, in the early days of prostaglandin analysis, most scientists in the field attempted to assay the prostaglandins as such in biological material, even blood plasma (*Figure 2*). After the first RIAs were developed for prostaglandins during the early 1970s, a large number of studies appeared claiming plasma levels of the primary prostaglandins ranging from several hundred pg/ml to several ng/ml.

The great discrepancies between the obtained values and the theoretically possible levels indicated that a substantial formation of the monitored compounds had occurred

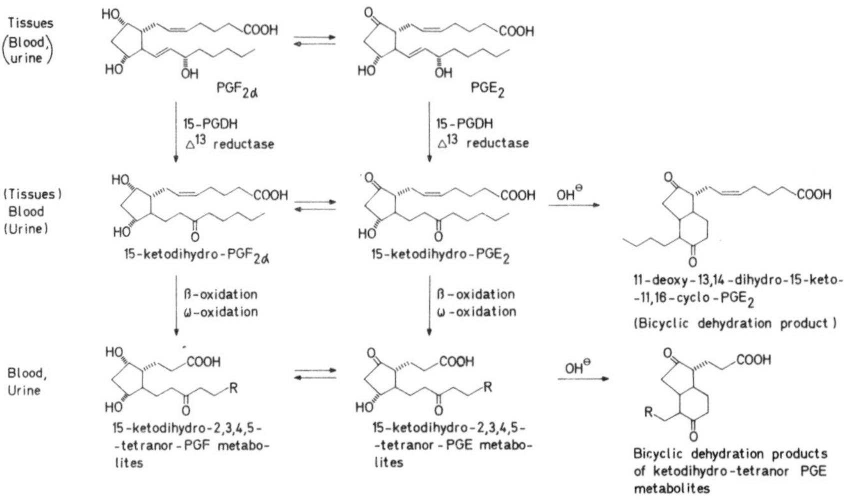

Figure 3. Metabolism of PGE$_2$ and PGF$_{2\alpha}$ with structures of major metabolites and stable degradation products, suitable as targets for measurement at different levels. Less suitable levels are indicated within parenthesis.

ex vivo during the collection and/or further processing of the blood samples. Several blood cell types are known to have a high capacity for eicosanoid formation, and mechanical stimulation or damage to a cell is a strong stimulus for this biosynthesis. In addition, the coagulation process contributes prostanoid amounts several orders of magnitude higher than those in plasma. This implies that even minor technical difficulties encountered during the blood sample collection may severely distort the picture.

The situation concerning measurement of the primary prostaglandins in blood has improved since these difficulties were recognized. Serum is now rarely analysed. Blood samples are now normally collected into tubes containing a potent inhibitor of the prostaglandin biosynthesis, in addition to the anti-coagulant. The samples are also usually cooled and further processed immediately. If blood is collected continuously over a longer time period, the cannula is usually rinsed with saline prior to sampling, etc. Following these measures, several laboratories now report levels of the primary compounds approaching the theoretical values, that is, in the low picogram range.

However, successful measurement of the primary compounds in plasma is hazardous. The formation *ex vivo* of prostanoids is difficult to prevent, since their biosynthesis is an extremely rapid process, whereas most preventive measures (inhibitors, cooling, etc.) require several minutes for full effect. Variations in obtained levels of the primary prostaglandins will thus always be difficult to interpret.

The earlier mentioned metabolic experiments however provided the solution to this difficulty. The rapid clearance of the prostaglandins from the blood stream is followed by the appearance of metabolites, which have longer half-lives and thus accumulate to levels considerably above those of the parent compounds. The initially formed metabolites, the 15-keto-13,14-dihydro compounds (*Figures 2* and *3*), appear within 1 min and are slowly removed from the blood stream with a half-life of about 10 min. Their formation is catalysed by two enzymes, 15-hydroxy prostanoate dehydrogenase and Δ^{13}-reductase, which occur in most tissues, but are particularly abundant in the liver, kidney and lung. Levels of these metabolites under basal conditions are around 20−50 pg/ml (humans) (1); thus, they are more easily detected than their elusive parent prostaglandins. However, the most important fact about these metabolites is that they are not formed as artifacts during sample collection or processing, and the obtained levels of these compounds thus faithfully mirror endogenous events only.

For analysis of prostaglandins in tissues (e.g. biopsies), it may be more pertinent in a clinical situation to try to establish the true *in situ* levels of the biologically active compound, that is the primary prostaglandin, than a metabolite. The same difficulty however applies to this problem: the great artifactual formation of the prostaglandins due to mechanical stimulation of the tissue when the sample is taken. It has been demonstrated that immediate snap-freezing of the biopsy in liquid nitrogen (within a few seconds) may prevent this biosynthesis.

If such a sampling technique cannot be used, for example if the biopsy is taken *in vivo* from an organ that is not easily accessible — the intestinal mucosa may serve as an example — it is perhaps better not to try to establish the endogenous levels of a prostaglandin, but rather to estimate the *biosynthetic capacity* of the tissue in question, by incubation with endogenous or exogenous precursor. This approach has been used successfully in a number of studies.

To avoid these difficulties, many scientists prefer to analyse urinary prostanoids instead. Usually, this fluid contains few viable cells, and uncontrollable formation of prostaglandins *ex vivo* should thus be negligible.

Different compounds may be monitored in urine, depending on the aim of the study. The primary prostaglandins, which are normally found in small amounts in urine, are generally believed to be of renal origin. Prostaglandins synthesized in other tissues are extensively degraded before being excreted by the kidney (see below). Monitoring these compounds may thus give information about the total body production of prostaglandins of a certain type. This may be of interest for example when evaluating the clinical efficacy of a drug interfering with prostaglandin biosynthesis.

When analysing urinary prostanoids, it should be kept in mind that there is a considerable lag of several hours, before a compound that has reached the blood stream has been completely metabolized and excreted. Thus, no rapid changes can be monitored by urinary analyses; for example, temporal endocrine relationships may be difficult to study with this approach. Furthermore, a small production of a compound at a limited site or during a limited period of time may not significantly influence the urinary levels of the finally excreted metabolites. With massive releases, on the other hand, there is no risk of missing even a short surge of prostaglandin production with urinary analyses — as can easily happen when blood levels of a compound are monitored — since the major part of a prostaglandin released *in vivo* will eventually reach the urine.

2.2 Individual metabolic fates of the prostaglandins

The vast majority of metabolic studies in this field, particularly in later years, have been done with the arachidonic acid metabolites. This chapter will thus mainly describe the metabolic fates of prostaglandins and thromboxanes of the 2-series and leukotrienes of the 4-series. Many metabolic reactions however seem to be common for compounds of either series, and in some cases the sequence of metabolic steps finally leads to the same end product, regardless of its origin. For example, certain highly degraded urinary metabolites of prostaglandins, the tetranor, ω-dinor-dioic acids (see *Figure 3*), may be formed from prostaglandins of either the 1-, 2- or 3-series. The implications of such metabolic convergence are discussed below.

2.2.1 *Metabolism of PGF$_{2\alpha}$*

After the compound has been metabolized to the biologically inactive 15-keto-13, 14-dihydro metabolite (*Figures 2* and *3*), several other metabolic processes degrade the molecule further into a large number of products, which are finally excreted into urine (1). These reactions include one or two steps of β-oxidation from the α-carboxyl end into dinor and tetranor compounds; ω-oxidation resulting in a hydroxyl or carboxyl group also at the ω-end of the molecule; and finally also β-oxidation from this end of the molecule into ω-dinor and even ω-tetranor dioic acid compounds. One more, rather unusual metabolic reaction takes place in some species: deoxygenation at C-15. This was first discovered in the human, where it is one of the major metabolic pathways (2), and later also in the monkey (3) and rabbit (E. Granström, unpublished). It has not been demonstrated in other commonly studied laboratory or domestic animal species.

The major metabolites finally excreted into urine are often tetranor compounds. In the human, 9α, 11α-dihydroxy-15-keto-2,3,4,5-tetranorprostane-1,20-dioic acid (previously designated 5α, 7α-dihydroxy-11-ketotetranorprostane-1,16-dioic acid) (see *Figures 2* and *3*) represents $20-25\%$ of the total urinary PGF metabolites (4), and is normally found in amounts about $5-50$ $\mu g/24$ h (5). In the guinea pig, the major urinary metabolite is the corresponding monocarboxylic acid (1). In the rat, several metabolites of comparable quantitative importance have been identified, such as the mono- and dicarboxylic tetranor metabolites mentioned above, as well as the ω-dinor (C_{14}) counterpart of the latter (1,6). In this animal, however, careful mapping of the metabolic profile as a function of age, sex and strain revealed pronounced differences (7). Similar metabolic differences may occur also in other species: this is not known at present.

Another metabolic fate of PGF$_\alpha$ compounds is dehydrogenation of the 9α-hydroxyl, resulting in E type metabolites (8). This reaction was first demonstrated in the rat but may occur also in other species; however, the human does not seem to utilize this pathway (1,4).

Knowledge of the structures and relative quantitative importance of PGF metabolites has made possible the development of several quantitative methods for such compounds. For a long time now, assay of the PGF$_{2\alpha}$ production *in vivo* has thus been done successfully by monitoring the initially formed metabolite, 15-keto-13,14-dihydro-PGF$_{2\alpha}$, in blood (e.g. 9), and a relevant tetranor metabolite in urine (e.g. 10, 11). For studies based on blood analyses of the 15-ketodihydro metabolites, however, it should be borne in mind that even its half-life of about 10 min may be too short if samples are taken with long intervals. A short-lasting prostaglandin release may thus be missed completely if samples are not taken frequently enough (12).

Recent, extended metabolic studies have, however, provided a solution to this problem. It was found that after injection or release of PGF$_{2\alpha}$ into the blood stream, the profile of circulating metabolites with time became closely similar to the urinary one (6,13). Thus, 15-keto-13,14-dihydro-PGF$_{2\alpha}$ was gradually replaced as the major blood metabolite by more degraded, urinary-type compounds, which could reach even higher concentrations and remained in the circulation long after the initial metabolite had returned to basal levels. Such late-appearing, long-lived metabolites may thus be preferable as targets for measurements, if blood samples are collected only infrequently (*Figures 2* and *3*).

2.2.2 *Metabolism of PGE₂*

The metabolism of PGE$_2$ has also been studied extensively in several species. Prostaglandins of the E type are degraded by similar metabolic pathways as the PGF compounds, that is, the 15-keto-13,14-dihydro metabolites initially dominate the blood metabolic profile (1), and the metabolites excreted finally in urine are then formed by various combinations of the metabolic reactions mentioned above: one or two steps of β-oxidation, and ω-oxidation (*Figure 3*). The major urinary metabolite in the human was identified as 11α-hydroxy-9,15-diketo-2,3,4,5-tetranorprostane-1,20-dioic acid (previously designated 7α-hydroxy-5,11-diketotetranor-prostane-1,16-dioic acid) (1). Numerous other metabolites have however also been identified.

A considerable reduction of the 9-keto group into F compounds has also been demonstrated in several species, including man (1). Generally, the formed products are of the F$_\alpha$ type; however, in the guinea pig and rat the corresponding β-epimers were identified. The tissue localization of this latter reductase has not been identified: the 9-keto reductase from guinea pig liver, for example, yields only F$_\alpha$ epimers *in vitro*, whereas the intact animal *in vivo* affords exclusively the β-epimer (1).

Several additional products of PGE degradation have been identified *in vivo* as well as *in vitro*. These include compounds epimeric at C-8 (8-iso compounds) as well as dehydrated products of the PGA and B type (1,14). Since compounds with the sensitive β-ketol system of the PGE ring are prone to dehydration, some of these products, or perhaps all, may have been formed non-enzymatically, possibly *ex vivo* during storage or processing of samples.

This non-enzymatic dehydration of PGE compounds is especially rapid in complex biological materials, particularly in the presence of albumin (15,16). This may be caused by the rapid removal of formed PGA compounds by addition of sulphhydryl groups or other nucleophiles at the activated carbon 11 (15,17). Such undesired side reactions long hampered attempts to assay 15-keto-13,14-dihydro-PGE$_2$ in plasma as an indicator of PGE$_2$ release *in vivo*. This analytical problem was finally solved by the discovery that all the dehydrated compounds could be converted by alkali treatment into one single stable, non-reactive end product, which can be monitored instead of the unstable parent metabolite, namely 11-deoxy-13,14-dihydro-15-keto-11,16-cyclo-PGE$_2$ (*Figures 2* and *3*) (15,18).

Although urine does not normally contain large amounts of albumin or thiol compounds, it may be advisable to convert also the urinary PGE metabolites into the corresponding bicyclic stable product(s). So far, only one assay has been developed for this kind of compound (19) (see *Figure 3*). Earlier methods were directed at the major metabolites retaining the E-ring (1).

To date, very few attempts have been made at studying the late profile of circulating PGE metabolites (6). It may however be assumed that the initially formed 15-ketodihydro metabolite, which dominates the early metabolic picture, is replaced by more degraded compounds with time, probably tetranor compounds, by analogy with the PGF metabolism (6,13). The considerable conversion of PGE into PGF in some species should also be borne in mind (1) (see also below).

2.2.3 *Metabolism of PGD$_2$*

The D type prostaglandins also possess a sensitive β-ketol system in the ring (*Figures 1* and *4*) and are consequently susceptible to dehydration, by analogy with PGE compounds (14). Epimerization of the C-12 side chain can also occur, due to keto−enol tautomerism of the C-11 keto group, corresponding to the formation of 8-iso-PGEs. In addition, PGD compounds can undergo other spontaneous degradation reactions, such as isomerization of the Δ^{13} double bond to the Δ^{12} position, and loss of water also from the C-12 side chain (20). In fact, PGs of the D type are even more unstable than PGEs, particularly in biological material containing albumin (16,20).

This feature of PGD$_2$ long hampered the efforts to determine its production *in vivo* and other biological systems, as well as elucidation of its metabolism. Remarkably few assay methods exist for PGD$_2$ itself (21,22), which probably reflects its rapid decomposition in biological material. Derivatization of the compound, for example into the 11-methoxime (23), or into a stable degradation end product (20) may be a safer approach to PGD$_2$ determinations.

Recent studies on the metabolism of PGD$_2$ in various biological systems have provided information which will no doubt facilitate the monitoring of PGD production *in vivo* as well as *in vitro*. A series of papers by the group at Vanderbilt describe the metabolism of PGD$_2$ *in vivo* in primates, including the human (24−26). Also PGD$_2$ was found to be metabolized via the common metabolic reactions described above for PGE and PGF compounds: β- and ω-oxidation, dehydrogenation of the C-15 hydroxyl group and reduction of the Δ^{13} double bond. As was the case with both PGEs and PGFs, a large number of urinary PGD$_2$ metabolites could be identified, formed by various combinations of these reactions (24−26). One of these, 9α-hydroxy-11,15-diketo-2,3,18,19-tetranorprost-5-ene-1,20-dioic acid (*Figure 4*), was considered a suitable target for measurement, and, using a g.c.−m.s. method, Roberts (27) found large amounts of this compound in urine from patients with mastocytosis. However, in a later metabolic study in a normal human volunteer, this metabolite was not detected at all (26), and its suitability as a parameter of PGD$_2$ production could thus be questioned.

A remarkable feature of PGD metabolism is that the vast majority ($\sim 70-80\%$) of the total metabolites in primates have been reduced to PGF compounds (24−26,28). Since the reduction of the 11-carbonyl of PGD by sodium borohydride is stereospecific and affords exclusively the α-isomer of the resulting 11-hydroxyl (29), it was originally believed that enzymatic reduction of PGD compounds by an 11-keto reductase also yielded the corresponding PGF$_\alpha$ compounds. Several studies have also been published claiming the identification of PGF$_{2\alpha}$ (or PGF$_\alpha$-metabolites) as the sole product of such a reaction: for example, PGF$_{2\alpha}$ in sheep blood (30) and in rabbit liver (31,32), 15-keto-13,14-dihydro-PGF$_{2\alpha}$ as the major circulating PGD$_2$ metabolite in the human (28) and a number of PGF$_\alpha$ metabolites in monkey urine (24). The choice of such a

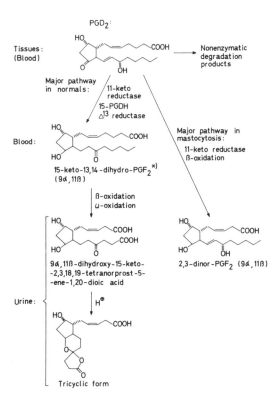

Figure 4. Simplified scheme for the metabolism of PGD$_2$ in the human. *The major circulating metabolite was earlier identified as 9α, 11α-dihydroxy-15-ketoprost-5-enoic acid, that is 15-ketodihydro-PGF$_{2\alpha}$ by pass spectrometry (37); however, at that time the reduction of the 11-keto group almost exclusively into an 11β-hydroxyl was not known (33).

compound as target for measurement would however lead to uncertainty concerning its origin.

However, recent metabolic studies have provided a solution to this analytical problem. Liston and Roberts discovered that, contrary to what was believed, the enzymatic reduction of the 11-keto group of PGD$_2$ yields almost exclusively the 11β-isomer, at least in the human (26,33). The major urinary metabolite, 9α, 11β-dihydroxy-15-keto-2,3,18,19-tetranorprost-5-ene-1,20-dioic acid (*Figure 4*), which can form a unique tricyclic structure by a combination of hemiketal formation and lactonization, can thus be quantitated as a specific PGD$_2$ metabolite without any contribution from PGF compounds (26).

2.2.4 *Metabolism of PGI$_2$, prostacyclin*

Measurement of prostacyclin in a system generating the compound *in vitro* is often done by immediate assay of its biologic activity, for example by measuring induced relaxation of vessels or by inhibition of platelet aggregation (34). Since its half-life is only about 2 min, this approach is generally not possible for measurement of the generation of prostacyclin *in vivo*. A stable break-down product has to be monitored instead.

For a long time, the immediate hydrolysis product, 6-keto-$PGF_{1\alpha}$, has been used for this purpose. Since it was found that PGI_2, in contrast to other prostaglandins, is not taken up and metabolized by the lung, it was once believed that prostacyclin was a circulating hormone (35). Plasma levels of 6-keto-$PGF_{1\alpha}$ were thus measured — and still are in many cases — and attempts were made to correlate obtained levels with various clinical conditions. Levels of several hundred pg/ml plasma were often reported (review, 36). It was however later found that also these measured levels almost completely reflected the artifactual formation of prostacyclin, for example by damaged endothelial cells or blood cells, when the blood sample was taken and/or processed. The true endogenous levels seem to be around $1-2$ pg/ml plasma, as with other prostaglandins (37), and the concept of prostacyclin as a circulating hormone was thus abandoned several years ago.

The metabolism of the compound was then elucidated in order to identify a more suitable assay parameter (review, 38). Certain similarities with, but also differences from, the metabolism of the other prostaglandins were found. Since the compound is so unstable chemically, it was at first assumed that the first step in PGI_2 metabolism was the non-enzymatic hydrolysis to 6-keto-$PGF_{1\alpha}$, and that further metabolism would proceed from there.

Studies on the degradation *in vivo* of 6-keto-$PGF_{1\alpha}$ revealed some fates in common with other prostaglandins, namely β-oxidation and ω-oxidation. Some differences were however also seen: biliary metabolite excretion was prominent, dehydrogenation at C-15 occurred only to a minor degree, and β-oxidation stopped at the dinor stage (38). The major metabolite of 6-keto-$PGF_{1\alpha}$ in several species was thus 2,3-dinor-6-keto-$PGF_{1\alpha}$ in urine as well as bile. Studies *in vitro* supported the finding that 6-keto $PGF_{1\alpha}$ was a poor substrate for 15-hydroxy-prostanoate dehydrogenase (38).

However, when labelled PGI_2 became available for metabolic studies, this compound was shown to be an excellent substrate for the enzyme, as well as for the Δ^{13} reductase. 6,15-Diketo-13,14-dihydro-$PGF_{1\alpha}$ was identified as a long-lived metabolite in human plasma during prostacyclin infusion (39) and, furthermore, at steady-state during such infusions, two related dinor metabolites also appeared as major circulating compounds, namely 2,3-dinor-6,15-diketo-13,14-dihydro-$PGF_{1\alpha}$ and its corresponding ω-carboxyl compound (40) (*Figure 5*).

Although PGI_2 is not taken up by the lung, thereby eliminating this organ as the site of these enzymatic reactions, other organs and tissues have been shown to have a high capacity for such conversions, for example the vessel wall and the kidney (38). The liver, in addition, efficiently β-oxidizes the compound. Furthermore, it has been shown that the differences in metabolism of PGI_2 itself and its hydrolysis product disappear when the compounds are administered by slow infusion at low concentration instead of by bolus injection, thereby mimicking the endogenous situation (41,42).

In addition to the major circulating prostacyclin metabolites, the major urinary breakdown products have also been identified in the human. These are 2,3-dinor-6-keto-$PGF_{1\alpha}$, 2,3-dinor-6,15-diketo-13,14-dihydro-20-carboxyl-$PGF_{1\alpha}$ and 2,3-dinor-6,15-diketo-13,14-dihydro-$PGF_{1\alpha}$ (42) (*Figure 5*). As is the case with the other prostaglan-

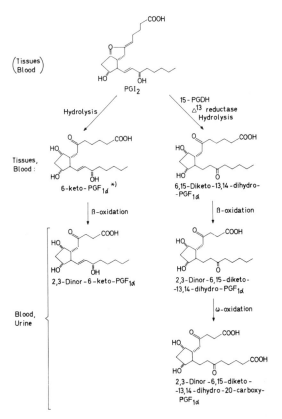

Figure 5. Simplified scheme of the metabolism of prostacyclin, PGI_2, in the human with structures of major metabolites, suitable for monitoring at different levels. *6-Keto-$PGF_{1\alpha}$ occurs as a major circulating metabolite of infused prostacyclin; however, its suitability as target for monitoring under other circumstances can be questioned.

dins, the urinary metabolite pattern seems similar to the late plasma profile after prostacyclin administration (40,42).

In summary, the best target for measurement of the prostacyclin formation *in vivo* is likely to be a metabolite different from 6-keto-$PGF_{1\alpha}$. Although this hydrolysis product may dominate in the circulation during a prostacyclin infusion (40), it has been repeatedly shown to be an unreliable indicator of prostacyclin biosynthesis, at least in plasma as was mentioned above. It may be more accurately determined in urine, where it is a minor metabolite of systemically administered prostacyclin (42); however, under most circumstances urinary 6-keto-$PGF_{1\alpha}$ may mainly reflect the renal PGI_2 biosynthesis (43).

A major metabolite, such as 2,3-dinor-6,15-diketo-13,14-dihydro-20-carboxyl-$PGF_{1\alpha}$, may be a better choice. This compound is prominent in blood as well as urine (40,42). A somewhat less prominent metabolite in both fluids is 2,3-dinor-6,15-diketo-13,14-dihydro-$PGF_{1\alpha}$, the corresponding monocarboxylic compound. 2,3-Dinor-6-keto-$PGF_{1\alpha}$ is the major urinary metabolite, as was mentioned above, and is

15

hence often monitored in urine; in plasma, however, it is probably an insignificant product (40).

The metabolic and practical problems encountered in assessment of the prostacyclin formation *in vivo* in the human were recently discussed by several leading scientists in the field (38,44−47).

3. METABOLISM OF THROMBOXANES

3.1 General comments

So far, much less has been uncovered about the metabolic fates of thromboxanes, particularly the highly unstable TXA_2. In attempts to assay the thromboxane production *in vivo*, the most common approach by far is to measure the stable hydrolysis product, TXB_2, in plasma. Several objections to this approach can however be raised. First, a considerable artifactual production may occur during the blood sample collection, by analogy with what was discussed above for the prostaglandins, since thromboxane is one of the major compounds synthesized by stimulated platelets, for example. Second, plasma TXB_2 is rapidly cleared from the circulation (48−50), leading to the same situation as for the prostaglandins: even if TXB_2 could be reliably measured in plasma, the concentration cannot be expected to exceed a few pg/ml (47,50). This is in contrast to most reported levels, which are often around 100 pg/ml or even higher. It has become increasingly clear that any technical difficulties encountered during collection and/or processing of the blood inevitably lead to high measured 'plasma TXB_2' (46,47,51).

Third, the compound of interest in biological studies is of course TXA_2, not TXB_2. It is known that TXA_2 can undergo a number of other metabolic fates than simple hydrolysis to TXB_2, such as binding to proteins in various ways, dehydrogenation and reduction to 15-keto-13,14-dihydro-thromboxane, and possibly others (reviews, 38, 52). Thus, plasma TXB_2 may reflect only a small fraction of the TXA_2 actually formed.

Urinary TXB_2 is sometimes monitored and is generally considered to be of renal origin (53) as is the case with the primary prostaglandins.

3.2 Metabolism of thromboxane B_2

The assay problems for thromboxane might be solved if a thromboxane metabolite could be identified, which represents a major and constant fraction of thromboxane A_2 formed *in vivo*, and which is not formed as an artifact during sample collection; thus, a compound analogous to the 15-ketodihydro metabolites or the tetranor dicarboxylic acids of the prostaglandins discussed above. In order to identify such a compound, extensive studies on thromboxane metabolism have recently been undertaken (49,51,54−57). Since it has not been possible to study the metabolism of TXA_2, all metabolic studies *in vivo* so far have employed TXB_2 as the starting material. Thus, if TXB_2 formed *in vivo* represents only a part of the actually synthesized TXA_2, any identified TXB_2 metabolite in blood and urine may be a quantitatively minor product.

The metabolic pathways in man have been extensively elucidated by Roberts *et al.* (56,57; review, 38). Twenty urinary metabolites of TXB_2 were identified, and the major one was found to be 2,3-dinor-TXB_2 (see *Figure 6*). Several quantitative methods

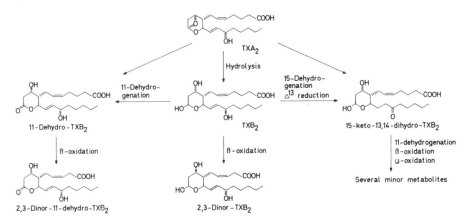

Figure 6. Simplified scheme of the metabolism of thromboxane in the human. Of the indicated C_{20} compounds, 11-dehydro-TXB_2 seems to be a reliable target for thromboxane monitoring in blood as well as urine. Dinor-TXB_2 is the major urinary compound; its concentration in blood is very low.

for this compound have been developed and successfully used for monitoring the thromboxane production *in vivo* in various clinical conditions (46,58,59). The normal daily amounts of this metabolite are much lower than those of major prostaglandin breakdown products: about 500 ng/day compared with $5-50$ μg for PGE or PGF metabolites. Under physiological conditions urinary 2,3-dinor-TXB_2 is considered to be mainly derived from platelets (60).

Until recently, far less has been known about circulating thromboxane metabolites. In attempts to identify major plasma metabolites of TXB_2, the tritium-labelled compound was administered by intravenous injection to man and rabbit, and the profile of circulating metabolites followed by analysis of frequently taken blood samples (49,51,54,55). The two species were found to metabolize TXB_2 differently. In rabbit, an extensive metabolism of the compound was seen with numerous metabolites appearing already at an early stage (49,54). As is the case with prostaglandins, the late blood profile was closely similar to the urinary one in this species. One of the most prominent products throughout the experiment was identified as 11-dehydro-TXB_2, which was also a major compound in urine (*Figure 6*).

In the human, the single most prominent compound in blood was the parent compound, TXB_2 (55). Very little polar metabolites were seen, in contrast to the urinary profile, where 2,3-dinor-TXB_2 dominated. This β-oxidized product was barely detectable in blood. One of the most prominent degradation products in the circulation was identified as 11-dehydro-TXB_2 also in the human, and it was also a relatively abundant product in human urine (51,55,57). Other circulating metabolites in the human were tentatively identified as 15-dehydro-13,14-dihydro-TXB_2 and 11,15-didehydro-13,14-dihydro-TXB_2 (55).

11-Dehydro-TXB_2 was not found to be formed as an artifact during collection of blood samples and can thus be expected to serve as a better thromboxane parameter than TXB_2. A recently developed RIA for this metabolite has confirmed this (49,54, 61).

4. INTERCONVERSIONS OF PROSTAGLANDINS AND RELATED COMPOUNDS

Interpretation of obtained quantitative data is, for many reasons, sometimes very difficult. Some of these difficulties were discussed above, such as the possible formation *ex vivo* of the monitored compound, as well as the uncertainty concerning its tissue origin.

An additional difficulty, which has more recently come into focus, concerns the metabolic interconversion of many compounds in this field; that is an additional ambiguity when evaluating data concerns the *biochemical* origin of the measured compound.

The formation of PGF compounds from PGE was first described by Hamberg and co-workers (review, 1). Enzymatic reduction of the 9-keto group resulted in either a 9α-hydroxyl, giving a PGF$_\alpha$ compound or, more rarely, a 9β-hydroxyl, yielding a PGF$_\beta$ metabolite (1). A corresponding formation of PGE compounds from PGFs has also been demonstrated, for example in the rat (8). A similar reaction is known for 6-keto-PGF$_{1\alpha}$ (and prostacyclin), which can be metabolized into 6-keto-PGE$_1$, although this reaction may not be prominent in the human (38).

Dehydrogenation of the 11α-hydroxyl of PGF$_\alpha$ compounds to PGDs is theoretically possible but has, to our knowledge, not been demonstrated. On the other hand, it has been shown that PGD$_2$ may be converted into PGF compounds to a great extent (24−26,28). In fact, the major metabolites in plasma as well as urine in man have F-ring structures, as was discussed above. Several studies in animals as well as the human claim that this reduction of the C-11 keto group stereospecifically yields the 11α-hydroxyl: in other words, the formed products are related to PGF$_\alpha$ (28,30−32). However, as was mentioned above, recent studies by Liston and Roberts showed that the PGF ring metabolites in the human are mainly of the 9α, 11β-type (26,33). This previously unknown pathway may also have contributed to the PGF formation detected in some of the earlier studies without being recognized.

If a PGF compound is converted into a metabolite of the E or D type, this conversion may go unnoticed (unless a specifically labelled PGF is used), since both E and D compounds are chemically unstable. The opposite phenomenon is more likely to be detected. Assay methods for PGF compounds are generally quite reliable in comparison with methods for E or D compounds. A large number of studies have shown elevated levels of PGF, measured as various metabolites in blood or urine, in a number of conditions. Increased levels of PGF are, for example, known to be associated with physiological conditions such as luteolysis, pregnancy and parturition, as well as a number of pathological conditions such as asthma, medullary carcinoma of the thyroid, cold urticaria, and so on. In view of the considerable reduction of other prostaglandins to PGF compounds, it is however by no means certain that such elevated levels really represent a release of the parent PGF itself, and that the biological condition in question is thus associated with PGF effects (see 47,62).

If stereospecific isomers of such metabolites could be identified as specific markers, typical of a certain metabolic pathway, the analytical situation might be somewhat improved. For example, the 9β-hydroxyl-PGF compounds may specifically originate in PGEs and the 11β-hydroxyl-PGF compounds in PGDs. However, even this may be misleading: a PGF$_\beta$ compound has in fact been identified in rat urine as a PGF$_\alpha$

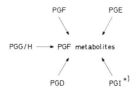

Figure 7. Known origins of PGF compounds. *$PGI_{1\alpha}$ is normally metabolized into 6-keto-$PGF_{1\alpha}$ derivatives, thus easily distinguished from other PGF compounds. However, one metabolite has been identified where degradation had eliminated the 6-keto group, that is pentanor-$PGF_{1\alpha}$ (48).

metabolite (63), no doubt formed by a two-step conversion involving a PGE compound as intermediate (see 20).

Figure 7 summarizes the known origins for PGF compounds.

Another difficulty in interpretation of quantitative data is that a measured increase in a certain compound does not necessarily reflect an increased biosynthesis and/or release of its parent compound. It might also be caused by a decreased metabolism into more 'distal' metabolites. A special case is the so-called 'spill-over' or 'shunting' effect, when selective inhibition of, for example, thromboxane synthetase leads to increased formation of prostaglandins, including prostacyclin, due to accumulation of the endoperoxides PGG_2 and PGH_2. The increase in lipoxygenase products sometimes seen during cyclo-oxygenase inhibition is also an example of this.

Some of these analytical difficulties will no doubt be solved when better profiling methods are developed, which allow the simultaneous measurement of many different metabolites. So far, most profiling assays have a somewhat lower sensitivity than most specific methods, which has somewhat limited their use to date.

An entirely different approach in prostaglandin assay was designed by Nugteren about 10 years ago (64). This approach to some extent eliminates the problem of interconversion of related compounds. Nugteren developed an assay method for urinary tetranor-prostaglandins which simultaneously measures all compounds with the tetranor skeleton in two groups: the mono- and dicarboxylic compounds. The method is based on extensive reduction of the molecule, which is thus stripped of all its substituents, including double bonds. Thus, all individual characteristics of the metabolites are removed, which normally suggest their origins from PGEs, Fs, Ds or Is (with the limitations discussed above), and also from which series they originate. A measure of total prostaglandins is thus obtained, which under certain circumstances may be more relevant than monitoring single pathways. A combination of this method with more specific assays may prove the best approach in prostaglandin measurement today. It may also be mentioned in this context that Nugteren's data on total tetranor prostaglandins in urine are considerably higher than can be explained by our present knowledge of these compounds.

No interconversion between prostaglandins and thromboxanes is known to date. It may however be mentioned in this context that two compounds sometimes believed to specifically reflect thromboxane biosynthesis, malondialdehyde (MDA) and 12-hydroxy-heptadecatrienoic acid (HHT) (*Figure 1*), are known also to be formed by direct decomposition of the endoperoxides.

5. METABOLISM OF LIPOXYGENASE PRODUCTS

5.1 **General comments**

A variety of compounds can be formed from polyunsaturated fatty acids in oxygenation reactions catalysed by different lipoxygenase enzymes. The substrate requirement for this reaction is a *cis*, *cis*-1,4-pentadiene structure in the substrate molecule (65). Thus, several oxygenated compounds with hydroperoxy groups at positions 5, 8, 9, 11, 12 or 15 can be formed from arachidonic acid.

The resulting hydroperoxy acids can be reduced enzymatically almost immediately yielding the rather stable corresponding hydroxy acids (hydroxyeicosatetraenoic acids, HETEs). However, it is not certain that all these enzymes occur in mammalian cells. It should be pointed out in this context that 11-hydroperoxyeicosatetraenoic acid (11-HPETE) as well as the corresponding 15-HPETE may be formed as by-products of cyclo-oxygenase action and do not necessarily indicate the presence of specific lipoxygenases (66).

Other conversions of the hydroperoxy acids are however also known, such as dehydration to form epoxides. From such intermediates, a large number of compounds can then be formed, among them the leukotrienes and the lipoxins (*Figure 1*) (67) (see also below).

The lipoxygenase-catalysed products thus constitute a very large and heterogenous group of compounds, the biochemistry of which has only recently been studied in detail. Thus, metabolic knowledge in this area is still limited and comparatively few assay methods for these compounds have been developed to date. In most cases assay of lipoxygenase products is based on chromatographic separation with u.v. detection of relevant compounds. Such techniques can be employed due to the presence of chromophores, consisting of conjugated double bonds, in many of these compounds. The majority of studies to date in this area have dealt with the formation of lipoxygenase products in various systems *in vitro*, generally leukocytes and blood platelets. Comparatively little is known about their occurrence *in vivo*. Thus, if not specifically pointed out, the studies referred to in this chapter were performed *in vitro*.

5.2 **Metabolism of hydroperoxy acids and monohydroxy acids**

The initial product of a lipoxygenase-catalysed reaction is a hydroperoxy acid, with the substituent in a specific position, as was mentioned above. Depending on the cell type, different products can be formed. 12-HPETE is the major compound in platelets but has also been detected in lung, spleen and other tissues (review, 66). 5-HPETE is predominantly formed by polymorphonuclear leukocytes (PMNL), basophils, macrophages and lymphocytes, 15-HPETE by PMNLs, eosinophils, macrophages, lung tissue and also other cell types (66).

Generally, these products are not assayed as HPETEs, due to their instability. Instead they are converted by reduction to their corresponding monohydroxy acids, which are more stable.

The further metabolism of the monohydroxy acids has so far not been extensively studied. No rapid degradation of HETEs to other derivatives has been reported, and thus, assay of these compounds usually reflects lipoxygenase activity rather reliably.

Again, it is important to keep in mind that monohydroxy acids derived via the cyclo-oxygenase pathway will contribute to the total amount of monohydroxylated compounds, and cannot be distinguished from the lipoxygenase-derived products.

However, in some biological systems, metabolic alteration of a HETE may occur. ω-Oxidation, a well-known catabolic step in prostaglandin and thromboxane metabolism, has been shown to occur with platelet-derived 12-HETE, which in the presence of neutrophils is converted to 12,20-dihydroxy-eicosatetraenoic acid (12,20-DHETE) (68): this may be of importance for correct interpretation of data when longer incubation times are used in relation to methods of analysis.

If a lipoxygenase reaction occurs twice in the same fatty acid molecule, that is a double oxygenation followed by reduction of the hydroperoxy groups, a dihydroxy acid is formed. 5(S), 12(S)-Dihydroxy-6-*trans*,8-*cis*,10-*trans*,14-*cis*-eicosatetraenoic acid, structurally related to LTB$_4$ (*Figure 1*), was first found in incubations with PMNLs (69), however, it has later been shown that the compound is likely to be formed via interaction between PMNLs and platelets (70). Note that this 5,12-dihydroxy acid is difficult to separate from LTB$_4$ if RP-h.p.l.c. (reversed phase high-performance liquid chromatography) is used for analysis of formed products. However, SP-(straight phase)-h.p.l.c. analysis will discriminate between these two arachidonic acid metabolites.

Another dihydroxy-acid formed in a similar way is the product 5,15-DHETE resulting from lipoxygenation at position 5 and 15 of arachidonic acid. This product has been reported in several leukocyte types, such as mononuclear cells, eosinophils and PMNLs (66). It has also been proposed that 8,15-DHETEs can be formed via double oxygenation (see Section 5.3).

Some trihydroxy acid derivatives have also been found. Both 8,9,12- and 10,11,12-trihydroxyeicosatetraenoic acids (THETEs) were found in platelets and an additional compound, 8,10,12-THETE, in the lung (71,72). They were all suggested to be formed from 12-HPETE via epoxy-hydroxy intermediates, 8-hydroxy-11,12 epoxy- and 10-hydroxy-11,12-epoxy-eicosatetraenoic acids. All these compounds have been isolated. Their biological importance is however unknown, and they may even be mainly formed non-enzymatically.

Recently a new group of compounds, the lipoxins, was discovered (*Figure 1*) (67). They all contain three hydroxyl groups and a conjugated tetraene structure. Two groups of compounds have so far been identified with the structures: 5,6,15-trihydroxy-7,9,11,13-eicosatetraenoic acid and 5,14,15-trihydroxy-6,8,10,12-eicosatetraenoic acid for isomers of lipoxin A (LXA) and lipoxin B (LXB), respectively. (*Figure 1*). The compounds were shown to be formed from 15-HPETE in Ca^{2+}-ionophore (A23187)-stimulated human PMNLs (67). More recent experiments showed that also 15-HETE can be converted to these metabolites (73,74). Several isomers of both compounds have been isolated and structurally identified (73,74). It is likely that the mechanism of formation involves an epoxide intermediate although the structure of this intermediate has not yet been clearly elucidated.

Of all the above-mentioned products, only the mono-HETEs are usually detected in larger quantities. However, it is important to keep in mind that some of the products may have strong biological activities at very low concentrations, thus, making even small amounts biologically relevant.

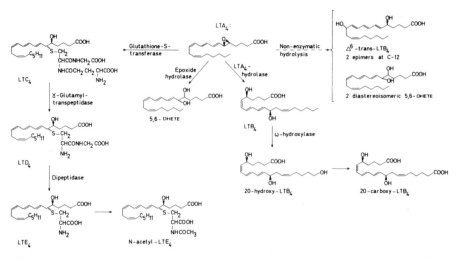

Figure 8. Conversion of leukotriene A_4 via enzymatic and non-enzymatic pathways mainly *in vitro*. Which pathways and compounds are relevant for a particular study will depend on the biological system, the time factor, employed stimulus, etc.

5.3 Metabolism of the epoxy intermediates, LTA$_4$ and 14,15-LTA$_4$

By far the most studied metabolic fate of monohydroperoxy acids is the conversion of 5-HPETE and 15-HPETE to epoxides: leukotriene A_4 (LTA$_4$) and 14,15-leukotriene A_4 (14,15-LTA$_4$), respectively. The further conversion of these metabolically reactive epoxides may give rise to many potent compounds (75).

The best known metabolism of the epoxide LTA$_4$ is the enzymatic conversion via addition of water to leukotriene B_4 in PMNLs (66,75) or via incorporation of a molecule of glutathione to form leukotriene C_4 in several cell types (66,75) (*Figure 8*). The conversion of LTA$_4$ to LTB$_4$ is catalysed by LTA$_4$-hydrolase, an enzyme which has been found to have a widespread occurrence, cellular as well as extracellular (83).

LTA$_4$ can also be non-enzymatically hydrolysed to two *all trans* isomers of 5,12-DHETE and two isomers of 5,6-DHETE (*Figure 8*) (66). One isomer of 5,6-DHETE has also been found to be formed enzymatically from LTA$_4$ via a cytosolic epoxide hydrolase, different from LTA$_4$ hydrolase, in the liver (*Figure 8*) (76). The occurrence of 5,6-DHETE in a biological system is thus difficult to interpret.

Another pathway for leukotriene biosynthesis has been demonstrated in human and porcine leukocytes and also other cell types (66,75). In this pathway the initial reaction is lipoxygenation of arachidonic acid at position C-15 instead of C-5, followed by an analogous dehydration. The so formed allylic epoxide, 14,15-LTA$_4$, can be converted to several isomers of 14,15-LTB$_4$ and of 8,15-LTB$_4$, by analogy with 5,6-LTA$_4$. A mechanism involving a 15-hydroperoxy radical was suggested, since the oxygen in the C-14 position in 14,15-DHETE was not exclusively derived from water (77). This means that not all of the 14,15-DHETE formed is derived from hydrolysis of an epoxide intermediate. Furthermore, 8,15-DHETE is to some extent believed to be generated from double lipoxygenation. The conversion of the epoxide or 15-HPETE to 14,15-

and 8,15-DHETEs has also been shown to be catalysed by haemoglobin (78). Finally, a compound with glutathione attached by a thioether linkage to C-14 was isolated, the 14,15-LTC$_4$, after incubation of the epoxide 14,15-LTA$_4$ with glutathione (93). This compound has however not been identified as a biologically occurring product in any system.

Obviously, this complexity of formed products adds to the uncertainty of what is actually a biologically relevant metabolic profile.

5.4 Metabolism of dihydroxy acids including LTB$_4$

Leukotriene B$_4$ (LTB$_4$), [5(S),12(R)-dihydroxy-6-*cis*, 8,10-*trans*-14-*cis*-eicosate-traenoic acid], has been shown to be metabolized by ω-oxidation to 20-hydroxy-LTB$_4$ in certain leukocyte types and also other tissues (66). In human leukocytes further metabolism to 20-carboxy-LTB$_4$ was also established (66) (*Figure 8*).

Both these ω-oxidized products of LTB$_4$ are less potent than LTB$_4$ as chemotactic agents but equipotent as constrictors of guinea pig lung parenchyma. Thus, this metabolism cannot be considered strictly as an inactivation of the leukotriene. It is also important to keep this metabolism in mind when LTB$_4$ is quantitated exclusively by bioassay.

The extent of ω-oxidation may be influenced by the incubation time, presence of stimuli, and other factors (66,80). Thus, measurement of LTB$_4$ alone may underestimate the products formed via this pathway.

In some studies small amounts of 19-hydroxy-LTB$_4$ have been identified (66, 80).

The other 5,12-dihydroxy acid, formed by double lipoxygenation [5(S), 12(S)-DHETE], has also been shown to be metabolized by ω-oxidation to the corresponding 20-hydroxy and 20-carboxy metabolites (66,80).

Attempts to determine the stability and/or conversion of LTB$_4$ *in vivo* were made in the rat in order to identify the most suitable assay target reflecting LTB$_4$ production (81). Disappearance and metabolism of LTB$_4$ were studied during carrageenan-induced pleurisy. The half-life of the radioactivity from the pleural exudate was about 45 min. The major breakdown product found was 20-hydroxy-LTB$_4$, which constituted about 10% of the radioactivity still present in the pleural exudate after 120 min.

The metabolism *in vivo* of LTB$_4$ was studied in the monkey after intravenous injection (82). This study showed that the major catabolism was by β-oxidation, since 70% of recovered urinary radioactivity was in the form of tritiated water. The major urinary metabolite only represented 0.8% of recovered radioactivity and was identified as 20-hydroxy-LTB$_4$.

5.5 Metabolism of the peptido-leukotrienes, LTC$_4$, LTD$_4$ and LTE$_4$

Metabolism of the cysteinyl-containing leukotrienes (*Figure 8*) has been studied quite extensively in the last few years. These studies have recently been reviewed (83). Studies *in vitro* showed step-wise enzymatic cleavage of the glutathione chain, attached to C-6 in LTC$_4$ [5(S)-hydroxy-6(R)-S-glutathionyl-7,9-*trans*,11,14-*cis*-eicosatetraenoic] to yield LTD$_4$ [5(S)-hydroxy-6(R)-S-cysteinylglycyl-7,9-*trans*-11,14-*cis*-eicosatetraenoic acid] and LTE$_4$ [5(S)-hydroxy-6(R)-S-cysteinyl-7,9-*trans*,11,14-*cis*-eicosatetraenoic acid], respectively (*Figure 8*). The same sequence of peptidase reactions were shown to occur in a variety of species.

Metabolism of LTC_4 was originally studied in rat basophilic leukaemia cells, where it was shown to be converted to $LTDb_4$ in a reaction catalysed by γ-glutamyl transpeptidase. In this reaction the glutamic acid moiety is removed from the glutathione chain attached to the fatty acid structure at C-6. This enzyme is inhibited by L-serine borate, however, in contrast, the conversion of LTC_4 to LTD_4 seems to be enhanced by L-cysteine (83).

Further metabolism to LTE_4 involves removal of the glycine resulting in a cysteine residue at C-6. This reaction is catalysed by dipeptidases and is known to be inhibited by L-cysteine (83).

These metabolic steps have later been shown to take place also in many other cell types and tissues, such as the kidney and lung (83).

The further metabolism of LTE_4 has also been investigated. First it was found that LTE_4 is transformed by γ-glutamyl transpeptidase to a compound with the same double bond structure but with the peptide substituent containing cysteine and glutamic acid. This compound was named LTF_4 (84), and it was later shown that it is only formed from LTE_4 in the presence of glutathione. No evidence has been reported so far for the existence of this compound *in vivo*. Its possible formation *in vitro* should however be borne in mind in studies aimed at quantitating leukotriene formation.

In rat liver microsomes, LTE_4 was converted to a novel compound (85). Structural identification revealed the compound to be N-acetyl-LTE_4. The enzyme catalysing the conversion was membrane bound in rat liver and was also found in rat kidney, spleen, skin and lung (85).

Several reports on LTC_4 metabolism in different cells and organs from different species have been published, mainly in attempts to elucidate which metabolite is the most suitable for monitoring LTC_4 release or production *in vivo*.

In cells and tissues from the airways, LTC_4 is also converted to LTD_4 and E_4. The metabolic spectrum depends on several factors, for example incubation time, but also on the specificity and sensitivity of the assay. Guinea-pig lung converted LTC_4 to D_4 and E_4 after antigen challenge (86). After 10 min mostly LTD_4 was present and shown to be the only leukotriene detectable with bioassay. Studies in our laboratory, however, showed that in the human lung both LTC_4, D_4 and E_4 could be detected, with h.p.l.c. analysis, 10 min after stimulation with ionophore or anti-IgE. Conversion was seen to less polar products with time, with LTE_4 being predominant after 30 min (87).

In eosinophils LTC_4 was found to be converted to isomers of LTB_4 (88). Furthermore, LTC_4, D_4 and E_4 could be converted to 6-*trans* isomers of LTB_4 together with sulphoxides of the peptido-leukotrienes. This metabolism was shown to be myeloperoxidase dependent in certain cell types (for review, see 89). However, evidence for occurrence *in vivo* is lacking for most of these observations.

Soybean lipoxygenase catalysed the formation of 15-hydroxylated metabolites of LTC_4, D_4 and E_4 (90). The 15-hydroxylated metabolite of LTC_4 was shown to be much less potent than LTC_4 in contracting the guinea pig ileum; the contractile activity was diminished about 90% by this transformation of the compound. This suggests that 15-hydroxylation acts as an inactivation of the biologically potent leukotriene. Although

15-lipoxygenase is known to be present in several tissues and cells, no evidence for formation of the 15-hydroxylated metabolites *in vivo* has been reported.

The metabolism *in vivo* of leukotrienes of the C-type was studied in guinea pig, monkey and mouse (for review, see 83). All these studies showed degradation of LTC compounds to LTDs and Es. Recently LTC_4 was administered intravenously to three human male subjects, and the major metabolite in urine was identified as LTE_4 (91), suggesting this compound to be the most suitable for monitoring leukotriene production *in vivo* in the human. In the rat, however, the major urinary and faecal metabolite of LTC_4 was N-acetyl-LTE_4 (92).

To date, a few studies are reported with measurements of leukotrienes in plasma using h.p.l.c. and RIA (93,94). One study showed successive degradation of LTC_4 to LTD_4 and LTE_4 by the same peptidase reactions shown in other biological systems (93). For measurements of endogenously formed cysteinyl-containing leukotrienes, RIA was used to detect plasma levels in human healthy volunteers (94).

6. CONCLUSIONS

Numerous compounds have been identified in the eicosanoid area to date, together comprising a highly complex metabolic picture (see *Figure 1*). For the scientist interested in quantitating the formation of a certain compound, or the biosynthesis of compounds belonging to a certain pathway, it is important to keep this complexity in mind. The metabolic profile is strongly influenced by the biological system under study, by the presence of different stimuli, by the time factor, and so on. Compounds from different pathways are sometimes known to be converted into each other, and to be able to influence the biosynthesis or metabolism of one another. Shunting or 'spill-over' effects are sometimes known to occur from one pathway to another. All these factors can profoundly influence the metabolic picture, which can all too easily be obscured by the additional contributions of various artifacts.

It is thus of greatest importance to begin a quantitative study by investigating the metabolic profile under the employed conditions, in order to select the best target molecule(s) for monitoring. A sadly common approach, when planning a project in this field, is instead to begin by investigating the commercial profile of available RIA kits.

7. REFERENCES

1. Samuelsson,B., Granström,E., Green,K., Hamberg,M. and Hammarström,S. (1975) *Annu. Rev. Biochem.*, **44**, 669.
2. Granström,E. and Samuelsson,B. (1972) *J. Am. Chem. Soc.*, **94**, 4380.
3. Sun,F.F. and Stafford,J.E. (1974) *Biochim. Biophys. Acta*, **369**, 95.
4. Granström,E. and Samuelsson,B. (1971) *J. Biol. Chem.*, **246**, 5254.
5. Hamberg,M. (1973) *Anal. Biochem.*, **55**, 368.
6. Granström,E. and Kindahl,H. (1982) *Biochim. Biophys. Acta*, **713**, 555.
7. Pace-Asciak,C.R. and Edwards,N.S. (1982) In *Methods in Enzymology*. Lands,W.E.M. and Smith,W.L. (eds), Academic Press, New York, Vol. 86, p. 552.
8. Pace-Asciak,C. and Miller,D. (1974) *Experientia*, **30**, 590.
9. Kindahl,H., Edqvist,L.-E., Granström,E. and Bane,A. (1976) *Prostaglandins*, **11**, 871.
10. Hamberg,M. (1974) *Life Sci.*, **14**, 247.
11. Granström,E. and Kindahl,H. (1976) *Prostaglandins*, **12**, 759.
12. Granström,E. (1978) *Prostaglandins*, **15**, 3.
13. Granström,E., Kindahl,H. and Swahn,M.-L. (1982) *Biochim. Biophys. Acta*, **713**, 46.

14. Stehle,R.G. (1982) In *Methods in Enzymology*. Lands,W.E.M. and Smith,W.L. (eds), Academic Press, New York, Vol. 86, p. 436.
15. Granström,E., Hamberg,M., Hansson,G. and Kindahl,H. (1980) *Prostaglandins*, **19**, 933.
16. Fitzpatrick,F.A. and Wynalda,M.A. (1981) *Biochemistry*, **20**, 6129.
17. Fitzpatrick,F.A., Aguirre,R., Pike,J.E. and Lincoln,F.H. (1980) *Prostaglandins*, **19**, 917.
18. Granström,E., Fitzpatrick,F.A. and Kindahl,H. (1982) In *Methods in Enzymology*. Lands,W.E.M. and Smith,W.L. (eds), Academic Press, New York, Vol. 86, 306.
19. Inagawa,T., Imaki,K., Masuda,H., Morikawa,Y., Hirata,F. and Tsuboshima,M. (1983) In *Advances in Prostaglandin, Thromboxane and Leukotriene Research*. Samuelsson,B., Paoletti,R. and Ramwell,P.W. (eds), Raven Press, New York, Vol. 11, p. 191.
20. Fitzpatrick,F.A. and Wynalda,M.A. (1983) *J. Biol. Chem.*, **258**, 11713.
21. Anhut,H., Peskar,B.A., Wachter,W. Gräbling,B. and Peskar,B.M. (1978) *Experientia*, **34**, 1494.
22. Narumiya,S., Ogorochi,T., Nakao,K. and Hayaishi,O. (1982) *Life Sci.*, **31**, 2093.
23. Maclouf,J., Corvazier,E. and Wang,Z. (1986) *Prostaglandins*, **31**, 123.
24. Ellis,C.K., Smigel,M.D., Oates,J.A., Oelz,O. and Sweetman,B.J. (1979) *J. Biol. Chem.*, **254**, 4152.
25. Roberts,L.J., II and Sweetman,B.J. (1985) *Prostaglandins*, **30**, 383.
26. Liston,T.E. and Roberts,L.J. II (1985) *J. Biol. Chem.*, **260**, 13172.
27. Roberts,L.J., II (1982) In *Methods in Enzymology*, Lands,W.E.M. and Smith,W.L. (eds), Academic Press, New York, Vol. 86, p. 559.
28. Barrow,S.E., Heavey,D.J., Ennis,M., Chappell,C.G., Blair,I.A. and Dollery,C.T. (1984) *Prostaglandins*, **28**, 743.
29. Granström,E., Lands,W.E.M. and Samuelsson,B. (1968) *J. Biol. Chem.*, **243**, 4104.
30. Hensby,C.N. (1974) *Prostaglandins*, **8**, 369.
31. Wong,P.Y.-K. (1981) *Biochim. Biophys. Acta*, **659**, 169.
32. Reingold,D.F., Kawasaki,A. and Needleman,P. (1981) *Biochim. Biophys. Acta*, **659**, 179.
33. Liston,T.E. and Roberts,L.J. II (1985) *Proc. Natl. Acad. Sci. USA*, **82**, 6030.
34. Moncada,S., Ferreira,S.H. and Vane,J.R. (1978) In *Advances in Prostaglandin and Thromboxane Research*. Frölich,J.C. (ed.), Raven Press, New York, Vol. 5, p. 211.
35. Moncada,S., Korbut,R., Bunting,S. and Vane,J.R. (1978) *Nature*, **273**, 767.
36. Pace-Asciak,C. and Gryglewski,R. (1983) In *Prostaglandins and Related Substances. New Comprehensive Biochemistry*. Pace-Asciak,C.R. and Granström,E. (eds), Elsevier, Amsterdam, Vol. 5, p. 95.
37. Blair,I.A., Barrow,S.E., Waddell,K.A., Lewis,P.J. and Dollery,C.T. (1982) *Prostaglandins*, **23**, 579.
38. Roberts,L.J., II, Brash,A.R. and Oates,J.A. (1982) In *Advances in Prostaglandin, Thromboxane and Leukotriene Research*. Oates,J.A. (ed.), Raven Press, New York, Vol. 10, p. 211.
39. Patrono,C., Ciabattoni,G., Peskar,B.M., Pugliese,F. and Peskar,B.A. (1981) *Clin. Res.*, **29**, 276A (abstract).
40. Rosenkrantz,B., Fischer,C. and Frölich,J.C. (1981) *Clin. Pharmacol. Ther.*, **29**, 420.
41. Sun,F.F., Taylor,B.M., Sutter,D.M. and Weeks,J.R. (1979) *Prostaglandins*, **17**, 753.
42. Rosenkranz,B., Fischer,C., Weimer,K.E. and Frölich,J.C. (1980) *J. Biol. Chem.*, **255**, 10194.
43. FitzGerald,G.A., Pedersen,A.K. and Patrono,C. (1983) *Circulation*, **67**, 1174.
44. Frölich,J.C., Rosenkrantz,B., Fejes-Toth,G., Naray-Fejes-Toth,A. and Frölich,B. (1985) In *Advances in Prostaglandin, Thomboxane and Leukotriene Research*. Hayaishi,O. and Yamamoto,S. (eds), Raven Press, New York, Vol. 15, p. 47.
45. Patrono,C. and Ciabattoni,G. (1985) In *Advances in Prostaglandin, Thomboxane and Leukotriene Research*. Hayaishi,O. and Yamamoto,S. (eds), Raven Press, New York, Vol. 15, p. 71.
46. FitzGerald,G.A., Lawson,J., Blair,I.A. and Brash,A.R. (1985) In *Advances in Prostaglandin, Thromboxane and Leukotriene Research*. Hayaishi,O. and Yamamoto,S. (eds), Raven Press, New York, Vol. 15, p. 87.
47. Dollery,C.T. and Barrow.S.E. (1985) In *Advances in Prostaglandin, Thromboxane and Leukotriene Research*. Hayaishi,O. and Yamamoto,S. (eds), Raven Press, New York, Vol. 15, p. 91.
48. Kindahl,H. (1977) *Prostaglandin*, **13**, 619.
49. Granström,E., Westlund,P., Kumlin,M. and Nordenström,A. (1985) In *Advances in Prostaglandins, Thromboxane and Leukotriene Research*. Hayaishi,O. and Yamamoto,S. (eds), Raven Press, New York, Vol. 15, p. 67.
50. Patrono,C., Ciabattoni,G., Pugliese,F., Pierucci,A., Blair,I.A. and FitzGerald,G.A. (1986) *J. Clin. Invest.*, **77**, 590.
51. Granström,E. (1986) *Progr. Lipid Res.*, **25**, 119.
52. Granström,E., Diczfalusy,U. and Hamberg,M. (1983) In *Prostaglandins and Related Substances. New Comprehensive Biochemistry*. Pace-Asciak,C.R. and Granström,E. (eds), Elsevier, Amsterdam, Vol. 5, p. 45.

53. Patrono,C., Ciabattoni,G., Patrignani,P., Filabozzi,P., Pinca,E., Satta,M.A., Van Dorne,D., Cinotti,G.A., Pugliese,F., Pierucci,A. and Simonetti,B.M. (1982) In *Advances in Prostaglandin, Thromboxane and Leukotriene Research*. Samuelsson,B., Paoletti,R. and Ramwell,P.W. (eds), Raven Press, New York, Vol. 11, p. 493.
54. Westlund,P., Kumlin,M., Nordenström,A. and Granström,E. (1986) *Prostaglandins*, **31**, in press.
55. Westlund,P., Granström,E., Kumlin,M. and Nordenström,A. (1986). *Prostaglandins*, **31**, 929.
56. Roberts,L.J., II, Sweetman,B.J., Payne,N.A. and Oates,J.A. (1977) *J. Biol. Chem.*, **252**, 7415.
57. Roberts,L.J., II, Sweetman,B.J. and Oates,J.A. (1981) *J. Biol. Chem.*, **256**, 8384.
58. Maas,R.L., Taber,D.F. and Roberts,L.J., II (1982) In *Methods in Enzymology*. Lands,W.E.M. and Smith,S.L. (eds), Academic Press, New York, Vol. 86, p. 592.
59. Vesterqvist,O. and Green,K. (1984) *Prostaglandins*, **27**, 627.
60. FitzGerald,G.A., Oates,J.A., Hawiger,J., Maas,R.L., Roberts,L.J., II and Brash,A.R. (1983) *J. Clin. Invest.*, **72**, 676.
61. Kumlin,M. and Granström,E. (1986) *Prostaglandins*, **32**, 741.
62. Roberts,L.J., II, Sweetman,B.J., Maas,R.L., Hubbard,W.C. and Oates,J.A. (1980) *Progr. Lipid Res.*, **20**, 117.
63. Brash,A.R. and Baillie,T.A. (1979) *Biochim. Biophys. Acta*, **572**, 371.
64. Nugteren,D.H. (1975) *J. Biol. Chem.*, **250**, 2808.
65. Axelrod,B. (1979) *Adv. Chem. Ser.*, **136**, 324.
66. Hansson,G., Malmsten,C. and Radmark,O. (1983) In *Prostaglandins and Related Substances. New Comprehensive Biochemistry*. Pace-Asciak,C.R. and Granström,E. (eds), Elsevier, Amsterdam, Vol. 5, p. 127.
67. Samuelsson,B., Hammarström,S., Hamberg,M. and Serhan,C.N. (1985) In *Advances in Prostaglandin, Thromboxane and Leukotriene Research*. Pike,J.E. and Morton,Jr.,D.R. (eds), Raven Press, New York, Vol. 14, p. 45.
68. Wong,P.Y.-K., Westlund,P., Hamberg,M., Granström,E., Chao,P.H.-W. and Samuelsson,B. (1984) *J. Biol. Chem.*, **259**, 2683.
69. Lindgren,J.-A., Hansson,G. and Samuelsson,B. (1981) *FEBS Lett.*, **128**, 329.
70. Maclouf,J., Fruteau de Laclos,B. and Borgeat,P. (1982) *Proc. Natl. Acad. Sci. USA*, **79**, 6042.
71. Walker,I.C., Jones,R.L. and Wilson,N.H. (1979) *Prostaglandins*, **18**, 173.
72. Pace-Asciak,C.R., Granström,E. and Samuelsson,B. (1983) *J. Biol. Chem.*, **258**, 6835.
73. Serhan,C.N., Hamberg,M., Samuelsson,B., Morris,J. and Wishka,D.G. (1986) *Proc. Natl. Acad. Sci. USA*, **83**, 1983.
74. Serhan,C.N., Nicolaou,K.C., Weber,S.E., Veale,C.A., Dahlen,S.E., Puustinen,T.J. and Samuelsson,B. (1986) *J. Biol. Chem.*, **261**, 16340.
75. Samuelsson,B. (1983) *Science*, **220**, 568.
76. Haeggström,J., Meijer,J. and Radmark,O. (1986) *J. Biol. Chem.*, **261**, 6332.
77. Maas,R.L. and Brash,A.R. (1983) *Proc. Natl. Acad. Sci. USA*, **80**, 2884.
78. Sok,D.-E., Ching,T. and Sih,C.J. (1983) *Biochem. Biophys. Res. Commun.*, **110**, 273.
79. Sok,D.-E., Han,C.-O., Sieh,W.-R., Zhou,B.-N. and Sih,C.J. (1982) *Biochem. Biophys. Res. Commun.*, **104**, 1363.
80. Claesson,H.-E., Lindgren,J.-A. and Gustafsson,B. (1985) *Biochim. Biophys. Acta*, **836**, 361.
81. Taylor,B.M. and Sun,F.F. (1985) *Biochem. Pharmacol.*, **34**, 3495.
82. Serafin,W.E., Oates,J.A. and Hubbard,W. (1984) *Prostaglandins*, **27**, 899.
83. Hammarström,S., Örning,L. and Bernström,K. (1985) *Mol. Cell Biochem.*, **69**, 7.
84. Bernström,K. and Hammarström,S. (1982) *Biochem. Biophys. Res. Commun.*, **109**, 800.
85. Bernström,K. and Hammarström,S. (1986) *Arch. Biochem. Biophys.*, **244**, 486.
86. Clancy,R.M. and Hugli,T.E. (1983) *Anal. Biochem*, **113**, 30.
87. Kumlin,M., Dahlen,S.-E. and Granström,E. (1987) In *Advances in Prostaglandin, Thromboxane and Leukotriene Research*. Samuelsson,B. and Paoletti,R. (eds), Raven Press, New York, Vol. 17, p. 1014.
88. Goetzl,E.J. (1982) *Biochem. Biophys. Res. Commun.*, **106**, 270.
89. Lewis,R.A. and Austen,K.F. (1984) *J. Clin. Invest.*, **73**, 889.
90. Örning,L. and Hammarström,S. (1983) *FEBS Lett.*, **153**, 253.
91. Örning,L., Kaijser,L. and Hammarström,S. (1985) *Biochem. Biophys. Res. Commun.*, **130**, 214.
92. Örning,L., Norin,E., Gustafsson,B. and Hammarström,S. (1986) *J. Biol. Chem.*, **261**, 766.
93. Köller,M., Schönfeld,W., Knöller,J., Bremm,K-D., König,W., Spur,B., Crea,A. and Peters,W. (1985) *Biochim. Biophys. Acta*, **833**, 128.
94. Beaubien,B.C., Tippins,J.R. and Morris,H.R. (1984) *Biochem. Biophys. Res. Commun.*, **125**, 97.

CHAPTER 3

Tissue sampling and preparation

CHIARA BENEDETTO and TREVOR F.SLATER

1. INTRODUCTION

The sampling of tissues and body fluids to provide accurate information on metabolites with short half-lives, is always accompanied by experimental difficulties. This is certainly true in relation to the sampling of tissues to obtain values for the so-called endogenous levels of eicosanoids but, additionally, a special problem exists. Tissue damage produced by cutting or penetration (as in venipuncture) activates phospholipase A_2 and rapidly changes the local content of eicosanoids. This particular point is discussed in Chapter 2 and in Section 2.1 of this chapter. An additional hazard of tissue sampling in this context is that tissue disruption is generally a good stimulus for peroxidative mechanisms (see Chapter 14), and lipid hydroperoxides can have profound effects on both the cyclo-oxygenase and lipoxygenase pathways. It is thus apparent, if we wish to obtain meaningful data on endogenous or steady-state levels, that the methods to be used should minimize not only conventionally recognized artefacts of sampling but also artefacts due to the rapidity of eicosanoid response to trauma and peroxidation. Problems associated with sampling become much easier, however, if the information required is on relative (or maximal) rates of eicosanoid synthesis, or on the tissue levels or intracellular localization of enzyme activities.

Techniques that help to minimize artefacts in relation to blood sampling are outlined in Section 2 below, and with solid tissues in Section 3. With tissues generally, the main emphasis of the sampling methods used is to work as quickly as possible in order to obtain values as near as possible to those occurring naturally prior to sampling. With animal models, and with studies *in vitro*, it is possible to sample very rapidly (see Section 3), but many of these fast techniques cannot be used in clinical situations.

2. SAMPLING BLOOD AND URINE

2.1 Blood

Blood must be always drawn with needles of the same size (for studies on adult humans we recommend butterfly needles No. 21) mounted on a polypropylene syringe and, if possible, without applying a tourniquet in order to avoid vascular stasis. However, because of the difficulties encountered in finding a vein in some subjects, the use of a tourniquet is sometimes necessary: if such a situation occurs we think it is better to apply the tourniquet in all cases under study so as to standardize that particular group of subjects. Furthermore, an imperfect vein puncture increases the likelihood of elevated prostaglandin levels; it is therefore recommended to discard the first 1 or 2 ml of blood.

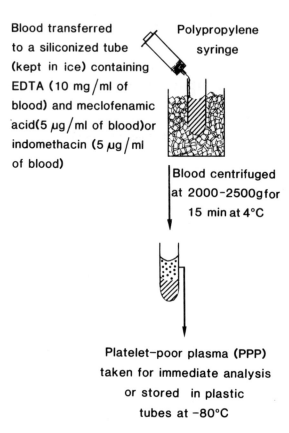

Blood transferred
to a siliconized tube
(kept in ice) containing
EDTA (10 mg/ml of
blood) and meclofenamic
acid(5 μg/ml of blood)or
indomethacin (5 μg/ml
of blood)

Polypropylene
syringe

Blood centrifuged
at 2000–2500g for
15 min at 4°C

Platelet–poor plasma (PPP)
taken for immediate analysis
or stored in plastic
tubes at −80°C

Figure 1. Standard method for the preparation of platelet-poor plasma (PPP) from whole blood for prostaglandin analysis.

If blood is collected continuously over a long period of time, the cannula must be flushed with heparinized saline prior to sampling and after each sampling.

In relation to the most suitable blood fraction for prostaglandin analysis it is preferable to collect platelet-poor plasma (PPP) (1) since prostaglandins are released during storage of platelet-rich plasma (PRP).

Blood samples should be transferred to siliconized tubes, kept in ice, containing an anti-coagulant (preferably EDTA; 10 mg/ml blood, equivalent to 28 mM final concentration) and potent inhibitors of the prostaglandin biosynthesis (e.g. meclofenamic acid and indomethacin 5 μg/ml blood, equivalent to ~17 and 14 μM final concentration respectively). The samples should be centrifuged as soon as possible in a refrigerated centrifuge (see *Figure 1*) and the PPP so obtained immediately analysed or stored at −20°C for 2−3 days and then at −80°C or in liquid nitrogen until required for analysis. It is recommended to keep the storage time to a minimum and if a complete analysis cannot be performed immediately it has also been suggested that the prostaglandins are extracted (see Chapter 4) and stored at −20°C in organic solvents, after any trace of acid has been removed by backwashing with water (1).

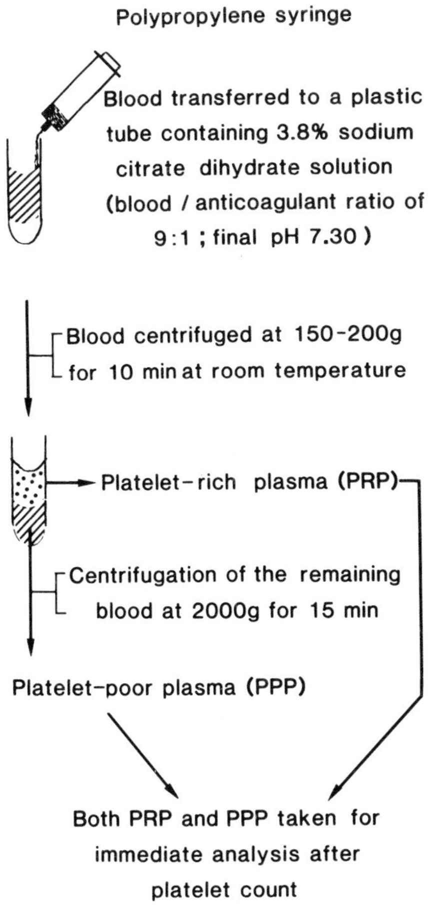

Polypropylene syringe

Blood transferred to a plastic
tube containing 3.8% sodium
citrate dihydrate solution
(blood / anticoagulant ratio of
9:1 ; final pH 7.30)

Blood centrifuged at 150-200g
for 10 min at room temperature

Platelet-rich plasma (PRP)

Centrifugation of the remaining
blood at 2000g for 15 min

Platelet-poor plasma (PPP)

Both PRP and PPP taken for
immediate analysis after
platelet count

Figure 2. Standard method for the preparation of platelet-rich plasma (PRP) and platelet-poor plasma (PPP) for studies on platelet aggregation.

Some experiments in the prostaglandin field require the preparation of plasma samples for studies on platelet aggregation. In these cases (see *Figure 2*) PRP can be obtained from citrated blood, carefully mixed and gently centrifuged ($150-200\ g$) at room temperature. PPP is then prepared by centrifugation of the remaining blood at 2000 g for 15 min (for alternative procedure see Chapter 9, Section 2.1.1). Since it has been demonstrated (2) that platelet aggregation, thromboxane B_2 (TXB_2) formation and platelet sensitivity to prostacyclin depend on the number of platelets in the PRP (*Figure 3*), once PRP and PPP have been pipetted it is advisable to make a platelet count. If a platelet counter is not available, the number of platelets must be estimated by standard procedures.

(i)   Suck up a small quantity of PRP to the mark 0.5 of a haemocytometer pipette and dilute 1:200 with ammonium oxalate (1% in water).

(ii)   After gentle mixing discard the distal fraction and lay the tip of the pipette on both chambers of the Bürker chamber. Platelets settle more slowly than erythro-

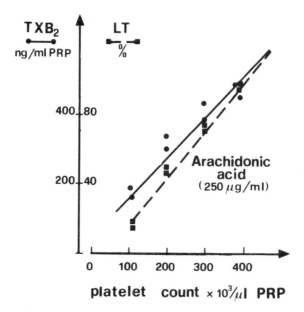

Figure 3. Influence of the number of the platelets in the PRP on thromboxane B$_2$ (TXB$_2$) formation and platelet aggregation (% light transmission, LT). The PRP was stimulated with arachidonic acid (modified from Siess *et al.*, 2).

cytes because of their low density; consequently, it is better to wait 10−20 min before counting them.

(iii)   Platelets look like small shining disks under the microscope; count them in a standard number of rectangles (usually 10) in each of the two chambers and calculate the final platelet counts by multiplying the mean obtained from the counts in both chambers by 20 000 (see legend to *Figure 4*).

In the case of PPP, the plasma should be initially diluted 1:100 with ammonium oxalate. Therefore, since the final calculation depends upon the dilution and the volume in which the count has been made, the mean obtained from the counts in both chambers should be multiplied by 10 000 in this case.

2.2 Urine

Urine should be collected in a bottle cooled in ice and kept at −20°C until assayed. In normal conditions it contains only a few viable cells, thus uncontrollable *ex vivo* formation of prostaglandins should be negligible.

For other body fluids (e.g. cerebrospinal fluid, semen, amniotic fluid, etc.) it is recommended to follow the general rules previously mentioned, that is

(i)   to reduce as much as possible mechanical and physical trauma during sampling;
(ii)   to keep the samples cool;
(iii)   to centrifuge them at 4°C if a sedimentation of red blood cells is required, and
(iv)   to store them at −80°C or in liquid nitrogen until assayed.

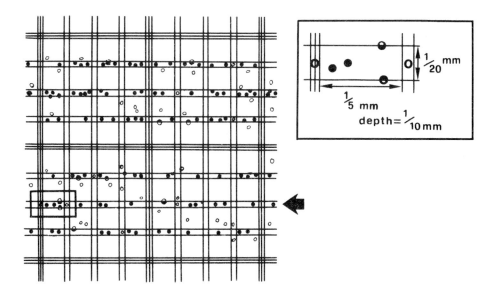

Figure 4. Platelet count in the Bürker chamber. Platelets should be counted in 10 or 20 rectangles in a particular row. The platelets to be counted are shown as black dots and those not to be counted as white circles. A platelet located on the outer line of the rectangle is given a value of 0.5. The volume of the counting rectangle is $1/5 \times 1/20 \times 1/10$ mm^3 = $1/1000$ mm^3. If 10 rectangles are counted this is equivalent to a volume of $1/100$ mm^3. With a dilution of 1:200 the number of platelets in the original suspension is equal to the number of platelets counted $(n) \times 200 \times 100$ mm^{-3}, that is $n \times 20\,000$.

3. SAMPLING SOLID TISSUES AND INTRACELLULAR FRACTIONS

3.1 Endogenous levels in solid tissue *in situ*

Typical examples here are experiments directed at measuring endogenous levels of eicosanoids in tissues such as lung, kidney, liver, tumours, etc. (see 3). As already mentioned, the sampling method used should effectively inhibit or destroy enzymic and non-enzymic processes that result in significant artefactual change. In practice, the main inhibitory procedures employed are very rapid cooling and the use of powerful inhibitors of phospholipase A$_2$, cyclo-oxygenase and/or lipid peroxidations. The main destructive procedures used are rapid microwave denaturation and acid precipitation. Comments on these different procedures are given below.

3.1.1 *Inhibitory procedures*

The simplest procedure is to freeze the sample as rapidly as possible: generally, the lower the temperature the better both for the initial inhibitory reaction and for subsequent storage. Speed is of the essence, as removing a piece of tissue from its location *in situ* can rapidly lead to anoxia, changes in co-enzyme levels and diverse metabolic disturbances with associated changes in substrate and metabolite contents. For example, in rat liver rapid sampling of tissue that had been ischaemic for 20 sec followed by 15 sec of re-perfusion gave ATP/AMP values of 0.82 and 8.5, respectively (4). An

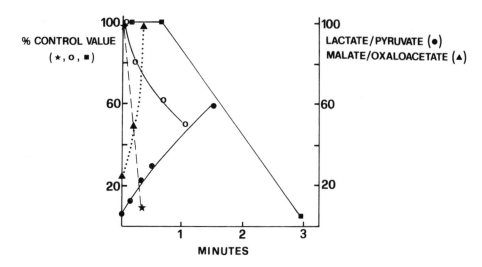

Figure 5. Some changes in rat liver that occur rapidly after the onset of ischaemic anoxia. Changes in ATP/AMP and in malate/oxaloacetate can be seen to be particularly rapid. The symbols used are: *, ATP/AMP; ▲, malate/oxaloacetate; ●, lactate/pyruvate; ■, bile flow; o, ATP. The figure is a modification of that in Slater (5) and used data from refs 4 and 7.

illustration of the rapidity of metabolite changes that can occur in the ischaemic interval following sampling is given in *Figure 5*.

Where it is possible to use the technique of freeze-clamping (see 6,7) this is to be preferred over the straightforward procedure of simply dropping a piece of excised tissue into liquid nitrogen. The reasons are as follows.

(i)   The freeze-clamping method produces a very thin layer of frozen powder in intimate contact with the conducting surfaces of the cold tongs (for description of experimental procedure see later). In consequence, all of the tissue in the sample is very rapidly cooled.

(ii) The rate of cooling of pieces of tissue dropped into liquid nitrogen is affected by the production of an enveloping bubble of nitrogen gas that does not ensure so rapid a cooling as with freeze-clamping.

Careful measurements (8) of the cooling of cubes of liver (2 mm^3) illustrate this effect clearly (*Figure 6*). Also shown is the fact that some solvents such as the Freons, can produce more rapid cooling than liquid N_2 itself. A rather good substitute for liquid N_2 cooling is hexane cooled by a bath of dry-ice in methanol (9). It is also important to note that the rate of cooling is affected by the size of the tissue sample, even with quite small sample sizes (see 8). Thus, where very rapid direct cooling of tissue samples is required it is necessary to work with samples of size about 100 mg wet weight or less.

The principle of freeze-clamping is illustrated in *Figure 7*. Substantial aluminium plates, about 3 cm × 3 cm × 1 cm are constructed to close in a pincer-like motion by the sudden manual compression of the insulated handles. (See safety aspects in the

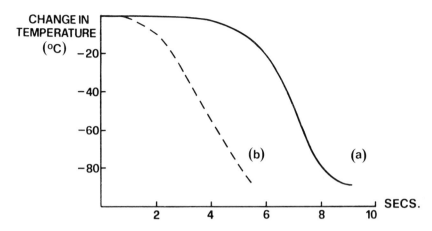

Figure 6. The time in seconds for a piece of tissue (2 mm³) to cool down when placed in **(a)** liquid nitrogen at $-196\,°C$ and **(b)** Freon 12 at $-77\,°C$. The data are taken from ref. 8.

legend to *Figure 7.*) Cool the plates thoroughly in liquid N_2 and expose the tissue to be sampled ready for freeze-clamping. With tissues *in situ* this entails prior anaesthesia. After clamping the tissue sample, return the securely closed clamps with the tissue sample quickly to liquid N_2. When properly applied the technique produces a thin layer of frozen powder; this can then be used for extraction by cold solvents or for acid precipitation (see Section 3.1.2).

If frozen tissue is to be stored for some time prior to extraction and analysis then it is best to store at temperatures of $-70\,°C$ or lower. It is known that samples maintained at $-20\,°C$ may still have some supercooled liquid phase that can have unexpected pH effects and cause metabolite disturbances (see 10). However, many enzymes and substrates are relatively stable when stored at $-20\,°C$; the stability of eicosanoids on storage is discussed in the Appendix.

Finally, in this short section on rapid freezing, it is important to emphasize the hazards of working with liquid N_2. The skin should be protected as far as possible from accidental splashes of liquid N_2, and the eyes should be shielded with safety glasses. Since oxygen is liquefied at a temperature somewhat higher $(-183\,°C)$ than that of liquid N_2 $(-196\,°C)$, appreciable quantities of liquid O_2 may accumulate with time in liquid N_2 containers. Liquid O_2 is a powerful explosive liquid and contact with any easily oxidizable material (especially fine powder such as charcoal dust as used in recrystallization procedures), should be avoided when the cold liquid is being poured out. For a full description of hazards with liquid N_2 see (12).

Although inhibitors of enzymic and non-enzymic processes (e.g. cyclo-oxygenase inhibitors and anti-oxidants) can also be considered under this section, they are of little use in practice with solid tissue samples due to slowness of penetration. They have a considerable application with tissue homogenates, tissue fractions and samples of biological fluids, and reference is made to the use of inhibitors in those specific contexts elsewhere in this chapter (see Section 5.1).

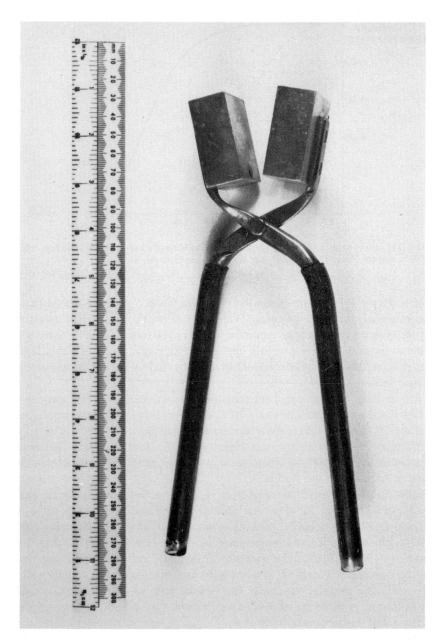

Figure 7. A pair of freeze-clamp tongs suitable for tissue samples of approximately 1 g wet weight. The large solid aluminium blocks are cooled in liquid nitrogen, and the exposed tissue is then rapidly clamped between the opposing faces of the tongs to yield a thin layer of rapidly frozen tissue. The tongs with frozen tissues can then be re-cooled in liquid nitrogen until the frozen powder is required for analysis. **Important:** note the insulation on the handles of the tongs; and remember the cautions already given about using liquid nitrogen in Section 3.1.1. In using the tongs it is best to wear thick insulated gloves to prevent any risk of the bare metal touching skin.

3.1.2 *Destructive procedures*

In these procedures the aim is either:

(i)   to rapidly destroy enzymes in the tissue sample that would otherwise cause metabolic perturbations of endogenous substrate and product contents;

(ii)   or to produce protein denaturation with acidic conditions that largely prevent further change in metabolite concentrations;

(iii)   or to rapidly homogenize and extract the sample with an organic solvent that results in the same stabilizing effect as in (ii).

An example of (i) is the use of focused microwave radiation to give localized protein denaturation in brain tissue prior to sampling for eicosanoid metabolites (see 13).

A much more widely used procedure is acid denaturation described in (ii) above. In this technique the tissue sample can be homogenized directly in cold acid, or tissue previously frozen in liquid N_2 can be transferred to cold acid and then homogenized. Techniques of homogenization are described by Graham (14) and in Section 5 below. A convenient acid for many purposes is 10% (v/v) perchloric acid used 1:1 with tissue; the cold acidic mixture can be centrifuged to obtain an essentially protein-free supernatant, and this can be neutralized with K_2CO_3 when necessary to produce a perchlorate-free solution as potassium perchlorate precipitates from the cold neutral solution. Although homogenizing in cold acid is often a convenient procedure, it does take an appreciable time (15−20 sec) between removing the sample, weighing and homogenizing. If weighing is considered inadvisable for reasons of speed then the amount of tissue taken can be estimated fairly accurately by measuring the DNA content of the acid-precipitated nucleoprotein pellet, and comparing this with the DNA content of a known weight of the same tissue (see 15) and *Figure 8.*

Homogenization of tissue samples directly into organic solvents is not nearly so widely practised as homogenization into acid and has a number of practical disadvantages and potential hazards. It is important *not* to use flammable solvents for homogenization procedures where local heating effects may exceed the flash-point of the solvent, or where electrostatic sparking may occur as with some blenders. In general, the use of organic solvents is best restricted to biphasic extractions of tissue samples already in a dispersed, homogenized form (see section below). In the context of hazards from the use of organic solvents it is important to remember that such substances are inevitably toxic, and therefore should be used under suitably safe conditions (for example, by doing all major manipulations in fume cupboards); also that flammable solvents should never be kept in refrigerators where sparking and subsequent explosions may occur. For safety procedures with organic solvents see (16).

3.2 Sampling cells and intracellular suspensions

The principles outlined above for use with solid tissue can be applied to cell and intracellular suspensions. Generally, manipulations are easier since the suspensions can be transferred quantitatively by pipetting directly into freezing-baths, into acid or into solvent. If rapid changes in metabolite concentrations are to be followed then rapid flow-quenching methods can be used whereby the reaction to be studied is initiated

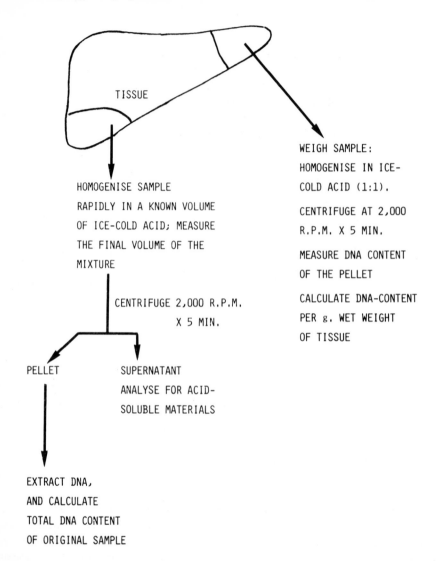

TISSUE

HOMOGENISE SAMPLE
RAPIDLY IN A KNOWN VOLUME
OF ICE-COLD ACID; MEASURE
THE FINAL VOLUME OF THE
MIXTURE

CENTRIFUGE 2,000 R.P.M.
X 5 MIN.

PELLET   SUPERNATANT
                ANALYSE FOR ACID-
                SOLUBLE MATERIALS

EXTRACT DNA,
AND CALCULATE
TOTAL DNA CONTENT
OF ORIGINAL SAMPLE

WEIGH SAMPLE:
HOMOGENISE IN ICE-
COLD ACID (1:1).

CENTRIFUGE AT 2,000
R.P.M. X 5 MIN.

MEASURE DNA CONTENT
OF THE PELLET

CALCULATE DNA-CONTENT
PER g. WET WEIGHT
OF TISSUE

Figure 8. A procedure whereby a tissue sample can be homogenized rapidly without weighing; the amount of tissue used is calculated subsequently by comparing the DNA content with that of a suspension of known tissue content. For further details see ref. 15.

by flowing component solutions together and thence into an acid-stop or freezing trap. Specialized rapid methods are described in (17).

4. TISSUE PREPARATIONS

Some standard procedures for studying the behaviour and activities of intact tissues and cells are described briefly in this section with reference to detailed descriptions.

4.1 **Perfused organs**

A number of well established procedures are available for studying the behaviour of whole perfused organs; a comprehensive review is by Ross (18). The use of perfused organs (for example, liver, kidney, heart, etc.) permits evaluations of multicellular organized cell assemblies, and where the perfusate compositions can be closely controlled to eliminate unwanted nervous and hormonal stimulations/suppressions. The perfusate and the perfused tissue can be sampled using methods described in Sections 2 and 3 above.

4.2 **Tissue slices and rings**

Much of the early classical work on metabolic pathways was done using tissue slices. This type of tissue preparation has a number of major advantages and some drawbacks. On the plus side are:

(i)   the ability to prepare many slices from a single piece of tissue, thereby allowing many controls and variations to be performed;

(ii)   a well prepared slice preserves cellular integrity in a large part of the sample, thus permitting studies with relatively undisturbed cellular architecture, and avoidance of cellular disintegration as occurs in homogenization.

On the debit side are:

(i)   difficulties in standardizing the amount of tissue added to each tube or flask;

(ii)   the inconvenience of not being able to pipette the tissue samples;

(iii)   the need to keep the sections sufficiently thin to permit adequate rates of diffusion of O_2 whilst thick enough to preserve a high proportion of intact cells.

Tissue slices are particularly useful for studying enzyme pathways, rates of metabolism, rates of uptake and secretion, etc.; a detailed practical account of work with slices and their preparation is given by Umbreit *et al.* (19).

4.3 **Isolated cells**

Isolated cell suspensions (for example, hepatocytes, myocytes) have the advantages outlined above for slices of maintaining cell integrity but, additionally, can be easily pipetted and conveniently manipulated. Among a number of disadvantages is the fact that the cells have been rather traumatically separated from their neighbours, usually by treatment with calcium-free medium and proteases. A comprehensive account of the practical problems associated with preparing and using hepatocytes is by Harris and Cornell (20).

Treatment of whole organs such as liver with enzymes, for example collagenase, to produce a disruption of tissue architecture often results in a suspension containing different classes of cells; these different cell types can be separated and studied. For example, in liver, the major class of cells (hepatocytes) can be separated from Kupffer cells and bile duct epithelial cells by centrifuging procedures (see 21); other methods that may be used for isolating different classes of cell from heterogeneous suspensions are elutriation (see 22) and flow cytometry (see 23,24).

5. HOMOGENIZING TISSUE SAMPLES

For many studies on enzymic activities, and for measuring and identifying products it is often very convenient to work with tissue homogenates and/or intracellular fractions such as microsomal suspensions or plasma membranes. The general principles of homogenizing, and of subcellular fractionation, are well described by Graham (14) in the Practical Approaches volume on 'Centrifugation', so it is inappropriate to review in detail here. However, a few comments are necessary in relation to eicosanoid metabolism.

5.1 Use of inhibitors

When so-called endogenous levels of eicosanoids in homogenates are to be determined then it is necessary to inhibit 'artefactual' production that may occur during homogenization and subsequent steps. Inhibition can be achieved by the inclusion in the homogenizing medium of substances such as indomethacin and meclofenamic acid together (final concentrations ~ 15 μM), BW755c (final concentration 10 μM), or TROLOX-c (final concentration 15 μM), for inhibiting cyclo-oxygenase, lipoxygenase or lipid peroxidation, respectively. The inclusion of such inhibitors is useful in studies on enzymes that would otherwise be affected by products of eicosanoid metabolism (for example, prostacyclin synthase by lipid hydroperoxides; 25). As far as endogenous levels are concerned it has to be remembered that these values will be strongly distorted, most probably by the rapid responses of cyclo-oxygenases and lipoxygenases to tissue trauma in sampling and in the initial stages of homogenization before the inhibitor(s) can become intimately mixed with the tissue.

5.2 Rapidity and cooling

Because of the rapidity of additional production of eicosanoid products, as already mentioned, it is important to work as fast as possible in sampling, in cooling to $0-2°C$, and in homogenizing with appropriate inhibitors. Homogenizing may also be done using material obtained by freeze-clamping; in this case, an appropriate weight of frozen tissue powder is added to cold medium and immediately homogenized. A clear description of a freeze-clamping technique, followed by rapid homogenizing and separation of intracellular organelles is by Eason and Zammit (26).

5.3 Homogenate complexity

Most tissues can be homogenized easily using a conventional Potter−Elvehjem type of homogenizer [it is worth noting that a similar procedure was described by Hagen in 1922 (27) but the technique has now become firmly associated with the names of Van Potter and Elvehjem, 28], and using a suspending medium of buffered sucrose or mannitol. The strength of the suspending medium that is often used is 0.25 M sucrose; this allows convenient centrifuging stages but also results in some abnormalities of the morphology of intracellular organelles [see Hogeboom *et al.* (29)]. For a general description of homogenizing techniques see Graham (14).

It is important to note that a homogenate of a tissue such as liver or lung includes components from many different cell types present in the tissue at the time of sampling.

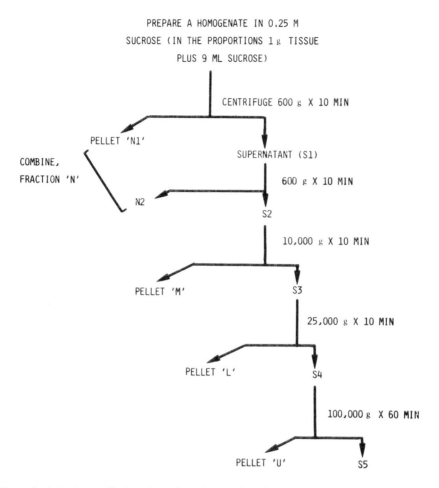

Figure 9. A simple centrifuging scheme for a tissue such as liver. In each case the pellet is indicated to the left of each centrifuging operation, and the corresponding supernatant is on the right. Fraction 'N' is a heterogeneous fraction containing unbroken cells, large debris, red blood cells and nuclei. Fractions M, L and U are the mitochondrial, lysosomal and microsomal fractions respectively. Supernatant fraction 'S5' is the cytosol or soluble fraction of the cell.

Moreover, experimental treatments, or different physiological states, can change the cellular content of a tissue sample and, thus, the content of the homogenate prepared from it. Simple illustrations are the influx of inflammatory cells, or changes in blood content.

5.4 Separation of intracellular organelles

It is very easy to obtain moderately 'clean' fractions of mitochondria, microsomes and cytosol from sucrose homogenates by simple differential centrifuging techniques [see Graham, (14)]. A standard scheme for liver homogenates is shown in *Figure 9*. Much more elaborate schemes are necessary if samples of much greater purity are needed,

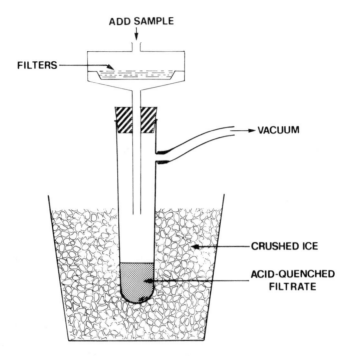

Figure 10. A method for obtaining acid-stopped soluble fractions of tissue homogenates (15). The tissue suspension is pipetted onto a filter assembly (see photograph) that retains all unbroken cells and intracellular organelles; convenient filters that can be used for this purpose are Millipore 5 μm and 0.2 μm, with the 5 μm filter on top. The filtrate is sucked through by negative pressure and goes directly into ice-cold acid.

usually requiring a combination of differential and density gradient centrifuging; for example, see Le Page *et al.* (30) for a centrifuging scheme for plasma membranes.

A point to emphasize is that the routine schemes such as that shown in *Figure 9* are very often those which have been originally worked out for liver. The centrifuging speeds and times may not be appropriate for other tissues (although in many cases they are); for instance, in rat mammary gland it was found necessary to vary considerably the centrifuging speeds used, compared with liver, in order to get good mitochondrial yields (31). Thus, the optimum conditions for centrifuging should be checked with any new tissue under study.

5.4.1 *Rapid separation of intracellular fractions*

It is possible to separate some major intracellular fractions within a few seconds – minutes of preparing the homogenate by using special centrifuging or filtration techniques.

For example, the homogenate can be layered on top of silicone oil that is itself layered on acid and then subjected to high-speed centrifugation for 25 min. Mitochondria pass through the silicone layer and are rapidly denatured ('fixed') by the acidic solution (32).

Another example concerns rapid filtration (15). In this technique, the homogenate is pipetted onto a cellulose acetate microfilter that retains all intracellular organelles but allows the cytosol to pass through directly into an acid fixative (*Figure 10*). In this way, cytosol fractions can be prepared within 20 sec of removing a tissue sample.

5.4.2 *Separation of small samples*

Normal methods for homogenizing and intracellular separations are not readily applicable with samples of less than $50-100$ mg. With smaller samples (for example, small biopsy samples) the rotor first devised by Beaufay and used with much effect on liver disease by Peters (33) is very useful.

6. ACKNOWLEDGEMENTS

We are grateful to our many collaborators for help in developing those practical procedures described here and that originated in our groups. We also thank the Association for International Cancer Research, and the National Foundation for Cancer Research who have generously supported our collaborative work over many years.

7. REFERENCES

1. Salmon,J.A. and Flower,R.J. (1980) In *Hormones in Blood. VI. Prostaglandins and Related Compounds.* 3rd edition, Gray,C.H. and James,V.H.T. (eds), Academic Press, New York, Vol. 2, p. 253.
2. Siess,W., Roth,P. and Weber,P.C. (1981) *Thromb. Haemostas.*, **45**, 204.
3. Bennett,A., Berstock,D.A., Carroll,M.A., Stamford,I.F. and Wilson,A.J. (1983) In *Advances in Prostaglandin, Thromboxane and Leukotriene Research.* Samuelsson,B., Paoletti,R. and Ramwell,P. (eds.), Raven Press, New York, Vol. 12, p. 299.
4. Bücher,T., Krejci,K., Rüssman,W., Schnitger,H. and Weseman,W. (1964) In *Rapid Mixing and Sampling Techniques in Biochemistry.* Chance,B., Eisenhardt,R.H.E., Gibson,Q.H. and Lonberg-Holm,K.K. (eds), Academic Press, New York, p. 255.
5. Slater,T.F. (1978) In *Biochemical Mechanisms of Liver Injury.* Slater,T.F. (ed.), Academic Press, London, p. 1.
6. Wollenberger,A., Ristau,O. and Schoffa,G. (1960) *Pflügers Arch.*, **270**, 399.
7. Faupel,R.P., Seitz,H.J., Tarnowski,W., Thiemann,V. and Weiss,C. (1972) *Arch. Biochem. Biophys.*, **148**, 509.
8. Cain,D.F. and Davies,R.E. (1964) In *Rapid Mixing and Sampling Techniques in Biochemistry.* Chance,B., Eisenhardt,R.H., Gibson,Q.H. and Lonberg-Holm,K.K. (eds), Academic Press, New York, p. 229.
9. Chayen,J., Bitensky,L. and Butcher,R.G. (1973) *Practical Histochemistry.* John Wiley and Sons, London.
10. Lowry,O.H., Passonneau,J.V. and Rock,M.K. (1961) *J. Biol. Chem.*, **236**, 2756.
11. Lowry,O.H. and Passonneau,J.V. (1972) *A Flexible System of Enzymatic Analysis.* Academic Press, New York.
12. Bretherick,L. (1979) *Handbook of Reactive Chemical Hazards.* Butterwick and Co. (Publishers) Ltd., London.
13. Cenedella,R.J., Galli,C. and Paoletti,R. (1975) *Lipids*, **10**, 290.
14. Graham,J. (1984) In *Centrifugation − A Practical Approach.* 2nd edition, Rickwood,D. (ed.), IRL Press, Oxford and Washington, DC, p. 161.
15. Delaney,V.B. and Slater,T.F. (1970) *Biochem. J.*, **116**, 299.
16. Health & Safety Executive (1986) *Storage and Use of Highly Flammable Liquids in Educational Establishments.* HSE Publication IAC L15. Bootle.
17. Chance,B., Eisenhardt,R.H., Gibson,Q.H. and Lonberg-Holm,K.K. (1964) *Rapid Mixing and Sampling Techniques in Biochemistry.* Academic Press, New York.
18. Ross,B.D. (1972) *Perfusion Techniques in Biochemistry: A Laboratory Manual.* Clarendon Press, Oxford.
19. Umbreit,W.W., Burris,R.H. and Stauffer,J.F. (1964) *Manometric Techniques.* 4th edition, Burgess Publishing Co., Minneapolis, MN.
20. Harris,R.A. and Cornell,N.W., eds (1983) *Isolation, Characterization and Use of Hepatocytes.* Elsevier Biomedical, New York.
21. Bodenheimer,H.C., Charland,C., Tente,W.E., McMillan,P.N. and Thayer,W.R. (1983) In *Isolation and Characterization and Use of Hepatocytes.* Harris,R.A. and Cornell,N.W. (eds), Elsevier Biomedical, New York, p. 99.
22. Brouwer,A., Barelds,R.J. and Knook,D.L. (1984) In *Centrifugation − A Practical Approach.* 2nd edition, Rickwood,D. (ed.), IRL Press, Oxford and Washington, DC, p. 183.
23. Horan,P. and Wheeless,L. (1977) *Science*, **198**, 149.

24. Darnell,J., Lodish,H. and Baltimore,D. (1986) *Molecular Cell Biology.* Scientific American Books, New York.
25. Moncada,S., Gryglewski,R.J., Bunting,S. and Vane,J.R. (1976) *Prostaglandins,* **12**, 715.
26. Easom,R.A. and Zammit,V.A. (1984) *Biochem. J.,* **220**, 733.
27. Hagan,W.A. (1922) *J. Exp. Med.,* **36**, 711.
28. Potter,V.R. and Elvehjem,C.A. (1936) *J. Biol. Chem.,* **114**, 495.
29. Hogeboom,G.H., Schneider,W. and Palade,G.E. (1948) *J. Biol. Chem.,* **172**, 619.
30. Le Page,R.N., Cheeseman,K.H. and Slater,T.F. (1987) *Cell. Biochem. Function,* in press.
31. Slater,T.F. and Planterose,D.N. (1960) *Biochem. J.,* **74**, 584.
32. Werkheiser,W.C. and Bartley,W. (1957) *Biochem. J.,* **66**, 79.
33. Cairns,S.C. and Peters,T.J. (1984) *Clin. Sci.,* **67**, 337.

CHAPTER 4

Extraction of eicosanoids from biological samples

SANTOSH NIGAM

1. INTRODUCTION

Since eicosanoids are normally not stored in the body as a pre-formed compound to any great extent, their release into the circulation reflects the local synthesizing capacity of the tissue. The lability and rapid degradation of eicosanoids during their passage through the circulation make their analysis very difficult. Although there have been several reports in the past of a direct assay for prostanoids in plasma and urine (1−5), the levels thus obtained were higher for prostaglandins (PG) and thromboxanes (TX) than those found when extraction and purification preceded the radioimmunoassay (RIA), reflecting the presence of both prostanoids and non-specific interfering plasma proteins. It is therefore preferable to extract biological samples before analysis. The easy extraction of eicosanoids into organic solvents in their protonated form is based on the weakly acidic character of eicosanoids.

2. METHODS OF EXTRACTION

2.1 Organic solvent extraction and open column chromatography

Analytical methods such as high-performance liquid chromatography (h.p.l.c.) or gas chromatography−mass spectrometry (g.c.−m.s.) require extensive purification of biological samples to prevent contaminants from interfering with the efficiency of the assay and to avoid the appearance of artifactual peaks. The most common methods used in the past for extraction of eicosanoids from body fluids (e.g. plasma and urine) and tissue or subcellular fractions were either to treat the acidified sample with organic solvents, such as diethyl ether, chloroform or ethyl acetate, after removing the neutral lipids with petroleum ether at a slightly alkaline pH (6), or to pass the sample through an XAD-2 column after acidification. Successive elution of the column with water and methanol resulted in extraction of eicosanoids into the methanol fraction. The large volumes of methanol thus obtained were then evaporated under reduced pressure, and the residue was subjected to open column chromatography on silicic acid to remove extraneous material prior to the final purification by h.p.l.c. One such extraction procedure without the XAD-2 column is used in our laboratory (7) and is described in *Table 1*.

The advantages of the above method are elimination of interfering proteins, specificity of the assay and improvement in sensitivity of the analysis. The above method does, however, involve many disadvantages, such as evaporation of large volumes of solvent

Table 1. Organic solvent extraction, open column- and reverse-phase (RP) h.p.l.c. of eicosanoids in biological samples.

1. Add the appropriate tritiated eicosanoid (~7000 d.p.m.) and 10 ng of deuterated eicosanoid (only for g.c.−m.s. assay) as internal standard to a 1 ml plasma or 10 ml urine sample.
2. Equilibrate the sample at 4°C for 10 min.
3. Acidify to pH 3.0−3.5 with 3% formic acid.
4. Extract twice with 3 vols of ethyl acetate:toluene (1:1).
5. Evaporate the combined organic phases under a stream of nitrogen and dry the residues under reduced pressure.
6. Add 1 ml of 0.05 M sodium borate buffer at pH 8.0 to the residue.
7. Prepare silicic acid columns (0.5 × 20 cm) of 0.5 g of non-activated silicic acid (100 mesh Mallinckrodt) equilibrated in 2 ml of solvent A (toluene:ethyl acetate:methanol/60:40:20).
8. Apply the sample (step 6) to the silicic acid column and wash once with 5 ml of solvent A and twice with 5 ml of solvent B (toluene:ethyl acetate/60:40).
9. Elute the eicosanoid fractions with 10 ml of solvent A.
10. Evaporate to dryness under nitrogen.
11. Reconstitute the residue in 100 μl of h.p.l.c. solvent (acetonitrile:water:acetic acid/33:67:0.1).
12. Separate the eicosanoids on a RP-h.p.l.c. C_{18}- column (4.6 × 250 mm; Nucleosil, 5 μm; Machery-Nagel, FRG) with mobile phase acetonitrile:water:acetic acid (33:67:0.1) at a flow-rate of 1 ml/min.
13. Collect the fractions every minute in siliconized glass tubes.
14. Localize the eicosanoids by counting aliquots of the fractions for ^{3}H-radioactivity.
15. Combine the tubes containing the same eicosanoid and evaporate the acetonitrile under nitrogen.
16. Extract the aqueous phase with 3 vols of ethyl acetate.
17. Evaporate the organic phase to dryness under nitrogen.
18. Reconstitute the residue either in buffer for RIA or in methanol for g.c.−m.s. analysis.

and low recovery due to multiple extraction steps; it is also very time consuming. Moreover, many solvents have a 'blank effect', raising basic levels in subsequent assays. The use of methanol in extraction of some prostanoids, for example 6-keto-PGF$_{1\alpha}$, may cause loss of immunoreactivity.

2.2 Powell method for extraction of eicosanoids other than peptido-leukotrienes from biological samples using octadecylsilyl (ODS)-silica

In 1980, Powell (8) developed a simple method for rapid extraction of eicosanoids from tissue homogenates and biological fluids using small columns containing the hydrophobic material ODS-silica. Several companies supply this material in the form of disposable minicolumns (see Section 4.2). In our laboratory we use Sep-Pak C_{18} cartridges from Waters Associates, USA.

Normally, the biological sample is applied to the ODS-silica column after acidification to pH 3.0−3.5. The eicosanoids are retained on the basis of hydrophobic interactions with the ODS-silica. The columns are then washed with water. Water mixed with small amounts of suitable organic solvent (e.g. methanol, ethanol or acetonitrile) removes the salts and polar components. Eicosanoids can then be eluted with an organic solvent of higher eluting strength, such as ethyl acetate or methyl formate. *Figure 1* shows the main steps for extraction of a biological sample on an ODS-silica column.

Furthermore, Powell observed that the ODS-silica column can also function as a straight-phase medium for chromatography, and so some separation can be accomplished for eicosanoids of differing polarity by varying the polarity of the eluting solvent. Figure

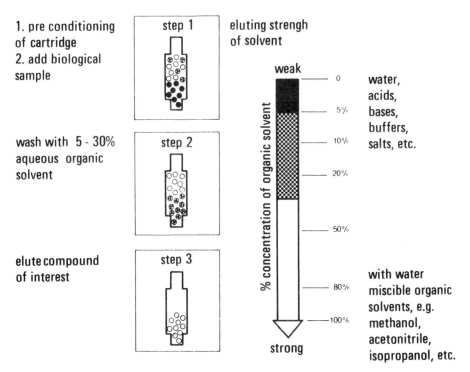

Figure 1. A general scheme for the extraction of eicosanoids from biological samples. **Step 1:** apply the sample onto a Sep-Pak C$_{18}$ cartridge and wash with water to eliminate inorganic salts, amino acids, hydrophilic proteins, etc. **Step 2:** elute the adsorbing polar substances, small peptides, etc. with 5–30% aqueous organic solvent of moderate eluting strength. **Step 3:** elute the retained substances, for example eicosanoids, with organic solvent of the desired eluting strength (e.g. methyl formate or ethyl acetate).

Table 2. Work-up procedure for extraction of eicosanoids other than leukotrienes using ODS-silica (Sep-Pak C$_{18}$) columns.

1. Add the appropriate tritiated (~7000 d.p.m.) and 10 ng of deuterated eicosanoid (only for g.c.–m.s. assay) as an internal standard to 1 ml of plasma, 1 ml of tissue homogenate or 10 ml of urine sample.
2. Equilibrate the samples at 4 °C for 10 min.
3. Add ethanol to the tissue homogenates, subcellular fractions and supernatants from cells to achieve a final concentration of 15% ethanol. Centrifuge the mixture at 375 *g* for 10 min at 4 °C. The supernatant is ready for applying to an ODS-silica column (Sep-Pak cartridge).
4. Attach the Sep-Pak cartridge to a 20 ml polypropylene syringe with Luerlok and wash with 20 ml of ethanol and 20 ml of water successively.
5. Apply the biological sample, after acidifying to pH 3.0 with 3% formic acid, to an ODS Sep-Pak cartridge.
6. Wash with 20 ml of water.
7. Wash with 20 ml of 15% aqueous ethanol.
8. Wash with 20 ml of petroleum ether.
9. Elute the eicosanoids with 10 ml of freshly distilled methyl formate or re-distilled ethyl acetate.
10. Evaporate the organic phase under a stream of nitrogen.
11. Reconstitute the residue in h.p.l.c. solvent (see *Table 1*).
12. Separate the eicosanoids on an RP-h.p.l.c. column as described in *Table 1*.

47

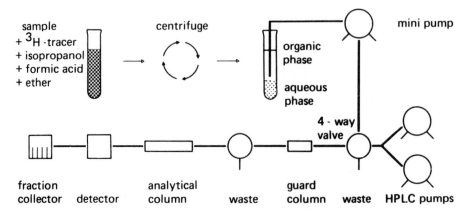

Figure 2. Schematic procedure for extraction of peptido-leukotrienes. First, the sample is combined with isopropanol and 5 M formic acid in a volume ratio of 1.0:0.5:0.03, respectively. After 5 min, 1.5 vol of ether is added, and the mixture centrifuged. The upper organic layer is pumped directly to a pre-conditioned guard column containing ODS-silica as the stationary material. The retained peptido-leukotrienes are then separated on a C_{18}-analytical column as described in *Table 3*.

1 in Chapter 6 shows such a scheme for extraction of eicosanoids other than peptido-leukotrienes. *Table 2* gives a complete work-up procedure for extraction of prostanoids and monohydroxy fatty acids.

2.3 Extraction of peptido-leukotrienes (LT)

The methods described above failed to extract conjugated peptido-leukotrienes LTC_4, LTD_4 and LTE_4 into organic solvents such as ether or chloroform. Furthermore, they could not be eluted from the ODS-silica column with methyl formate. Powell therefore developed a direct method for loading the biological sample onto the h.p.l.c. guard column without prior extraction (see Chapter 6). The chromatograms obtained revealed no difference compared with the chromatograms of eicosanoids obtained using the conventional method.

Clancy and Hugli (9) described a simple two-step extraction method for isolating peptido-leukotrienes C_4, D_4 and E_4 from lung tissues. The advantage of the method lies in the fact that it eliminates the effect of vasoamines and the platelet-activating factor (PAF). We have modified this method in our laboratory with the help of h.p.l.c. The schematic set-up of the extraction method has been depicted in *Figure 2*. A complete work-up procedure for extraction of LTC_4, LTD_4 and LTE_4 is described in *Table 3*.

3. RECOVERIES OF STANDARD EICOSANOIDS FROM BIOLOGICAL SAMPLES

The recoveries of tritiated 6-keto-$PGF_{1\alpha}$ and TXB_2 added to human plasma ($n = 6$) after extraction according to the procedure described in *Table 1* were approximately 35% and 55%, respectively.

Powell (10) reported recoveries of between 84 and 97% for PGD_2, PGE_2, $PGF_{2\alpha}$, 6-keto-$PGF_{1\alpha}$, TXB_2 13,14-dihydro-15-keto-$PGF_{2\alpha}$ and 13,14-dihydro-15-keto-PGE_2

Table 3. Work-up procedure for extraction of peptido-leukotrienes C_4, D_4 and E_4 from biological samples.

1. Add the appropriate tritiated peptido-leukotrienes (~ 7000 d.p.m.) to 1 ml of plasma or 1 ml of tissue homogenate.
2. Equilibrate the sample at 4°C for 10 min.
3. Add isopropanol and formic acid (5.0 M) to the sample in a volume ratio of 0.5:0.03:1.0, respectively and keep at 4°C for 5 min.
4. Add 1.5 volume of cold ether, shake and centrifuge.
5. Add two drops of 30% ammonia and rapidly pump the upper organic phase onto a guard column of h.p.l.c. containing ODS-silica as the stationary material.
6. Pump 5 ml of 20% methanol through the guard column. The effluent from the column is rejected using a three-way valve.
7. The peptido-leukotrienes retained by the guard column are then separated isocratically on an RP-h.p.l.c. C_{18} column (4.6 × 250 mm; Nucleosil, 5 μm; Macherey-Nagel, FRG) with mobile phase methanol: water:EDTA (75:25:0.1) having a pH of 5.6 at a flow-rate of 1 ml/min.
8. Collect the isolated leukotrienes with the help of a fraction collector.

after solid-phase extraction (see *Table 2*) from spiked bovine lung homogenate. The recoveries for PGE_2 and $PGF_{2\alpha}$ from spiked plasma and urine samples ranged between 96 and 102%.

The recoveries for 5-, 12- and 15-hydroxyeicosatetraenoic acid (HETE), LTB_4, LTC_4, LTD_4 and LTE_4 from human plasma ($n = 6$) according to the extraction method described in *Table 3* were between 90 and 98% for HETEs and 97%, 85%, 74% and 49% for LTB_4, LTC_4, LTD_4 and LTE_4, respectively.

4. GENERAL CONSIDERATIONS ON THE EXTRACTION OF EICOSANOIDS

4.1 **Materials required**

The commercial suppliers of the eicosanoids are listed in the Appendix of this book. Cartridges containing ODS-silica can be obtained as Sep-Pak C_{18} cartridges (Waters Associates, Milford, USA), Bond-Elut columns (Jones Chromatography, Llanbrodach, UK) or Supelclean LC-18 tubes (Supelco, Inc., PA, USA). ODS-silica can also be prepared by treating BioSil HA (Bio-Rad Labs., USA) with octadecyltrichlorosilane, as described by Bennett *et al*. (11). Cartridges of ODS-silica can be used several times after regeneration with 20 ml of 75% ethanol, 20 ml of ethanol and 20 ml of water successively. In our laboratory, we use Sep-Pak C_{18} cartridges three times for extraction of eicosanoids from body fluids.

4.2 **Extraction device and dry-down apparatus**

Several commercial sample preparation systems, such as Sep-Pak multisampler (Waters Associates, USA) or SPE vacuum manifold plus (Supelco, Inc., USA), are available for extracting up to 12 samples at a time.

We have developed a semi-automatic extraction device (*Figure 3*) in our laboratory for preparation of 10 samples at a time. We use normal polypropylene syringes with Luerlok, which permits mechanical filling with the required organic solvent and pressing of the eluting solvent through the Sep-Pak C_{18} cartridges. The flow-rate of the solvent can be adjusted to between 0.1 and 10 ml per min. A recently introduced

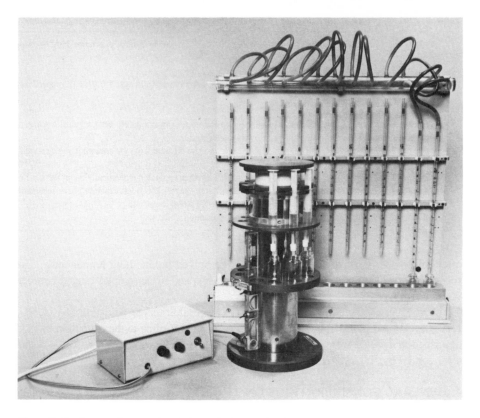

Figure 3. Semi-automatic extraction device and nitrogen dry-down apparatus.

modified system (not shown here) allows automatic changing of organic solvents and simultaneous evaporation of the eluting solvent containing eicosanoids under a stream of nitrogen. The whole process is controlled by a microprocessor. This simplifies the sample preparation method and reduces the time required to 30 min.

4.3 **Preparation of the sample**

Acidified plasma and urine samples can be applied directly to a pre-conditioned Sep-Pak C_{18} cartridge.

(i)   Wash the cartridge with water and aqueous ethanol, as already described.

(ii) As very low normal levels of eicosanoids in plasma have been reported in the literature, it is advisable to extract at least 5 ml of plasma and 10 ml of urine. Larger volumes of urine (30−50 ml) after acidification can be extracted twice with an equal volume of chloroform.

(iii) Dry the combined extracts under nitrogen, reconstitute to at least twice the original urine volume, and then apply to an ODS-silica column.

(iv) Homogenize tissue samples in 0.1 M Tris-HCl buffer (5 ml/g tissue), pH 7.4, with a Polytron homogenizer at 4°C, and add 3 vols of ethanol.

(v)   After adding known amounts of ^{3}H- or ^{14}C-labelled standards dissolved in ethanol for calculating the recovery of eicosanoids, allow the mixture to stand at room temperature for 5 min.

(vi)   Add water to attain a final concentration of 15% ethanol; centrifuge the mixtures at 400 g for 10 min.

(vii)   Collect the supernatant, acidify to pH 3.0 and pass it through the Sep-Pak cartridge as described above.

4.4 Influence of pH on the extraction

Eicosanoids, being weak acidic lipids, are readily extracted into organic solvents in their protonated form. The recovery of a particular eicosanoid depends on the pH and the type of biological specimen involved. Using ethyl acetate as the solvent, Goswami *et al.* (12) reported pH 4.5 as an optimum for extraction of prostanoids (recoveries between 91 and 98%) from different tissues. Ramwell *et al.* (13) observed the dehydration of PGE_2 to form PGA_2 at pH 3.0. 2,3-Dinor-6-keto-$PGF_{1\alpha}$, a urinary metabolite of prostacyclin, exists in different isomeric forms depending upon the pH conditions of the medium. At a low pH, this metabolite favours the γ-lactone form, whereas at a high pH the ketone form of the free acid is dominant. This property permits extraction of 2,3-dinor-6-keto-$PGF_{1\alpha}$ in a sufficiently pure form with organic solvents from a mild aqueous base medium, for example pH 8.0 (see Chapter 7).

Powell (10) observed no difference in solid-phase extraction of $PGF_{2\alpha}$, 19-OH-$PGF_{2\alpha}$ or acid-labile prostanoids, such as prostacyclin, PGG_2 and PGH_2, at a neutral or mild basic pH.

Which acid should be used to acidify the biological sample is still a matter of discussion. It is preferable to use an organic acid with a relatively high pK_a. Formic acid $(1-3\%)$ and citric acid $(0.5-2.0$ M) have frequently been used, because their volatility allows easy removal.

4.5 Precautions required for assaying eicosanoids in biological samples

It is advisable to analyse the samples for eicosanoids as early as possible. A biological sample should be stored in adequate small portions at $-70°$C to $-80°$C to avoid thawing of the whole sample for analysis. In RIA, the maximum binding value observed with plasma increased with successive cycles of freeze/thawing of stored samples. The storage at $-70°$C to $-80°$C should not take place abruptly. The sample should initially be stored at $-20°$C for 2 h and then into storage at lower temperatures for longer periods. Morris *et al.* (14) have reported a shift in the binding of plasma after long storage at $-20°$C.

Pipettors and/or pipettes should deliver the required volumes accurately and precisely. Pipettes and/or pipette tips used to transfer diluted standards, tracer or samples should be made of polypropylene or siliconized glass. While handling solid eicosanoids, it is absolutely necessary to take the precaution of wearing a mask over the nose and mouth, because eicosanoids such as PGE_1, PGE_2, PGD_2, $PGF_{2\alpha}$-tromethamine salt and leukotrienes cause asthma, coughing, reddening, irritation, swelling of eyes and headache. It is advisable to handle them carefully in a fume hood. Oily prostanoids and monohydroxy fatty acids should not come into contact with skin. Gloves should be worn while handling these materials.

5. ACKNOWLEDGEMENTS

The author wishes to thank the Research Workshop of Klinikum Steglitz, Berlin, for constructing the extraction apparatus and Dr J.Weirowski for reviewing the manuscript. The technical assistance of Barbara Steiger and Sybille Fröhlich is gratefully acknowledged. This work was generously supported by the Association for International Cancer Research, UK.

6. REFERENCES

1. Brummer,H.C. (1973) *Prostaglandins, 3*, 3.
2. Youssefnejadian,E., Walker,E., Sommerville,I.F. and Craft,I. (1974) *Prostaglandins, 6*, 23.
3. Strickland,D.M., Brennecke,S.P. and Mitchell,M.D. (1982) *Prostaglandins Leukotrienes Med., 9*, 491.
4. Starczowski,M., Voigtmann,R., Peskar,B.A. and Peskar,B.M. (1984) *Prostaglandins Leukotrienes Med., 13*, 249.
5. Korteweg,M., De Boever,J., Vandevivere,D. and Verdonk,G. (1980) *Adv. Prostaglandin Thromb. Res., 6*, 201.
6. Salmon,J.A. and Flower,R.J. (1982) In *Methods in Enzymology.* Lands,W.E.M. and Smith,W.L. (eds), Academic Press, New York, Vol. 86, p. 477.
7. Nigam,S., Becker,R., Rosendahl,U., Hammerstein,J., Benedetto,C., Barbero,M. and Slater,T.F. (1985) *Prostaglandins, 29*, 513.
8. Powell,W.S. (1980) *Prostaglandins, 20*, 947.
9. Clancy,R.M. and Hugli,T.E. (1983) *Anal. Biochem., 133*, 30.
10. Powell,W.S. (1982) In *Methods in Enzymology.* Lands,W.E.M. and Smith,W.L. (eds), Academic Press, New York, Vol. 86, p. 467.
11. Bennett,H.P.J., Hudson,A.M., McMartin,C. and Purdon,G.E. (1977) *Biochem. J., 168*, 9.
12. Goswami,S., Mai,J., Bruckner,G. and Kinsella,J.E. (1981) *Prostaglandins, 22*, 693.
13. Ramwell,P.W. and Daniels,E.G. (1969) In *Lipid Chromatographic Analysis.* Marinetti,G.V. (ed.), Dekker, New York, Vol. 2, p. 313.
14. Morris,H.G., Sherman,N.A. and Shepperdson,F.T. (1981) *Prostaglandins, 21*, 771.

CHAPTER 5

Thin-layer chromatography (including radio thin-layer chromatography and autoradiography) of prostaglandins and related compounds

JOHN S.HURST, STEPHEN FLATMAN and ROBERT G.McDONALD-GIBSON

1. INTRODUCTION

There is no doubt that the modern era of prostaglandin research, beginning in the early 1960s, was greatly facilitated by the introduction and development of thin-layer chromatography (t.l.c.) techniques at around the same time. Indeed it is probably true that no other single separative analytical technique has been used so extensively in the study of arachidonic acid metabolites throughout the last 20 years or more. The original t.l.c. systems described by Green and Samuelsson (1), and modifications of these, are still widely used and of course many others have been developed. The theory of t.l.c. is beyond the scope of this chapter. We have attempted to describe some of the basic t.l.c. procedures that, over the years, we ourselves have found to be useful. Reference to others is made where appropriate. We have included a section on radio-t.l.c. since this technique is becoming increasingly popular, aided, perhaps, by recent technical advances in instrumentation. As well as describing the basic methodologies involved we draw attention to the merits and limitations of the various procedures, since these are not always fully appreciated.

2. EQUIPMENT

2.1 Thin-layer plates

Silica gel is the preferred adsorbent for the t.l.c. of prostaglandins and related compounds. Commercially pre-coated t.l.c. plates are available from a number of UK sources: Alltech (Carnforth), Anachem (Luton), BDH (Poole), Gelman (Northampton), Pierce (Cambridge), Sigma (Poole) and Whatman (Maidenhead). These plates are superior to those prepared in the laboratory (2–4) but are more expensive. The humidity, thickness and quality of the silica layer is more strictly controlled during industrial coating which results in low batch to batch variation with consequent increased reproducibility of chromatographic separation.

   In our laboratory we use 20 × 20 cm glass-backed silica gel 60 plates ('Merck' No.5721) which have a silica layer thickness of 0.25 mm without impregnated fluorescent indicator, obtained from BDH. LKD plates (Whatman) have been recommended for prostaglandin research (5) but are more expensive. These have similar sorbent to the 'Merck' plates but have pre-scored sample channels or lanes, the number varying with the size of plate (19 for 20 × 20 cm) and a concentration or pre-adsorbent zone that speeds and facilitates sample application. BDH also supply plates with a similar concentration zone but these cost approximately twice as much as the regular plates. Flexible plates (plastic or aluminium backed) are commercially available and are convenient for scintillation counting (Section 7.3), when zones of interest are to be excised, as they can easily be cut with scissors and material may be recovered from the gel as described (Section 5). The plastic plates are supplied either as individual sheets or as a roll from which the required length may be cut. The thickness of the coating of the flexible plates does not exceed 0.2 mm and would thus not be suitable for large-scale preparative t.l.c. (purification of material) which requires a thicker sorbent layer (1.5−2 mm), although we have successfully used glass plates with a silica coating of 0.25 mm to purify 1−2 mg of lipoxygenase metabolites of arachidonic acid.

2.2 **Applicators**

We apply samples by glass micro-syringes which have a stainless steel plunger and replaceable needle. It is essential to have a 1−10 μl micro-syringe for the spot-application of standards (reference compounds) or samples smaller than 10 μl for which we recommend the SGE series (SGE, Milton Keynes, UK) and Shandon−Terumo series (Shandon Southern, Runcorn, UK). The SGE series (1−50 μl and 1−100 μl) are also suitable for the application of samples larger than 10 μl which are streaked on to the plate as narrow bands (Section 3.4.2).

Clean the syringe before and after each use by flushing through at least 10 volumes of ethanol or a volatile solvent, such as ethyl acetate, that does not react with or attack any part of the syringe.

Different types of automated and semi-automated sample delivery systems are commercially available, for example, 'Camag' (BDH) and 'Desaga' (Whatman). These are labour-saving and give more reproducible results than manual application but are very expensive (£2000−7000). The sample capacity (20 nl−10 μl) will vary with the model.

2.3 **Solvents**

The solvent mixtures (Section 4) used to develop t.l.c. plates require constituents of high purity and 'Analar' or h.p.l.c. (generally more expensive) grades are suitable and may be obtained from BDH, Fisons (Leicester, UK), Koch-Light (Haverhill, UK) and May and Baker (Dagenham and Manchester, UK). We have not found a need to re-distil solvents before use for our purposes.

2.4 **Development chambers (tanks)**

These may be obtained from the same sources as the t.l.c. plates and are made of thick-walled glass. There are two principal designs; rectangular (for 20 × 20 cm plates) and cylindrical (for flexible and small diameter plates). The tank is covered by a flush-fitting lid. The edges at the top of the tank and usually under the lid have ground glass and are lubricated with stop-cock grease, before use, to provide an air-tight fit. There is frequently a raised ridge, running lengthwise, that bisects the flat bottom of the rectangular tank. This assists the optimum positioning of plates in the tank (Section 3.5).

2.5 **Reagent-sprayers**

A finely atomized spray is required to homogeneously coat the chromatogram (developed plate) with reagent in order to detect separated material of interest (Section 3.6). These are of two designs; spray guns and glass atomizers and are available from the above t.l.c. specialists (Section 2.1). Spray guns use inert, non-toxic, non-flammable propellant as aerosol in a can which fits into the spray-head connecting the glass jar containing reagent. Atomizers are glass flasks connected via reducing valves to compressed nitrogen or air. The rubber bulb attachment as an alternative to compressed gas is not favoured as uniform finely atomized sprays are rarely produced. Many generally used reagents, such as phosphomolybdate (Section 3.6.2) are also commercially available ready-prepared in aerosol spray cans. These are convenient but frequently the spray nozzles do not produce a fine enough mist.

2.6 **U.v. cabinets**

These generally contain two u.v. lamps, one of short wavelength (254 nm) and one of long wavelength (350−378 nm) fixed in a light-tight portable cabinet. The fluorescence of separated compounds detected by spraying (Section 3.6.2) may be viewed by placing the plate in the cabinet in a darkened room and illuminating with the appropriate lamp.

3. PROCEDURES

3.1 **Concentration and preparation of the sample**

(i)   Adjust the pH of the sample (tissue extract or biological fluid) to within the range 3−4 and extract 2−3 times with 2−4 volumes of ethyl acetate [more than one sample may be shaken by 'SMI' Multi-Tube Vortexer (Alpha Laboratories, Eastleigh, UK)].

(ii)   The pooled extract is too dilute to be applied to the t.l.c. plate and must be concentrated. Dry the extract by passing oxygen-free nitrogen over it. Evaporation of the solvent may be assisted by gently warming the extract on an electrically-heated hot-plate, ensuring that the surface temperature never exceeds 30°C to prevent decomposition of compounds of interest. A blow-down manifold with multi-outlets, that can be closed when not in use, is convenient for processing more than one sample and may be easily constructed by a competent glass-blower. The dried extracts may be stored desiccated at −20°C for long periods (weeks to several months).

(iii)   Reconstitute the dry extract in 20−50 µl of ethyl acetate before use, mix thoroughly for 1−2 min and store on ice. Ethyl acetate is preferred because it is non-toxic, readily solubilizes arachidonic acid and its metabolites and will facilitate sample application and limit diffuse movement of the sample band or spot during development because of its relative volatility and low polarity.

3.2 **Preparation of the plate**

We have not found that activation, by heating at 110°C for 30−60 min, of 'Merck' plates before use improves chromatographic separation nor have we found it useful to wash plates in development solvent before use as we have not encountered problems related to contaminant impurities within the silica sorbent.

3.2.1 *Impregnation of the plate*

(i) *Impregnation with silver nitrate.* Silver nitrate impregnated plates are of use in differentiating prostaglandins such as PGE_1 and PGE_2 on the basis of the degree of unsaturation (5). Commercially impregnated plates are generally unsatisfactory as they rapidly deteriorate. To impregnate the plates dissolve 5 g of silver nitrate in 5 ml of distilled water and add to 95 ml of methanol, mix rapidly and pour into a flat dish. Immerse the plate for 1 min, remove it then dry in air and use immediately.

(ii) *Impregnation with ferric chloride.* This is useful for the separation of prostaglandins A, B and C (6). Dip the plates twice in 10% ferric chloride in acetone, dry in air after each rinse. Activate the layers at 100°C for 90 min before use.

3.3 **Marking of the plate**

The samples and standards are applied to the plate in specific zones or lanes defined within vertically ruled lines. The manner in which the plate is sectioned depends upon the purpose for which it is to be used, whether for routine analysis or for preparative/semi-preparative work.

3.3.1 *Sectioning of the plate for analytical t.l.c.*

A sectioned plate, ready for sample application, is shown in *Figure 1* and the procedure is as below.

(i)   Mark a point along the edge of the plate 1–1.5 cm from one side with a sharp soft pencil then mark another parallel to it the same distance on the opposite side. Gently draw a line between these points. This indicates the origin or starting line along which material is to be applied. The sorbent layer is stably bound to commercial plates and should not be damaged by soft marking.

(ii)   Similarly rule a parallel horizontal line 1 cm from the opposite edge to indicate the solvent front or the extent to which the solvent will ascend the plate.

(iii)   Mark two parallel points, one on the origin and the other on the solvent front 2 cm from the left-hand edge of the plate and draw the vertical line between them.

(iv)   At a distance of 1 cm from this line draw another parallel to it. The area enclosed is the first sample lane.

(v)   Continue ruling lanes as above, but leave spaces of 1.5–2 cm between lanes. The plate will be divided into six sample lanes if the inter-lane space is 2 cm.

Scoring may be automated by a relatively cheap adjustable device such as the t.l.c. plate scriber (Alltech) which scoops the required number of narrow channels (up to 20, ~1 cm wide) in the adsorbent.

3.2.2 *Sectioning of the plate for preparative/semi-preparative t.l.c.*

Divide the plate into three areas by following steps (i)–(iii) above (Section 3.3.1). Apply the standards to the outer sectors and the preparation along the remainder of the origin (Section 3.4).

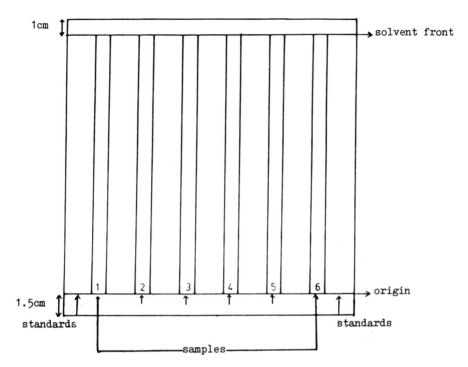

Figure 1. Silica gel t.l.c. plate divided into sectors for the application of standard (reference) compounds and samples.

3.4 Application of standards and sample

R_f values (ratios between distances travelled by the substances separated and the solvent front from the origin) are frequently cited to confirm the presence of a particular compound. In our experience exactly reproducible values are difficult to obtain as they tend to vary from one chromatographic run to another and even between two plates of the same type simultaneously developed in the same tank. They are influenced by variables which include; size of the sample, temperature, changes in the solvent composition during chromatography and especially relative humidity. It is for these reasons R_f values should not be considered decisive in confirmation of the identity of material separated. This is especially relevant to examples of poor resolution, where compounds have closely migrated. Therefore it is always good practise to run known standards, together with samples, to assist in qualitative analysis. Depending upon the purpose the standards may be unlabelled (usual mode) or radio-labelled, which should be restricted to preparative/semi-preparative t.l.c., where enhanced sensitivity of detection is relevant for the elution and recovery of the compound of interest (Section 5). Unlabelled arachidonic acid may be obtained from Sigma. Unlabelled prostaglandins, leukotrienes and hydroxyeicosatetraenoic acids (HETEs) may be purchased from: Cayman (Ann Arbor, USA), Upjohn (Kalamazoo, USA), Seragen (Boston, USA), and Metachem (Northampton, UK). [^{14}C] and [^{3}H]arachidonic acid are available from Amersham International (Amersham, UK) and NEN (Dreieich, FRG). Only tritiated prostaglandins, HETEs and leukotrienes are currently commercially available from these sources. [^{14}C]15-HETE may be prepared in the laboratory according to the method of Crawford *et al.* (7), [^{14}C]12-HETE may be synthesized according to the method of McGuire *et al.* (8) and [^{14}C]5-HETE may be prepared according to the method of Corey *et al.* (9).

3.4.1 *Application of standards*

Apply 2−5 μl of appropriate standards (1 mg/ml stock solutions in ethanol, stored desiccated at −20°C) in duplicate by solvent-cleaned 10 μl micro-syringe as a series of small spots to the same position on the origin within two reference lanes on both sides of the plate (e.g. either in the middle of the left hand and right hand zones immediately preceding and following the first and last sample lanes, respectively or between two pairs of corresponding lanes, such as 1 and 2 and 5 and 6). Take care not to damage the silica surface by pressing the needle too hard on the plate. Clean the syringe with ethanol as recommended (Section 2.2) and dry each spot with cold air from a hairdryer before application of the next standard. The alternative procedure is to mix equal amounts of standards and apply to the plate in the same manner as the extract (Section 3.4.2).

3.4.2 *Application of the sample*

The same sample is equally apportioned between two plates developed in different solvent systems (Section 4) in order to confirm the presence of a particular compound.

Hold the 50 μl or 100 μl micro-syringe, containing the extract, at an acute angle to the plate, without disturbing the surface, in the allocated sector and gently push in the plunger until a continuous narrow stream or streak of material (1 cm long, 2−3 mm wide) is released and repeat on the other plate. Dry the streaked material as above (Section 3.4.1) before the next release of sample and continue application to both plates until the syringe is fully discharged. The width of the sample band should be restricted since as the chromatography develops the areas occupied by the separated zones tend to increase and the bands widen due to diffusion. In practice it is frequently difficult to regulate the streak as appreciable contamination of the extract with viscous polar and lipid material other than that of interest will cause a broadening of the initial streak. The load applied is critical and will affect the size and shape of the zone after development. Over-loaded sample applications produce 'comet-like' vertical streaks and the rate of development will be slowed with consequent poorer resolution of separated material.

The chromatographic resolution of radiolabelled compounds may be improved by dilution with unlabelled standards. Dissolve a mixture of appropriate standards (∼1 μg each) in the radiolabelled sample and apply as above. Satisfactory chromatography may be achieved without this option, which if exercised routinely becomes expensive.

3.5 **Development**

Plates are developed by the ascending technique: the separated compounds will migrate with solvent up the plate and the eventual destination will relate to relative polarity in the selected solvent. Polar material such as phospholipids and peptidyl-leukotrienes will generally remain on or close to the origin, whereas the least polar material including arachidonic acid and neutral lipids will migrate farthest.

With certain solvents the development may be uneven such that the zones of the same compound are not at the same level and R_f values progressively increase from the centre towards both edges of the t.l.c. plate, the 'edge effect' which is related to solvent evaporation may sometimes be eliminated by saturating or equilibrating the tank with solvent vapour as described below.

(i)   Line the back and side walls of the dry tank with filter or blotting paper, leaving the front side open so that the plate is visible.

(ii)   Grease the ground glass under the lid and at the top of the tank with silicone stop-cock grease.

(iii)   Pour $80-100$ ml of solvent into the tank ensuring that the paper dips into solvent.

(iv)   Cover the tank and allow it to equilibrate with solvent vapour ($40-60$ min).

(v)   Weight down the lid so that it is not dislodged by the vapour pressure and heat generated by the solvent so that the constant environment and equilibrium within the system may be maintained.

Saturation has the additional advantage that development times are reduced by about one third. Solvents should be used for one development only as changes in composition due to evaporation will occur with time.

With certain solvents, however, chromatographic separation is impaired if the tank is saturated. This is the case with solvent system A9 (Section 4) and development in this solvent should always occur in a non-equilibrated tank.

After sample application incline the plate at an angle of 45° (optimum position for development) to the surface of the solvent in the tank. Two 20×20 cm plates may be simultaneously developed in the tank with their silica layers facing each other inwards, in a 'v'-shaped conformation. Remove the plate when the solvent has reached the solvent front and dry in air ($10-20$ min). The development time will vary according to the nature of the solvents. It will be faster in ether/petroleum ether/acetic acid than either A1 or A9 (Section 4). Development at $0-4$°C may be advisable for such purposes as the separation of unstable hydroperoxides of arachidonic acid (9).

3.6 Detection

The two principal methods for the detection or location of separated compounds on the plate are physical: u.v. absorbance (non-destructive, i.e. the chemical nature of the compound is unchanged), and chemical using combination with iodine or other reagent to produce a coloured complex. This may be destructive or non-destructive depending upon the reagent.

3.6.1 *U.v. detection*

This is relatively unimportant, with limited application, since all prostaglandins absorb u.v. maximally at 192.5 nm and only PGA, 15-keto-PGE and PGB compounds are differentiated on the basis of additional absorbance at 217, 228 and 278 nm, respectively. These can be detected *in situ* by u.v. scanning spectroscopy (10) and the sensitivity is reported to surpass that of chemical methods. PGE and PGA on the plate may be converted to PGB by spraying with alkali (10) and this may be used to quantitate PGE by scanning the chromatogram before and after treatment. However additional restraints imposed are the absorbance between 270 and 280 nm of the leukotrienes and the diene conjugation at 234 nm of 12-L-hydroxyheptadecatrienoic acid (HHT) and the HETEs.

3.6.2 *Chemical methods*

These are the methods most generally used. The chromatogram is exposed to reagent to reveal stained areas which coincide with separated compounds. However caution should be exercised with regard to these methods as in certain circumstances the resulting information may be misleading. Samples are frequently contaminated with non-arachidonic acid derived material which co-migrate with authentic standards including cholesterol, diglycerides and 12-HETE and this confusion may be compounded when t.l.c. systems are unable to resolve chemically and biologically distinct metabolites such as TXB_2 and PGE_2.

(i) *Iodine*. This is the simplest method and is carried out as follows.

(1)   Place a few crystals of iodine in a closed dry t.l.c. tank in a fume cupboard (iodine is very harmful) and after a brief interval it will be filled with the purple-blue haze of iodine vapour.

(2)   Place the plate in the tank, cover and small quantities of material (eg. μg-amounts) will stain yellow brown to dark brown on a pale background on exposure to the vapour (1−10 min). The intensity of staining progressively increases with exposure time.

(3)   Outline the stained areas in pencil as they spontaneously fade with time, the process is partly reversible.

The method is less sensitive for compounds containing only one double bond, such as 6-keto-$PGF_{1\alpha}$ which stain more faintly. This technique is generally regarded as non-destructive but the possibility that the chemical character of compounds such as HETEs is changed cannot be neglected as iodine will add to double bonds. The method does not work on silver nitrate-impregnated plates and is non-specific as non-related lipids will also stain.

(ii) *Reagent-spraying*. Many of the reagents used are harmful or toxic and should be used in a fume cupboard. It may be convenient to contain the plate within a box to avoid spraying elsewhere. Remove the top and one side of a suitable carton and line it with filter paper. Most of the commonly used reagents are general rather than specific.

(a) *Phosphomolybdate*. Spray the chromatogram with 5−10% (w/v) phosphomolybdic acid dissolved in ethanol or propanol and heat with a hairdryer for several minutes. Material will stain blue on a yellow background. Ammonia vapour may intensify the spots and lighten the background. The method is destructive and comparable in sensitivity to iodine.

(b) *Antimony pentachloride*. Heat the plate to 120°C and dip into a 1% (w/v) solution of antimony pentachloride in carbon tetrachloride/ethylene chloride (6:1, v/v). PGF compounds initially revealed as red turn dark grey−brown, PGEs appear brown with a red tinge, PGAs change from green to brown and PGBs stain lemon−yellow. Minimum detection limit is 2−5 μg.

(c) *Vanillin-phosphoric acid*. 1% (w/v) vanillin in 85% phosphoric acid in ethanol. PGEs stain yellow and PGFs blue.

(d) *Charring*. Heat the plate at 110−120°C for a few minutes and spray immediately with sulphuric acid (50% or concentrated). Compounds are disclosed as brown or black areas.

(e) *Ferrous thiocyanate*. Organic peroxides including PGG_2 and hydroperoxy-eicosatetraenoic acids (HPETEs) may be visualized by spraying with solutions freshly prepared as below.
Dissolve 0.7 g of ferrous ammonium sulphate hexahydrate in 10 ml of 5% (w/v) ammonium thiocyanate containing 1 ml of concentrated sulphuric acid. Hydroperoxides appear as red spots that fade within a few minutes.

(f) *Cupric acetate−phosphoric acid*. 3% (w/v) cupric acetate in aqueous orthophosphoric acid. PGFs appear purple, PGEs and PGAs green, PGBs yellow, whilst 6-keto-$PGF_{1\alpha}$ will stain pale grey after prolonged heating, dihydro-PGI_2 appears blue whilst methyl-PGI_2 turns red−brown.

(g) *Anisaldehyde-sulphuric acid*. Add 2 ml of concentrated sulphuric acid to 20 ml of ice-cold absolute ethanol, mixing after each addition to dissipate the heat evolved and add 2 ml of anisaldehyde similarly. The reagent is stable at −20°C for several days. Similar reagents may be prepared by substituting other aromatic aldehydes such as cinnamic, etc. This is a very sensitive (0.1 μg) and relatively specific method (11) for detecting 6-keto-$PGF_{1\alpha}$ and PGI_2 which appear as intensely yellow areas (stable for 1 month) on a white background within less than 30 sec of spraying on an unheated plate. The yellow colour will intensify on heating. Other PGs stain differently but will be revealed only after activation of the plate at 85°C for several minutes.
PGE and PGA appear orange−red, PGD turns orange−brown, PGE stains brown and PGF appears blue−violet. Similar results are obtained with reagents prepared with substituted aromatic aldehydes. Compounds exposed to the reagent will fluoresce differently when viewed under u.v. (375 nm): for example, 6-keto-$PGF_{1\alpha}$ (ochre) and PGI_2 (green−yellow). 6-keto-$PGF_{1\alpha}$ also fluoresces distinctly with substituted aromatic aldehydes e.g. cinnamaldehyde (dark yellow).

(h) *Rhodamine B*. Spray with 0.2% (w/v) rhodamine B in absolute ethanol either before sample application (for lipid class separation of tissue extract) and activate at 100°C, or after development for routine detection of standards as above. Lipids will fluoresce

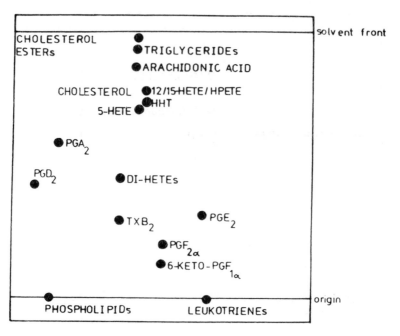

Figure 2. Separation of arachidonic acid and metabolites on silica gel t.l.c. plate developed in solvent A9. HETE, hydroxyeicosatetraenoic acid; HHT, 12-L-hydroxyheptadecatrienoic acid; HPETE, hydroperoxy-eicosatetraenoic acid; PG, prostaglandin; TX, thromboxane.

under u.v. (375 nm) as pink−orange areas on a pale background. The method is non-destructive and material may be recovered (Section 5) from the gel unchanged.

4. SOLVENT SYSTEMS

The solvent system is selected to suit the particular requirements of the separation, whether it is to analyse polar or less polar products. The two systems that we routinely use to separate prostaglandins are the A1 (12) and the A9 (1) and an ether-based solvent for lipoxygenase metabolites. Solvent mixtures are stored in stoppered brown glass bottles and are stable for several weeks.

4.1 A9 system

This is probably the most widely used solvent.

(i)   Mix ethyl acetate/trimethyl pentane/distilled water/acetic acid (55:25:50:10, by vol.) in a separating funnel and allow phases to separate (5−10 min).

(ii)   Discard the lower aqueous layer, add a little anhydrous sodium sulphate to the organic phase, shake and filter.

(iii)   Pour the filtrate into a non-equilibrated tank.

Development at 20−22°C is approximately 2 h. The sequence in which material separates is shown (*Figure 2*). 6-keto-PGF$_{1\alpha}$ is well resolved from PGF$_2$ but TXB$_2$ and PGE$_2$ frequently co-chromatograph (when they are resolved it is TXB$_2$ that precedes PGE$_2$). Leukotrienes (except LTB$_4$) and phospholipids are retained on the origin.

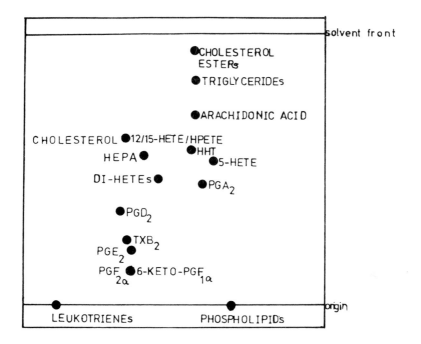

Figure 3. Separation of arachidonic acid and metabolites on silica gel t.l.c. plate developed in solvent A1. HEPA, hydroxyepoxy arachidonic acid; HETE, hydroxyeicosatetraenoic acid; HHT, 12-L-hydroxy-eicosatetraenoic acid; HPETE, hydroperoxyeicosatetraenoic acid; PG, prostaglandin; TX, thromboxane.

4.2 **A1 system**

The tank is equilibrated with benzene/dioxan/acetic acid (60:40:2, by vol.). The order in which compounds separate is shown (*Figure 3*) and is similar to A9 however $PGF_{2\alpha}$ and 6-keto-$PGF_{1\alpha}$ co-migrate and on those occasions when TXB_2 and PGE_2 are resolved the latter is more polar.

4.3 **Systems for lipoxygenase metabolites**

These are ether-based, for example diethyl ether/petroleum ether/acetic acid (50:50:1, by vol.) and the tank is saturated before use. Chromatograms are rapidly developed (35−60 min) in this volatile solvent of low polarity. Polar material (e.g. leukotrienes, phospholipids and prostaglandins) is retained on the origin. HHT is well resolved from 5-HETE and 12/15-HETEs can be distinguished from their hydroperoxides as shown (*Figure 4*). Similar separations may be obtained with modifications of the solvent ratios and when hexane substitutes petroleum ether (e.g. diethyl ether/hexane/acetic acid, 60:40:1, by vol.). Diethyl ether/hexane/acetic acid (20:80:2, by vol.) may be used to separate the major lipid classes (e.g. di- and triglycerides, cholesterol, cholesterol esters, fatty acids, phospholipids etc.) detected by rhodamine B (Section 3.6.2).

4.4 **Other solvent systems**

Tanks saturated with chloroform/methanol/acetic acid/water (90:9:1:0.65, by vol.) (13) and related systems have been used for prostaglandin analysis but are not as satisfac-

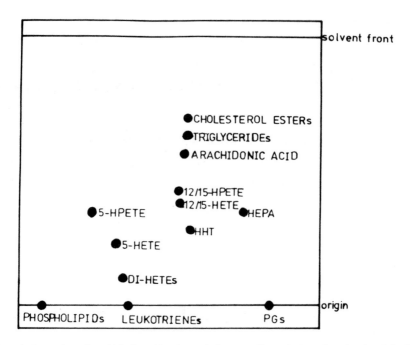

Figure 4. Separation of arachidonic acid and metabolites on silica gel t.l.c. plate developed in diethyl ether/petroleum ether/acetic acid (50:50:1, by vol.). HEPA, hydroxyepoxy arachidonic acid; HETE, hydroxy-eicosatetraenoic acid; HHT, 12-L-hydroxyeicosatetraenoic acid; HPETE, hydroperoxyeicosatetraenoic acid.

tory as A1 and A9 described above and it has been reported (14) that extracted 6-keto-$PGF_{1\alpha}$ chromatographs at not one but several distinct loci in this solvent and that authentic non-extracted standard will co-migrate with PGE_2. These systems are however useful for the separation of phospholipids.

5. ELUTION AND RECOVERY

If the compounds of interest are to be analysed later by another technique (e.g. h.p.l.c., RIA, etc.) they have to be eluted from the silica gel into water or polar solvent and extracted as below.

(i)   Locate the standards by scanning if radiolabelled (Section 7.2) or otherwise by the methods described above (Section 3.6.2).

(ii)   Outline the relevant area, with pencil, by reference to the positions of the appropriate standard applied to both sides of the plate, allowing for uneven solvent flow, if appropriate.

(iii) Extend the corners of the outlined sector vertically and horizontally by 2 mm (to account for any spreading of this zone during development).

(iv)   Score the outlined sector with the blade of a micro-spatula and carefully scrape off the gel (lightly spraying the area with water or buffer may facilitate this).

(v)   Tip the scrapings into a small piece of paper folded in half and carefully pour the contents into a graduated siliconized glass conical centrifuge tube, pulverize the silica, extract with 4 vol of methanol, and mix for $1-2$ min, using the Multi-Tube Vortexer (Section 3.1) if appropriate.

(vi) Centrifuge for $5-10$ min ($600-1500$ g), remove the supernatant with a glass Pasteur pipette into another conical tube, retain the silica precipitate and re-extract with methanol as above. The extraction may be repeated once more to maximize recovery.

(vii) Pool the methanol extracts and concentrate with nitrogen evaporation (Section 3.1). The extract may be completely dried (prolonged because of the aqueous content of the methanol).

(viii) Add 0.5 ml of acidified distilled water (pH 4.0) and extract twice with 2 ml of diethyl ether, mix well and centrifuge as above to separate the phases. Remove and pool the ether supernatant into a conical centrifuge tube, concentrate to dryness with nitrogen evaporation and store desiccated at $-20°C$. Alternatively concentrate the methanol extract from step (vii) to 0.5 ml, acidify to pH $3-4$ and extract with diethyl ether and concentrate as above. The ether extraction removes contaminant silica from the material which might interfere with subsequent assay techniques.

Elution of material from gel into methanol and extraction with ether has yielded reported recoveries of $80-90\%$ (1). More than 80% recoveries of PGs eluted from gels into acetone/water (95:5, v/v) and acetone/0.2 M glycine buffer (95:5, v/v) have been reported (11). Approximately 70% recovery has been reported from elution into buffer (10) which may be convenient for RIA analysis.

To eliminate the loss of silica gel, by spillage or blowing, re-useable gel collectors based on vacuum suction have been developed (e.g. the Alltech). These are very practical for the management and containment of radioactive material. 'Stripmix' (Alltech) is another convenient alternative and binds the adsorbent into a single flexible film that may be peeled from the plate. The film is completely porous so that material may be extracted with solvents or buffer.

6. OTHER THIN-LAYER CHROMATOGRAPHY TECHNIQUES

6.1 Two-dimensional t.l.c.

Conventional t.l.c., that is, chromatographic separation in one solvent mixture in one direction, frequently fails to discriminate between compounds of related polarity. To improve resolution, in such circumstances, a complementary separation procedure at 90° to the original direction of development in a second solvent system, two-dimensional chromatography, may be employed. Examples of this technique are described (15). In order for the compounds to be resolved they must have different mobilities in each of the solvent systems. If the solvents are of similar polarity, information may be obtained over a narrow range of products such as the prostaglandins. If, however, it is different then investigation over a wider spectrum is possible.

6.2 High performance thin-layer chromatography (h.p.t.l.c.)

The recent introduction of h.p.t.l.c. was made possible by the development of silica gel particles of finer quality and smaller size than those in conventional thin layers. The maximum sample loading on h.p.t.l.c. plates (preferably with a concentration zone) is approximately one tenth that of the regular plates, but development is much more rapid and the resolution superior. Promising results have been obtained from the present few applications to prostaglandin research (16).

In the future, h.p.t.l.c. with the complementary even newer over pressure-layer chromatography technique (o.p.l.c.) which regulates h.p.t.l.c. development within a closed system and has analogies to h.p.l.c. (17) may play a progressively important role. The 'Chompres' o.p.l.c. system is available from Newman—Howells Associates (Winchester, UK).

7. RADIO-T.L.C.

7.1 Experimental details

The availability of radiolabelled substrates has proved an invaluable tool for research into eicosanoid metabolism. The use of carbon-14 and tritium isotopes has been described extensively and, together with the detection methods outlined in the following sections, has led to the discovery of metabolites involved in the prostaglandin and lipoxygenase pathways in a variety of tissues.

Procedures for t.l.c. are as described in Section 3.3. Additional attention must be paid to the precautions normally associated with the handling of low energy β-particle emitters. Various radiolabelled eicosanoids are available (Section 3.4). Here we concentrate on the use of radiolabelled arachidonic acid which has been studied most extensively. ^{14}C-Labelled arachidonic acid is routinely used in preference to the tritiated derivative. The energy of the β-particle emitted from the ^{14}C atom is greater than that of the tritium atom and therefore more easily detected. Secondly the ability of tritiated compounds to undergo proton exchange with the surrounding aqueous environment is not a problem. [1-^{14}C]Arachidonic acid is supplied (Amersham International or NEN) with a specific activity of approximately 60 mCi/mmol in either ethanol or toluene with or without antioxidant. [^{14}C(U)]Arachidonic acid (400 mCi/mmol) is available but at a much higher cost and has no advantage over the single-labelled derivative for most purposes. Arachidonic acid stored dissolved in toluene at $-20°C$ undergoes insignificant oxidation ($<1\%$) over a period of 3 months.

Experiments using tissue slices, cells or homogenates require a minimum of 0.1 μCi per incubation. Lower amounts of radioactivity (0.05 μCi) may be used in incubations with subcellular fractions and enzyme preparations where the recovery of material from the extraction procedure (Section 3.1) is more reliable. The required amount of toluene is evaporated under nitrogen and the dried-down arachidonic acid re-dissolved in a minimum volume of ethanol plus ice-cold 0.2% (w/v) sodium carbonate. This solution is mixed with a solution of non-radioactive sodium arachidonate, if necessary, prior to aliquoting into assay tubes. Following the extraction of completed assays and the concentration of extracts, apply the samples to silica gel t.l.c. plates with at least 1.5 cm separating each lane; this prevents the overlapping of radioactive areas due to the spreading of bands during development of t.l.c. plates.

7.2 Instrumentation

The three types of instrument principally used for the detection of radioactive regions on t.l.c. plates are the linear analyser, the radiochromatogram scanner and the spark

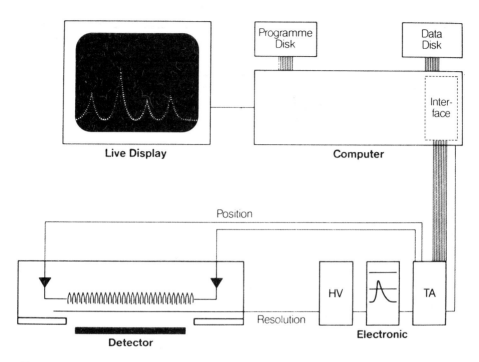

Figure 5. Diagramatic representation of the Isomess radioactivity intelligent thin-layer analyser (RITA).

chamber. In our laboratory we have extensively used a linear analyser manufactured by Isomess (Straubenhardt, FRG; supplied by Lablogic, Sheffield, UK) and a Berthold LB2723 (Wildband, FRG) radiochromatogram scanner. Both instruments are based on modified proportional counters.

7.2.1 *The linear analyser*

The system (*Figure 5*) consists of a moving head assembly (30 × 10 × 10 cm) containing an open window (1.5 × 20 cm) on the underside exposing a suspended fine gold wire of uniform thickness, running the length of the window, across which a potential is applied. Above the wire is a multicoiled delay-line. The function of the wire is to detect the number and intensity of ionization events caused by the β-particles emitted from a source. The delay-line locates the position of these events at points along the wire. By selecting only events of low intensity (low energy electrons), using a discriminator, this limits the recorded β-particles to those emitted perpendicular to the wire and so provides excellent resolution of different point sources. In practice there is a balance between resolution and counting efficiency which also affects the uniformity of efficiency (linearity) at all points on the wire. Linearity and resolution are parameters best checked at regular monthly intervals using a standardized test plate containing a number of regions of known activity at set distances. Counting is performed in an atmosphere of methane:argon (90:10, v/v). Including methanol or ethanol vapour in the gas mixture improves resolution and efficiency but is not recommended for routine use as the alcohol content is critical and must therefore be very carefully controlled. The open window may be covered with thin aluminium foil ('Mylar' supplied by Isomess) which lowers the background counts by reducing static build up on the plate.

Tritiated compounds are only detected using an open window because of the low energy of the β-particle. The counting efficiency for tritium (0.5%) is less than that for ^{14}C; however, resolution is particularly good even without the use of the discriminator as the distance between the detection wire and the t.l.c. plate can only be transversed by electrons perpendicular to the wire.

The Isomess machine has facilities for four standard t.l.c. plates (20 $\times$ 20 cm). One and two plate versions are available where laboratory space is limited. The efficiency of the analyser is proportional to the potential across the wire and varies according to the degree of resolution required but generally is approximately 5%. Analysers are supplied interfaced to a computer for compilation and rapid evaluation of data.

7.2.2 The radiochromatogram scanner

The radio-t.l.c. scanner has now been outdated by modern linear analysers due to a 100-fold decrease in the amount of time to record a measurement with equal accuracy. The scanner consists of a proportional counter with an open slit window (10 $\times$ 0.5 – 2.0 mm) which moves along the length of each lane at speeds ranging from 12 to 12 000 mm/h recording counts continually. Data are accumulated using a computer or presented graphically on an integrated plotter. The Berthold thin-layer scanner has been used most extensively. At a fixed pressure of methane the counting efficiency is constant at all points along each lane at approximately 13%. In practice the scanner has given more reproducible measurements than the linear analyser following day to day use over a period of months. The efficiency of the scanner is higher as all counts entering the window are registered and not just those of a certain energy. The cost of the scanner (£7000) is less than half that of the analyser (£20 000).

7.2.3 The spark chamber

The spark chamber is a rapid method for detecting radioactive areas which has special advantages for two-dimensional work giving an image of the whole plate. Quantitation is possible by scintillation counting of radioactive regions or by densitometry of polaroid prints. We have no practical experience of this machine and recommend Filthuth (18) as a suitable source of information on its capabilities.

7.3 **Quantitation**

Analysers and scanners are usually interfaced to a computer and supplied with suitable software for data evaluation. Traces are visualized on a monitor and regions set by cursor movement. Values are presented as counts per region and as a percentage of the total counts per lane. Knowing the concentration of one metabolite allows calculation of the absolute amount of all others.

An alternative to the above detection methods is to scrape silica gel off glass plates, or cut up plastic or aluminium plates, and count in a suitable scintillation fluid. This is either done on selected regions following autoradiography or by removing sequen-

Table 1. Comparison of measurements of radioactivity made on a single t.l.c. track using different methods of detection.

Region	Scintillation counting		Linear analyser		Radiochromatogram scanner	
	d.p.m.	%	c.p.m.	%	c.p.m.	%
1	1012	1.5	40	2.0	97	1.8
2	7738	11.6	253	12.4	635	11.8
3	4536	6.8	151	7.4	360	6.7
4	5182	7.7	176	8.6	398	7.4
5	5716	8.5	167	8.2	452	8.4
6	1420	2.1	41	2.0	91	1.7
7	5864	8.8	178	8.7	479	8.9
8	35 486	53.0	1036	50.7	2867	53.3

^{14}C-labelled metabolites of arachidonic acid were monitored using: (a) an Isomess linear analyser, (b) a Berthold radiochromatogram scanner and (c) scintillation counting of silica gel by sectioning into regions corresponding to peaks of radioactivity identified following (a) and (b). Results are expressed as d.p.m. or c.p.m. per region and as a percentage of the total activity.

tial sections of silica at intervals along a lane. The interval distance $(1-10$ mm) will determine the degree of resolution. Intervals of 5 mm are recommended when manually cutting sections for routine work. Sections should be 15 mm wide for samples applied as a 10 mm streak to allow for possible spreading during development.

Metabolites must be completely extracted from silica gel into the liquid phase of the scintillant for accurate quantitation. A mixture of ethanol:toluene:PPO:POPOP (200 ml: 800 ml:5 g:0.3 g) is a good liquid scintillant for the counting of eicosanoids. The ethanol facilitates complete elution of eicosanoids but at the same time reduces counting efficiency due to quenching. Add the powdered silica gel to the scintillant and mix by vortex for 30 sec to ensure a good extraction of metabolites from the silica into the liquid phase. A quench correction curve must be determined to calculate the number of d.p.m. per fraction (19) and amount of each metabolite. The method is very sensitive and relatively inexpensive if a scintillation counter is readily accessible. However the time required for sectioning plates, counting and evaluating data may be a problem for extensive studies. Also resolution is limited by the interval distance between sections.

Table 1 demonstrates the variation in counting efficiency between the linear analyser, the radiochromatogram scanner and scintillation counting and also the close agreement, in terms of the relative amounts of each metabolite, achieved using the different methods for measurement.

7.4 **Limitations**

7.4.1 *Qualitative*

Positive identification of metabolites is not possible by t.l.c. alone even in the presence of authentic standards. The use of specific inhibitors can supply substantial evidence as to the possible identity of a compound but definite identification is only achieved using other techniques such as RIA, h.p.l.c., g.l.c. and, most importantly, mass spectrometry. There are numerous examples of metabolites which co-chromatograph. We

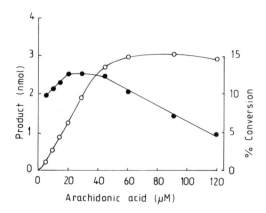

Figure 6. The effect of increasing substrate concentration on enzyme activity as measured by radio-t.l.c. A purified extract of human cervix 12-lipoxygenase was assayed with increasing concentrations of sodium [1-^{14}C]arachidonate and enzyme activity measured by radio-t.l.c. The percentage conversion to 12-H(P)ETE was determined (•——•) and the amount of product (○——○) calculated from the initial substrate concentration.

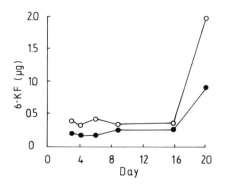

Figure 7. The effect of endogenous substrate levels on arachidonic acid metabolism. Uterus homogenates prepared from rats at various days of pregnancy were incubated at 37°C for 30 min with 15 μM sodium [1-^{14}C]arachidonate and the conversion to 6-keto-PGF$_{1\alpha}$ (6-KF) measured by radio-t.l.c. The amount of 6-KF synthesized was calculated based on the concentration of only exogenous arachidonate (•——•) and secondly taking into account the endogenous (○——○). Endogenous arachidonic acid levels were determined by capillary gas chromatography.

have encountered a lipoxygenase metabolite, possibly a tri-HETE (20) which chromatographs in the same position as thromboxane B$_2$ in all the solvent systems we have used. Diglycerides of arachidonic acid migrate very close to 12- and 15-H(P)ETE in the hexane/ether solvent systems used routinely to separate HETEs from other metabolites.

7.4.2 *Quantitative*

The amount of material applied to the t.l.c. plate is dependent on the efficiency of the extraction procedure used to prepare the sample. The efficiency may vary from sample to sample, therefore the amount of each metabolite within a sample is best expressed as a proportion of the total. Knowing the initial concentration of the substrate in an

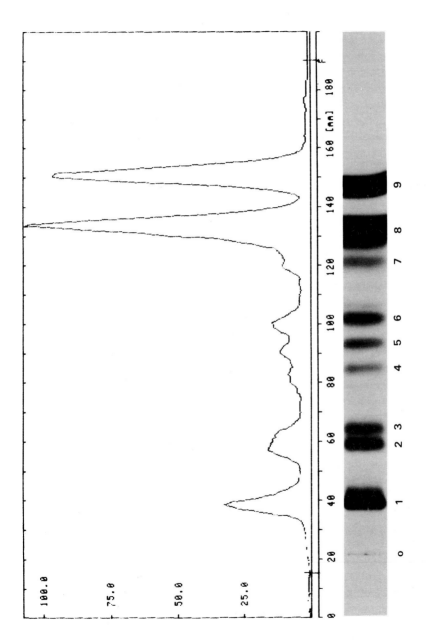

Figure 8. The resolution achieved by autoradiography compared with a trace of the same track obtained using the Isomess linear analyser. O, Origin; 1, 6-keto-$PGF_{1\alpha}/PGF_{2\alpha}$; 2, PGE_2; 3, TXB_2; 4, PGD_2; 5, DIHETE; 6, DIHETE; 7, HHT; 8, 12-HETE; 9, arachidonic acid.

assay or the amount of one metabolite by other means we are able to calculate the amount of all labelled metabolites.

The percentage conversion at various substrate levels using a purified enzyme system is shown in *Figure 6*. At substrate concentrations above the saturation level the percentage conversion decreases as expected. In assays with tissue homogenates, slices and subcellular fractions the percentage conversion may not reflect the actual amounts of synthesized metabolites, or the true level of enzyme activities, as the endogenous substrate concentration may be high or change during the assay. *Figure 7* shows the amounts of 6-keto-$PGF_{1\alpha}$ (the stable decomposition derivative of PGI_2) synthesized by rat uterine tissues at various stages of pregnancy during incubations with [^{14}C]arachidonate for 30 min at 37°C, estimated by radio-t.l.c. taking into account (a) only exogenous and (b) also endogenous arachidonic acid. The synthesis of a given metabolite may be much higher than that observed by radio-t.l.c.

7.5 Autoradiography

Autoradiography is generally used as a qualitative method of detection. Quantitation is possible by densitometry of exposed films using a Gelman ACD-18 automatic computing densitometer (Gelman Instrument Company, Michigan, USA) or by scintillation counting of identified regions (Section 7.3). The advantage of autoradiography over the other methods is the high degree of sensitivity and resolution achieved by this technique. The type of result possible is shown in *Figure 8*. The autoradiograph resolves adjacent areas of label difficult to separate on a trace of the same lane obtained using an Isomess linear analyser. Autoradiographs are produced by the following method.

(i)   Place the t.l.c. plate in contact with X-ray film (Kodak X-Omat R or AR, Kodak Ltd, Hemel Hempstead, Hertfordshire, UK), cover completely with black polythene in order to exclude all light and store at room temperature in a shaded area for 1 − 30 days, depending on the amount of radioactivity on the plate and sensitivity required.

(ii) Develop the exposed film in Kodak D19 (according to the manufacturer's instructions) for 5 min at 20°C or until the required contrast is reached.

(iii) Rinse the film in running water and then fix in Kodak Unifix for 10 min at 20°C.

(iv) Finally wash the film in running water for 30 min and hang dry.

Exposure times are decreased, low levels of ^{14}C detected and tritium detected by fluorography. A suitable fluor is En^{3}hance^{TM} supplied by NEN. Spray the plates with the fluor and expose the film at −70°C. At this temperature a single silver atom produced by a single photon striking a silver halide crystal is more stable in the absence of further photons striking the same crystal. Thus the enhancing effect is more efficient and sensitivity increased.

Normal X-ray film is not suitable for autoradiography of tritiated compounds because of the low energy of the β-particle emitted. In addition to fluorography with the aid of enhancers, non-plastic coated film is available for this purpose ([^{3}H]ultro film, LKB, Stockholm, Sweden). However this film has proved less sensitive than fluorography using normal X-ray film.

8. REFERENCES

1. Green,K. and Samuelsson,B. (1964) *J. Lip. Res.*, **5**, 117.
2. Stahl,E. (1969) In *Thin-layer Chromatography*. Stahl,E. (ed.), Springer-Verlag, New York, p. 5.
3. Touchstone,J.C. and Dobbins,M.F. (1983) In *Practice of Thin-layer Chromatography*. John Wiley and Sons, New York, p. 18.
4. Kirchner,J.G. (1978) In *Thin-layer Chromatography*. Perry,E.S. (ed.), John Wiley and Sons, New York, p. 15.
5. Flower,R.J. and Salmon,J.A. (1982) In *Methods in Enzymology*. Lands,W.E.M. and Smith,W.L. (eds), Academic Press, New York, Vol. 84, p. 477.
6. Wickramasinghe,J.A.F. and Shaw,S.R. (1974) *Prostaglandins*, **4**, 903.
7. Crawford,C.G., Van Alphen,G.W., Cook,H.M. and Lands,W.E.M. (1978) *Life Sci.*, **23**, 1255.
8. McGuire,J.C., Kelly,R.C., Gorman,R.R. and Sun,F.F. (1978) *Prep. Biochem.*, **8**, 147.
9. Corey,E.J., Albright,J.O., Barton,A.E. and Hashimoto,S.-I. (1980) *J. Am. Chem. Soc.*, **102**, 1435.
10. Shaw,J.E. and Ramwell,P.W. (1968) In *Methods of Biochemical Analysis*. Glick,D. (ed.), John Wiley and Sons, New York, Vol. 17, p. 325.
11. Ubatuba,F.B. (1978) *J. Chromatogr.*, **161**, 165.
12. Hamberg,M. and Samuelsson,B. (1966) *J. Biol. Chem.*, **241**, 257.
13. Pace-Asciak,C.R. and Wolfe,L.S. (1971) *Biochemistry*, **10**, 3657.
14. Mitchell,M.D. (1978) *Prostaglandins Med.*, **13**, 389.
15. Granstrom,E. (1982) In *Methods in Enzymology*. Lands,W.E.M. and Smith,W.L. (eds), John Wiley and Sons, New York, p. 493.
16. Beneytout,J., Greuet,D., Tixier,M. and Rigaud,M. (1984) *J. High Resol. Chromatogr.*, **7**, 538.
17. Newman,J. (1985) *Lab. Equip. Dig.*, **23**, 78.
18. Filthuth,H. (1982) In *Advances in Thin-layer Chromatography*. Touchstone,J.C. (ed.), John Wiley and Sons, New York, p. 89.
19. Kobayshi,Y. and Maudsley,D.V. (1969) In *Methods of Biochemical Analysis*. Glick,D. (ed.), John Wiley and Sons, New York, Vol. 17, p. 55.
20. Sun,F.F., McGuire,J.C., Morton,D.R., Pike,J.G., Sprecher,H. and Kunau,W.H. (1981) *Prostaglandins*, **21**, 333.

CHAPTER 6

High-pressure liquid chromatography in the analysis of arachidonic acid metabolites

WILLIAM S.POWELL

1. INTRODUCTION

Arachidonic acid is a key biological intermediate that can be converted to many highly active substances. The spectrum of arachidonic acid metabolites formed by different cells can be quite different, depending on the enzymes that are present. High-pressure liquid chromatography (h.p.l.c.) has been instrumental in the identification of many of these products and in the analysis of complex mixtures of cyclo-oxygenase and lipoxygenase products. In this chapter, h.p.l.c. on three types of stationary phases will be discussed: normal-phase (NP)-h.p.l.c. on silica, argentation (Ag)-h.p.l.c. on silver ion-loaded cation-exchange columns and reversed-phase (RP)-h.p.l.c. on octadecylsilyl (ODS) silica. Of these, the latter is the most commonly used for the separation of eicosanoids.

The major advantage of h.p.l.c. is that stationary phases with very small particle sizes can be used, reducing Eddy diffusion (which is caused by unequal path lengths through the column) to a minimum. This results in very narrow peaks and good resolution of components. In order to achieve maximum resolution, the particle size should be as small as possible, the limiting factor being the resultant increase in back pressure. Columns containing stationary phases with particle diameters of 10 μm have often been used in the past, but it is now becoming much more common to use particle sizes of 5 μm or even smaller. Another advantage of h.p.l.c. is that the column eluate can be continuously monitored by a flow-through detector, enabling products to be rapidly detected and quantitated in a variety of ways. H.p.l.c. lends itself to the use of solvent gradients, which facilitates the separation of mixtures of components of very different polarities.

Although h.p.l.c. has replaced open column and thin-layer chromatography to a large extent, these techniques are also useful for some applications because they are much less time-consuming, since many chromatographies can be carried out concurrently. Moreover, with h.p.l.c. it is necessary to spend considerable amounts of time preparing the column between chromatographies. We normally equilibrate the column with the mobile phase for 10 min at a flow-rate of 2 ml/min before injection of each sample. Following each chromatography, the column should be purged for a similar period of time with a strong solvent (e.g. acetonitrile in the case of RP-h.p.l.c.). This removes retained material which has not been eluted by the mobile phase.

2. CHROMATOGRAPHIC BEHAVIOUR OF ARACHIDONIC ACID METABOLITES

Arachidonic acid metabolites can be divided into four main groups on the basis of their chromatographic behaviour. These include:

(i)   monohydroxy products such as 12-HETE;
(ii)   dihydroxy products such as LTB_4;
(iii)   prostaglandins, TXB_2, and other trihydroxy products; and
(iv)   peptido-leukotrienes.

Some cyclo-oxygenase products exist in tautomeric forms, which are in equilibrium with one another during the chromatography, giving rise to broad or multiple peaks (see below). This is true for both TXB_2 and 6-oxo-$PGF_{1\alpha}$, which are observed as broad peaks upon NP-h.p.l.c. TXB_2 also appears as a broad peak when it is chromatographed by RP-h.p.l.c.

The presence of a peptide moiety drastically alters the chromatographic behaviour of eicosanoids. The strategies used for the separation of mixtures containing peptido-leukotrienes are therefore different from those for mixtures which do not contain these products. Of the types of h.p.l.c. described above, only RP-h.p.l.c. has proved useful for the analysis of peptido-leukotrienes. The latter products are quite sensitive to acid and can be adsorbed by untreated glass. When dealing with mixtures containing these products it is advisable to reduce the manipulation of the sample to a minimum.

3. PREPARATION OF SAMPLES

3.1 **Eicosanoids other than peptido-leukotrienes**

We have developed a rapid method to extract eicosanoids from biological media using cartridges containing ODS-silica (1,2) as follows.

(i)   Add ethanol to supernatants from cells, homogenates, or particulate fractions, or to biological fluids to give a final concentration of 15% (*Figure 1*).
(ii)   Centrifuge the sample and acidify the supernatant to a pH of about 3, and then pass it through a cartridge containing ODS-silica. We routinely apply samples of up to about 50 or 60 ml. Before use, the ODS-silica must be treated with an organic solvent such as ethanol, followed by water. We normally use Sep-Pak C_{18} cartridges (Waters Associates), but other brands may also be used.
(iii)   Once the sample has been applied, wash the cartridge with 15% ethanol (20 ml), water (20 ml) and petroleum ether (20 ml), and then elute the eicosanoids with methyl formate (10 ml; re-distilled), or another similar solvent such as diethyl ether or ethyl acetate.
(iv)   Evaporate the methyl formate under a stream of nitrogen and dissolve the residue in an appropriate solvent and analyse the sample by h.p.l.c.

The advantages of this approach are that almost all eicosanoids can be extracted with high recoveries in a small volume of a very volatile organic solvent which can be rapidly removed under nitrogen. Many contaminating materials are removed, minimizing interference and overloading of the h.p.l.c. column. The capacity of the ODS-silica is very high, and incubations with homogenates of up to 5 g of tissue can easily be extracted with a single cartridge. We routinely re-use ODS-silica cartridges up to five times,

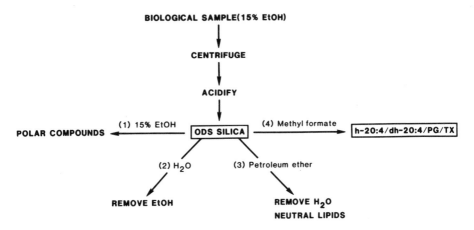

Figure 1. Procedure for the solid-phase extraction of arachidonic acid metabolites using cartridges of ODS-silica. The ODS-silica should be washed with ethanol (10 ml) and water (10 ml) prior to use. Taken from ref. 16.

provided they have not been used to extract large samples. Before re-use, they should be washed with 80% ethanol (20 ml), ethanol (20 ml) and water (10 ml).

3.2 Precolumn extraction of samples containing peptido-leukotrienes

The method described above cannot be used to extract peptido-leukotrienes. These substances will be retained by the ODS-silica, but will not be eluted by methyl formate. It is possible to modify the procedure, so that after washing the ODS-silica with 15% ethanol, eicosanoids are eluted with 80% methanol or 80% acetonitrile in ammonium acetate buffer at pH 6. The solvent is then evaporated, and the residue analysed by RP-h.p.l.c.

It has been found that considerable losses of peptido-leukotrienes can be incurred using the above approach, and it is better to use the following procedure.

(i)   Load the biological samples directly on to a precolumn (guard column) containing ODS silica (3) as shown in *Figure 2*. The apparatus consists of a 6-port switching valve coupled to: a precolumn, an analytical column, a solvent delivery system for the analytical column, and an auxiliary pump (e.g. a Milton Roy minipump), which is used to load the sample on to the precolumn.

(ii)   Add methanol to the sample to give a final concentration of 15%. For example, if incubations are carried out in volumes of 1 ml, they can be terminated by the addition of 0.75 ml methanol, followed by 3.25 ml water.

(iii) Remove any particulate matter by centrifugation.

(iv)   Using the auxiliary pump, equilibrate the precolumn (e.g. a Pierce RP-18 guard cartridge or a Waters μBondapak C_{18} Guard-PAK precolumn insert, both of which are end-capped) with 8 to 10 ml of 15% methanol in 2.5 mM phosphoric acid (precolumn solvent) with the switching valve in the 'load' position as indicated in *Figure 2*.

(v)   Equilibrate the analytical column with the starting solvent for the h.p.l.c. at the same time.

77

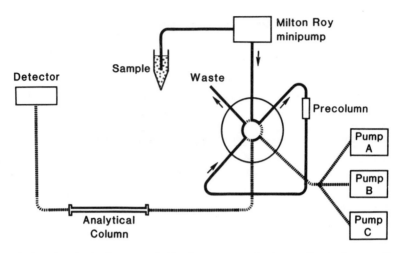

Figure 2. Procedure for loading a sample directly on to a guard column without prior extraction. In the first step, the sample is pumped on to the guard column with a Milton Roy minipump, and the eluate from the guard column is directed to waste. After the guard column is washed using the Milton Roy pump, a gradient formed by pumps A, B and, if necessary C is used to analyse the material retained by the guard column on the analytical column.

(vi)   Pump the sample on to the precolumn with the switching valve in the same position.

(vii) Transfer the solvent line from the auxiliary pump back to the precolumn solvent, pump the remainder of the sample in the solvent line on to the precolumn and wash the precolumn with the precolumn solvent (5 to 6 ml).

(viii) Introduce the sample on to the analytical column by changing the position of the switching valve to the 'inject' position.

(ix)   After completion of the chromatography, purge the precolumn with a strong solvent such as acetonitrile with the switching valve in the 'load' position.

The sample can be loaded on to the precolumn at neutral pH without compromising recoveries significantly. Using the conditions described above, recoveries of prostaglandins, including 6-oxo-PGF$_{1\alpha}$, TXB$_2$, LTB$_4$, 20-hydroxyLTB$_4$, peptido-leukotrienes, and HETEs are all between 80% and 100%. The recovery of 6-oxo-PGF$_{1\alpha}$ can be improved slightly by acidification of the sample to pH 3, but this results in slightly lower, although still acceptable, recoveries of HETEs (3). This procedure is much more convenient than conventional liquid-liquid or solid phase extraction procedures, since extraction and h.p.l.c. are combined in a single step. This reduces manipulation of the sample to a minimum, thereby minimizing the possibilities for loss of sample and contamination. The procedure can readily be automated using an automatic injector coupled to an auxiliary pump and an automatic switching valve (e.g. Waters WAVS) (3).

An automated procedure similar to that described above has been reported for the extraction and chromatography of some specific metabolites of arachidonic acid (14). Borgeat and co-workers use a similar approach, except that the sample is loaded directly on to an analytical column (15).

4. DETECTION OF EICOSANOIDS

4.1 U.v. absorbance

Most lipoxygenase products can be detected on the basis of u.v. absorbance due to the presence of conjugated double bonds. There are two main groups of these compounds: monohydroxy (or monohydroperoxy) products with conjugated diene systems, which have absorption maxima between about 232 and 237 nm (see *Table 4* in Section 8, below); and leukotrienes and their isomers containing conjugated triene systems which have three absorption maxima between 260 and 290 nm. LTB_4 and its isomers have absorption maxima at about 260 nm, 270 nm and 280 nm, whereas peptido-leukotrienes have similar u.v. spectra, but with each absorption maximum shifted upwards by about 10 nm. Lipoxins have u.v. spectra resembling leukotrienes, except that each of the absorption maxima occurs at a higher wavelength (287, 301 and 316 nm) due to the presence of four conjugated double bonds (6). For routine analysis of monohydroxy products and leukotrienes we normally monitor u.v. absorbance at 235 nm and 280 nm simultaneously using a Waters model 490 programmable multiwavelength u.v. detector.

Unlike lipoxygenase products, most products formed by the action of cyclo-oxygenase do not absorb u.v. light, except at low wavelengths. Although it is possible to detect these products in biological samples by monitoring absorbance at low wavelengths (195−205 nm), due to the presence of unconjugated double bonds (7,8), this method is limited to samples containing relatively large amounts of eicosanoids because of interference from many other unrelated compounds. An alternative approach is to convert prostaglandins and related compounds to suitable u.v.-absorbing derivatives. Phenacyl bromide and its *p*-bromo and *p*-nitro derivatives have been used to convert prostaglandins to their corresponding phenacyl ester derivatives, which can be detected using a fixed wavelength detector at 254 nm (9,10). Eicosanoids can also be converted to fluorescent derivatives by treatment with 4-bromo-7-methoxycoumarin (11), 9-anthryldiazomethane (12,13) or panacyl bromide [*p*-(9-anthroyloxy)phenacyl bromide] (14).

4.2 Radioactivity

Eicosanoids formed from radioactive substrates can be monitored using a radioactivity detector. The substrates can be incubated either directly with preparations containing cyclo-oxygenase or lipoxygenases, or can be incorporated first into cellular phospholipids: Cells pre-labelled with radioactive arachidonic acid are washed and then treated with an appropriate agent to stimulate the release of the substrate, which is then converted to products.

Most radioactivity detectors have two types of cells. The first utilizes a solid scintillator, such as cerium-coated glass beads, for heterogeneous counting. This has the advantage of allowing all of the sample to be collected. Although this method is reasonably sensitive to ^{14}C (efficiences of 30−40%), it is not very sensitive to tritium (efficiency <1%). Recently, solid scintillators have become available that have considerably higher efficiencies (>5%) for ^3H, but unfortunately carboxylic acids may bind to these materials, giving increasingly high background radioactivity. The second type of cell, for homogeneous counting, consists of a coiled Teflon tube. In this case, the column eluate is mixed with scintillation fluid and passed through the counting cell.

The efficiencies for homogeneous counting range from 50% for tritium to 90% for ^{14}C. This is therefore the best method to detect tritium-labelled products. If it is necessary to collect samples, the column eluate can be split using a stream splitter prior to the addition of liquid scintillant.

The volumes of the cells used for both heterogeneous (cell volume typically 0.2−0.6 ml) and homogeneous (cell volume 0.5−2.5 ml) detection of radioactivity are quite large. This results in considerable losses in resolution, especially at low flow-rates. A compromise must therefore be reached between good resolution, which is favoured by a small cell, and sensitivity, which is increased by using a large cell. For the chromatograms shown in this chapter, radioactivity was monitored using a Berthold detector equipped with a 0.2 ml solid cell containing cerium-coated glass beads.

5. NORMAL-PHASE HIGH-PRESSURE LIQUID CHROMATOGRAPHY

Normal-phase (straight-phase) h.p.l.c., which is usually carried out on columns of silica, can be used for all eicosanoids except peptido-leukotrienes. The major advantages of NP-h.p.l.c. are:

(i)   it has a relatively high capacity;
(ii)   the solvents used are volatile, and can be rapidly removed; and
(iii)   the solvents generally have low viscosities, resulting in low back pressures.

One problem with NP-h.p.l.c. is that many organic solvents which give good separations absorb u.v. light, making detection on the basis of u.v. absorbance impossible. This is generally not a drawback with prostaglandins and thromboxanes, since they only absorb at very low wavelengths in any case. For chromatography of u.v.-absorbing eicosanoids, u.v.-transparent solvents such as hexane and isopropanol can be used. It should be noted that methanol, ethanol and acetonitrile are not completely miscible with hexane, but can be made so by the addition of 5% propanol. Another problem with NP-h.p.l.c. is that the recoveries can occasionally be rather low. In addition, the chromatographic behaviour of products can be markedly altered by the injection medium, as discussed below.

5.1 Separation of cyclo-oxygenase products by NP-h.p.l.c.

A method that we have developed to separate cyclo-oxygenase products by NP-h.p.l.c. is illustrated in *Figure 3*. This shows a radiochromatogram of a mixture of radioactive products obtained by incubating [1-^{14}C]arachidonic acid separately with a bovine lung homogenate and a suspension of human polymorphonuclear leukocytes. The products were extracted as described above using ODS-silica, and then analysed by h.p.l.c. The mobile phase consisted of a gradient between hexane/toluene/acetic acid (50:50:0.5) and toluene/ethyl acetate/acetonitrile/methanol/acetic acid (30:40:30:2:0.5) as described in the legend to *Figure 3*. We originally used benzene in the mobile phase (1), but subsequently found that substitution of toluene for benzene gave identical results. This method completely separates PGD_2, PGE_2, $PGF_{2\alpha}$, 6-oxo-$PGF_{1\alpha}$, and TXB_2, as well as 20-hydroxyLTB$_4$. Both TXB_2 and 6-oxo-$PGF_{1\alpha}$ are observed as broad peaks due to the presence of tautomeric forms of each of these compounds.

The mobile phase in *Figure 3* is not as satisfactory for lipoxygenase products as it is for cyclo-oxygenase products, however. The dihydroxy-products, 6-*trans*-LTB$_4$

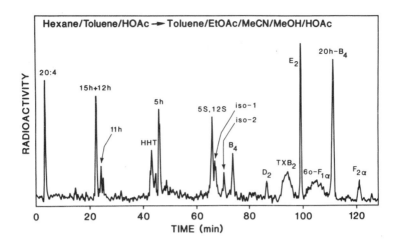

Figure 3. Separation by NP-h.p.l.c. of a mixture of arachidonic acid metabolites obtained by incubating [1-^{14}C]arachidonic acid separately with a bovine lung homogenate and a suspension of human polymorpho-nuclear leukocytes. The products were extracted with ODS-silica prior to analysis. ^{14}C-labelled 11-HETE and 15-HETE were also added to the mixture. The mobile phase consisted of a gradient formed from solvent A (hexane/toluene/acetic acid, 50:50:0.5) and solvent B (toluene/ethyl acetate/acetonitrile/methanol/acetic acid, 30:40:30:2:0.5) as follows: 0 min, 4% B; 25 min, 4% B; 40 min, 25% B; 76 min, 25% B; 81 min, 47% B; 131 min, 80% B. The flow-rate was 2 ml/min. Abbreviations: 5S, 12S, 6-*trans*-8-*cis*-12-epi-LTB$_4$ (5S,12S-dh-20:4); iso-1, 6-*trans*-LTB$_4$; iso-2, 6-*trans*-12-epi-LTB$_4$; B$_4$, LTB$_4$; D$_2$, PGD$_2$; E$_2$, PGE$_2$; F$_{2\alpha}$, PGF$_{2\alpha}$; 6o-F$_{1\alpha}$, 6-oxo-PGF$_{1\alpha}$; 20h-B$_4$, 20-hydroxyLTB$_4$. Taken from ref. 17.

(iso-1) and 6-*trans*-8-*cis*-12-epi-LTB$_4$ (5S, 12S) are not completely resolved. Neither are the 12- and 15-monohydroxy metabolites of arachidonic acid separated under these conditions. Although this mobile phase is very useful for the separation and analysis of cyclo-oxygenase products, it cannot be recommended for lipoxygenase products, because detection by u.v. absorbance is not possible.

5.2 Separation of lipoxygenase products by NP-h.p.l.c.

A mobile phase which has often been used for the separation of both the free acids and the methyl esters of monohydroxy and dihydroxy metabolites of arachidonic acid is hexane/isopropanol/acetic acid (15,16). This system separates both types of products very well and is transparent to u.v. light. The separation of a mixture similar to that described above is shown in *Figure 4*. The mobile phase consisted of a gradient between hexane/isopropanol/acetic acid (99.4:0.6:0.1) and hexane/isopropanol/acetic acid (85:15:0.1). Although this system separates mono- and di-hydroxy products very well, TXB$_2$ and 6-oxo-PGF$_{1\alpha}$ give very broad peaks, which are not resolved from PGE$_2$ and PGF$_{2\alpha}$. These conditions therefore cannot be recommended for the separation of cyclo-oxygenase products. The choice of mobile phases therefore depends on the type of products to be separated.

5.3 Effects of injection medium on chromatographic behaviour

One drawback with NP-h.p.l.c. is that the chromatographic behaviour of solutes is markedly affected by the polarity of the injection medium. Ideally, one should always

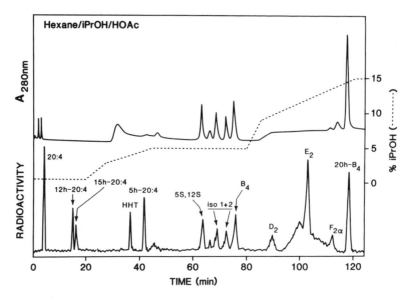

Figure 4. Separation by NP-h.p.l.c. of a mixture of arachidonic acid metabolites similar to that described in the legend to *Figure 4* (except that 11-[1-¹⁴C]HETE was not added). The mobile phase consisted of a gradient between solvent C (hexane/isopropanol/acetic acid, 99.4:0.6:0.1) and solvent D (hexane/isopropanol/acetic acid, 85:15:0.1) as follows: 0 min, 0% D; 20 min, 0% D; 28 min, 17% D; 45 min, 31% D; 80 min, 31% D; 85 min, 51% D; 120 min, 100% D. The flow-rate was 2 ml/min. Abbreviations are defined in the legend to *Figure 3*. Taken from ref. 17.

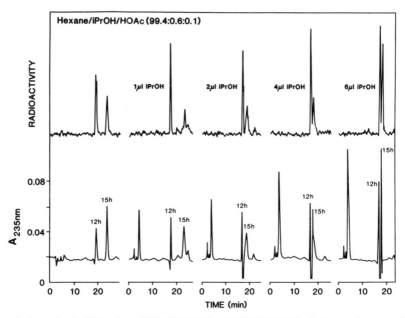

Figure 5. Separation by NP-h.p.l.c. of 12-HETE (12 h) and 15-HETE (15 h) using hexane/isopropanol/acetic acid (99.4:0.6:0.1) at a flow-rate of 2 ml/min as the mobile phase. The samples were injected in 20 μl of mobile phase (extreme left) or 20 μl of mobile phase containing different amounts of isopropanol. Taken from ref. 17.

dissolve the sample either in the mobile phase alone, or in a weaker solvent. When a mixture of polar (e.g. prostaglandins or ω-oxidation products of LTB$_4$) and non-polar (e.g. monohydroxyeicosanoids) products is to be chromatographed, the mobile phase is generally insufficiently polar to dissolve all of the polar products, resulting in low recoveries. This problem can be overcome by the addition of a few microlitres of a polar solvent such as isopropanol to the injection medium. Unfortunately, the addition of as little as 1 μl of isopropanol can have noticeable effects on the chromatography (16). This is illustrated by *Figure 5*, which shows the separation of 12-hydroxyeico-satetraenoic acid (12-HETE) and 15-HETE, which were injected in 20 μl mobile phase [hexane/isopropanol/acetic acid (99.4:0.6:0.1)] containing different amounts of isopropanol. The isopropanol in the injection medium modifies the mobile phase in a small segment of the column, making it stronger, and causes the negative peak at about 18 min. This markedly affects the chromatographic behaviour of products such as 12-HETE and 15-HETE, the retention times of which are about the same as that of isopropanol. The retention times of these products are thus reduced and multiple peaks are observed for 15-HETE. The chromatographic behaviour of more polar eicosanoids is not affected significantly by the presence of small amounts of isopropanol in the injection medium, however.

5.4 NP-h.p.l.c. of methyl esters

Methyl esters of eicosanoids often give better results than free acids when they are chromatographed by NP-h.p.l.c. However, chromatograms of mixtures containing 6-oxo-PGF$_{1\alpha}$ can be difficult to interpret due to the presence of multiple sharp peaks due to different tautomeric forms of this compound. In general, mobile phases similar to those described above, except that acetic acid can often be omitted, are used for methyl esters (cf. *Figure 7A* in Section 6 and refs 18 and 19).

6. ARGENTATION HIGH-PRESSURE LIQUID CHROMATOGRAPHY

6.1 Preparation of stationary phase

Argentation h.p.l.c. (Ag-h.p.l.c.) can conveniently be carried out using cation-exchange columns loaded with silver ions. This can be accomplished by washing a column of RSil CAT (Alltech Associates, Deerfield, IL) with water, followed by silver nitrate as shown in *Table I*. The excess silver nitrate is removed by washing with water, and the column is then washed with a series of organic solvents (20,21).

6.2 Mechanism of Ag-h.p.l.c.

The stationary phase described above interacts with solutes by two mechanisms:

(i)   interactions between polar groups of the solute and polar groups on the stationary phase, and
(ii)   interactions between olefinic double bonds of the solute and silver ions of the stationary phase (*Figure 6*).

The relative contributions of these two mechanisms depends on the nature of the mobile phase (20). If acetonitrile is added to the mobile phase, it competes with the solute for the silver ions of the stationary phase, and the order of elution of solutes is similar

Table 1. Preparation of a silver ion-loaded cation-exchange column[a] for argentation-high pressure liquid chromatography[b].

The following solvents should be pumped through the column:
   Water (300 ml)
   1 M silver nitrate (150 ml)
   Water (300 ml)[c]
   Methanol (300 ml)
   Acetone (200 ml)
   Ethyl acetate (200 ml)
   Chloroform (200 ml)
   Hexane (200 ml)
The column should be kept in hexane when not in use.

---

[a]We used a column of 5 μm particle size RSil CAT (4.6 × 350 mm) (Alltech Associates).
[b]See refs 20, 21.
[c]The water should remove all of the silver ions not bound by the stationary phase. At the end of this wash, the column eluate should therefore not turn cloudy when added to a solution of sodium chloride.

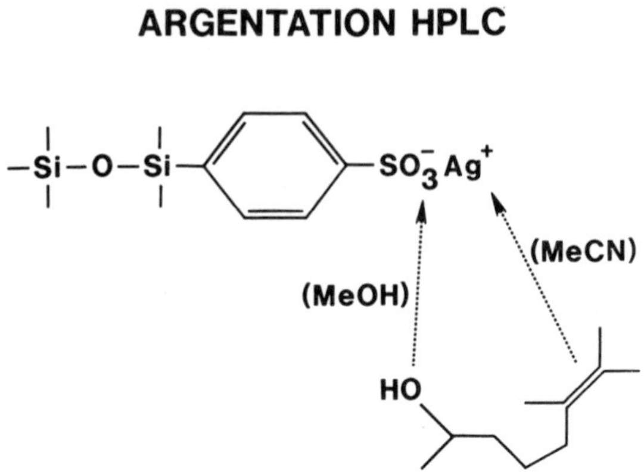

ARGENTATION HPLC

Figure 6. Interactions between solutes and the stationary phase in Ag-h.p.l.c. on a silver ion-loaded cation-exchange column. Methanol in the mobile phase competes with polar groups of the solute for polar sites on the stationary phase. Acetonitrile in the mobile phase competes with olefinic groups of the solute for silver ions on the stationary phase.

to that observed in NP-h.p.l.c. With a mobile phase consisting of methanol/acetonitrile/chloroform/acetic acid (2:18:80:0.5), for example, the order of retention times of some standards is: $PGF_{2\alpha} > PGE_2 > 12$-HETE $>$ arachidonic acid (*Table 2*). On the other hand, mobile phases containing high concentrations of methanol tend to suppress polar interactions, so that the number of double bonds becomes a much more important factor in determining the retention time. This can be illustrated by comparing the retention times of 12-HETE and $PGF_{2\alpha}$ in *Table 2*. With a mobile phase containing 18% acetonitrile and only 2% methanol, the ratio of the retention time of 12-HETE to that of $PGF_{2\alpha}$ is 0.16. If the composition of the mobile phase is changed to 1% acetonitrile and 19% methanol, the ratio is increased to 1.2, and if the mobile phase is almost entirely methanol, the ratio is 2.3.

Table 2. Retention times of some eicosanoids on a silver ion-loaded cation-exchange column.

Mobile phase	Retention time (min)						
	$20{:}3^a$	$20{:}4^b$	12-HETE	PGE_1	PGE_2	$PGF_{1\alpha}$	$PGF_{2\alpha}$
MeOH:MeCN:CHCl$_3$:HOAc (2:18:80:0.5)	–	4.0	4.9	10.5	11.5	23.8	30.2
MeOH:MeCN:CHCl$_3$:HOAc (19:1:80:0.5)	–	>50	48.9	5.2	8.4	10.2	40.6
MeOH:HOAc(99.8:0.2)	19.0	65.0	25.1	3.1	5.1	3.8	10.8

^{a}8,11,14-Eicosatrienoic acid.
^{b}Arachidonic acid.

6.3 Applications of Ag-h.p.l.c.

Because the retention times of eicosanoids in Ag-h.p.l.c. do not correspond very well to the different classes of eicosanoids (i.e. monohydroxy products, dihydroxy products, prostaglandins, etc.) the chromatograms of complex mixtures of these substances can be difficult to interpret. For example, the retention time of $PGF_{2\alpha}$ is much longer than that of 6-oxo-$PGF_{1\alpha}$ in methanol, but nearly identical to that of 15-HETE (20). Another problem is that the column has a rather low capacity, causing deterioration in peak shapes when the amount of a solute injected exceeds $15-20$ μg.

Argentation-h.p.l.c. can be very useful for certain specific applications, however, as illustrated by *Figure 7A* and *B*. *Figure 7A* shows the separation by NP-h.p.l.c. of metabolites of 8,11,14-eicosatrienoic acid formed by aorta (18,22). One of the peaks has a retention time identical to that of PGE_1. Re-chromatography of this peak by Ag-h.p.l.c. revealed that the major component was not PGE_1, however, but another metabolite (product X), which was identified by mass spectrometry as 8,11,12-tri-hydroxy-9-heptadecenoic acid (18). This product had been formed from 12-hydroper-oxy-8,10-heptadecadienoic acid, which in turn had been formed from PGG_1 by the action of prostacyclin synthase.

The above example clearly illustrates that one must be very cautious in attempting to identify metabolites on the basis of their retention times on h.p.l.c., or any other type of chromatography. In order to provide more conclusive evidence as to the nature of a particular product, one can demonstrate that it co-chromatographs with an authentic standard with a second system which interacts with solutes by a different mechanism. In the case described above, NP-h.p.l.c. and Ag-h.p.l.c. have been used. Another possibility would have been to use RP-h.p.l.c. as the second step.

6.3.1 *Separation of isotopically-labelled eicosanoids from unlabelled eicosanoids*

Another application of Ag-h.p.l.c. is the separation of isotopically-labelled eicosanoids from the corresponding unlabelled compounds (23). This can be very useful if deuterium or tritium-labelled products are prepared by incubation of labelled arachidonic acid with various tissue fractions or cells which contain endogenous arachidonic acid. This is illustrated by *Figure 8*, which shows the separation by Ag-h.p.l.c. of products in the monohydroxy fraction obtained after incubation of a mixture of

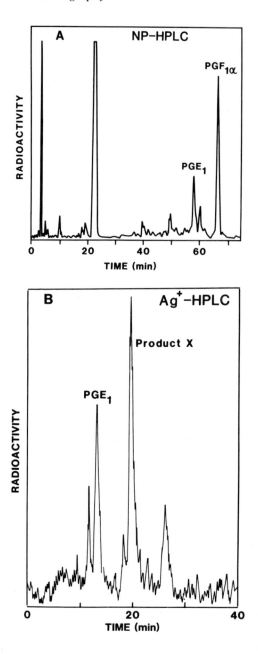

Figure 7. (**A**) Normal phase high-pressure liquid chromatography of the methylated products formed after incubation of 8,11,14-[1-^{14}C]eicosatrienoic acid with a particulate fraction from fetal calf aorta. The mobile phase consisted of a gradient between solvent E [hexane/benzene (1:1)] and solvent F [benzene/ethyl acetate/acetonitrile/methanol (30:40:30:2)] as follows: 0 min, 2% F; 30 min, 2% F; 80 min, 100% F. The flow-rate was 2 ml/min. Toluene can be substituted for benzene in this mobile phase. Taken from ref. 22. (**B**) Re-chromatography by Ag-h.p.l.c. of the peak labelled PGE$_1$ in *Figure 7A*. The mobile phase was methylene chloride/methanol/acetonitrile (90:9.75:0.25). The flow-rate was 1 ml/min. Taken from ref. 18.

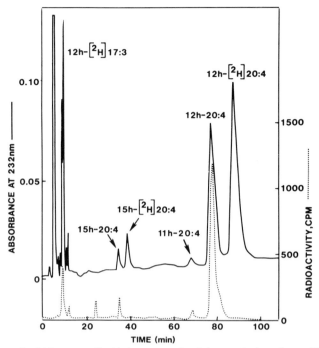

Figure 8. Argentation-high-pressure liquid chromatography of the monohydroxy fatty acid fraction obtained by incubating a mixture of [1-^{14}C]arachidonic acid and [5,6,8,9,11,12,14,15-^{2}H]arachidonic acid with a rat spleen homogenate. The mobile phase was methanol/acetic acid (99.8:0.2) and the flow-rate, 1 ml/min. Solid line, absorbance at 232 nm; broken line, radioactivity. Taken from ref. 23.

[5,6,8,9,11,12,14,15-^{2}H] arachidonic acid and [1-^{14}C]arachidonic acid with a rat spleen homogenate (23). The products were first extracted with ODS-silica and partially purified by NP-h.p.l.c. The components of a fraction containing all of the monohydroxy products were then separated by Ag-h.p.l.c. Deuterium-labelled 15-HETE and 12-HETE were completely separated from the corresponding unlabelled products, formed from the large amount of endogenous arachidonic acid in the spleen homogenate. The ^{14}C-labelled monohydroxy products, on the other hand, co-chromatographed with their unlabelled counterparts. Tritium-labelled products have retention times still longer than their deuterium-labelled analogs (23).

The mechanism for the separation of unlabelled, deuterium-labelled, and tritium-labelled products is due to the fact that the length of the carbon—hydrogen bond decreases in the order C-^{1}H > C-^{2}H > C-^{3}H. If the deuterium or tritium atoms are present on olefinic carbons, the shorter bond length permits a greater degree of interaction between the olefinic group and silver ions of the stationary phase, resulting in a longer retention time. We have used this technique to increase the isotopic purity of a variety of ^{2}H- and ^{3}H-labelled prostaglandins as well as LTB$_4$ derived from octadeuterated and octatritiated arachidonic acid (23).

7. REVERSED-PHASE HIGH-PRESSURE LIQUID CHROMATOGRAPHY

Reversed-phase-h.p.l.c. on ODS-silica is the most frequently used type of h.p.l.c. for the separation and analysis of eicosanoids. Recoveries are generally very good, and most of the solvents commonly used (water, methanol, acetonitrile and tetrahydrofuran) are transparent to u.v. light, permitting detection at wavelengths as low as $190-200$ nm. The injection medium does not normally interfere with the chromatography, as may be the case with NP-h.p.l.c. Samples can either be injected in the mobile phase or in water-miscible solvents such as ethanol or isopropanol. Injection of up to 30 μl of these solvents does not normally affect either the retention times or peak shapes. An alternative method of applying samples in RP-h.p.l.c. is to load the sample directly on to the column, as discussed in Section 3.2.

It is important that the water used for RP-h.p.l.c. should be pure, especially if gradients are to be used. If the water contains organic contaminants, they can be adsorbed at the top of the column during the first part of the gradient, and then be eluted as sharp peaks as the strength of the mobile phase increases. We use glass-distilled water which we pass through either a cartridge containing ODS-silica (Waters C_{18} Sep-Pak) or a Millipore Norganic cartridge in order to remove any organic contaminants.

Reversed-phase-h.p.l.c. is a more universally applicable technique than NP-h.p.l.c., since it can also be used for the chromatography of peptido-leukotrienes. It also gives better results than NP-h.p.l.c. for 6-oxo-PGF$_{1\alpha}$ which is observed as a single sharp peak with mobile phases consisting primarily of water and acetonitrile. TXB$_2$ still usually appears as a broad peak with RP-h.p.l.c., however.

7.1 Separation of mixtures of eicosanoids not containing peptido-leukotrienes

As with NP-h.p.l.c., the choice of mobile phases will depend on the natures of the products to be chromatographed. The mobile phases most commonly used for RP-h.p.l.c. of eicosanoids consist of water/acetonitrile or water/methanol, along with an acid such as acetic acid, phosphoric acid (5,7) or trifluoroacetic acid (TFA) (24). In our experience, each of these acids gives exactly the same results for eicosanoids not containing amino acids. We therefore normally use acetic acid for chromatography of mixtures of these products, since it is the weakest acid and is volatile.

The selectivity of the stationary phase can be altered markedly, depending on whether acetonitrile or methanol is used in the mobile phase. Both acetonitrile and methanol can be used to separate monohydroxy eicosanoids, but only acetonitrile is capable of

Table 3. Retention times of some dihydroxyeicosatetraenoic acids on a 5 μm Ultrasphere ODS-silica column (4.6 × 250 mm) with various mobile phases.

	Mobile phase		
Compound	$H_2O/MeOH^a$	$H_2O/MeCN^b$	$H_2O/MeOH/MeCN^c$
6-*trans*-LTB$_4$	31.1	21.2	21.3
6-*trans*-12-epi-LTB$_4$	36.4	21.5	23.7
5,15-dihydroxy-20:4^d	34.7	19.5	22.5
LTB$_4$	43.0	21.9	26.7
6-*trans*-8-*cis*-12-epi-LTB$_4$ (5S,12S-dh-20:4)	43.0	26.0	29.0

^{a}Water/methanol/acetic acid (38:62:0.05); flow-rate, 1.5 ml/min.
^{b}Water/acetonitrile/acetic acid (62:38:0.05); flow-rate, 2 ml/min.
^{c}Water/methanol/acetonitrile/acetic acid (45:30:25:0.05); flow-rate, 2 ml/min.
^{d}5,15-Dihydroxy-6,8,11,13-eicosatetraenoic acid.

separating TXB_2 and all of the major prostaglandins derived from arachidonic acid.

Neither water/acetonitrile nor water/methanol alone can be used to separate all of the major dihydroxy metabolites formed from arachidonic acid by human polymorphonuclear leukocytes (*Table 3*). Methanol/water/acetic acid separates LTB_4 from its two 6-*trans* isomers, but does not separate LTB_4 from the double lipoxygenase product, 6-*trans*-8-*cis*-12-epi-LTB_4 (5S,12S-dh-20:4). Neither are 6-*trans*-LTB_4 and 5,15-dihydroxy-6,8,11,13-eicosatetraenoic acid completely separated by this mobile phase. On the other hand, water/acetonitrile/acetic acid can be used to separate the above two pairs of isomers, but does not adequately separate LTB_4 from its 6-*trans* isomers (*Table 3*). In order to separate all of these products completely by RP-h.p.l.c., it is advisable first to separate LTB_4 from its two 6-*trans* isomers using water/methanol/acetic acid, and then to re-chromatograph the second and third peaks containing dihydroxy products using water/acetonitrile/acetic acid. Alternatively, use a mixture of water, acetonitrile, methanol and acetic acid to separate all five of the dihydroxy products shown in *Table 3*.

7.2 High-pressure liquid chromatography of peptido-leukotrienes

The chromatographic behaviour of peptido-leukotrienes (LTC_4, LTD_4, LTE_4 and LTF_4) is quite different from that of other eicosanoids due to the presence of amino acid residues. Unlike other eicosanoids, the retention times of peptido-leukotrienes are strongly dependent upon the pH of the mobile phase and the nature of the acid it contains. Retention times can also differ markedly with different brands of ODS-silica stationary phases, depending on the degree of coverage with ODS and end-capping. When attempting to reproduce a published procedure for h.p.l.c. peptido-leukotrienes, it is therefore very important to use exactly the same type of column as that described in the paper.

7.2.1 *Effect of pH on retention times of peptido-leukotrienes*

The retention times of peptido-leukotrienes are generally lowered as the pH of the mobile phase is increased. With a 5 μm Nucleosil C_{18} column, for example, the retention time of LTC_4 (31.0 min) was reported (25) to be longer than that of LTB_4 (28.8 min) with a mobile phase consisting of water/methanol/acetic acid (35:65:0.02) (pH 4.0). When the pH was raised to 5.7 by the addition of ammonium hydroxide, the retention time (t_R) of LTB_4 was only slightly lowered (27.0 min), whereas those of peptido-leukotrienes were considerably shortened (t_R of LTC_4, 10.0 min) (25). It should be noted, however, that metal ions can interfere with the h.p.l.c. of peptido-leukotrienes when mobile phases containing acetic acid are used, and it has therefore been recommended to wash the column with EDTA before use (26). Since EDTA is poorly soluble in methanol, it is important to wash the column with water prior to equilibration with mobile phases containing methanol (27). An alternative to washing the column with EDTA is to either inject oxalic acid as a bolus, or to incorporate oxalic acid (0.5 mM) into the mobile phase (28).

An advantage of using acetic acid in the mobile phase is that it is a weak acid which is volatile, and can therefore easily be removed. For preparative applications, it is therefore probably preferable to use mobile phases containing acetic acid for all

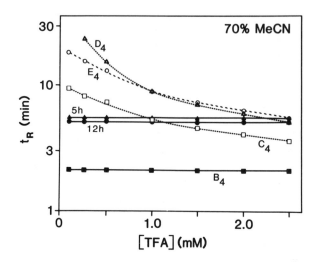

Figure 9. Effects of the concentration of trifluoroacetic acid in 70% acetonitrile on the retention times of leukotrienes B_4, C_4, D_4 and E_4, and 5-HETE and 12-HETE. A column of 5 μm Ultrasphere ODS and a flow-rate of 2 ml/min were used. Taken from ref. 24.

eicosanoids. One of the problems with such mobile phases is that peptido-leukotrienes are not separated as a group from other products, such as LTB_4, which absorb at 280 nm.

For analytical applications, stronger acids such as phosphoric acid and TFA give better chromatography and more reproducible results. Borgeat and co-workers found that with a gradient containing 0.02% phosphoric acid (pH 3.0), peptido-leukotrienes are not eluted from a Waters radial-pak C_{18} column. They can subsequently be eluted by employing a pH gradient using a third solvent at pH 5.5. In this way, peptido-leukotrienes can be eluted as a group after arachidonic acid (and the calcium ionophore, A23187) (5).

7.2.2 Effects of trifluoroacetic acid on retention times

TFA is a strong acid and ion-pairing reagent which is used extensively for the h.p.l.c. of peptides (29). We make up a stock solution of 2% TFA, which we pass through a cartridge containing ODS-silica in order to remove contaminants.

The effects of TFA on the retention times of peptido-leukotrienes cannot be explained purely in terms of alterations in the pH of the mobile phase. We found that with a 5 μm Beckman Ultrasphere ODS column, the retention times of leukotrienes C_4, D_4 and E_4 are much longer than those of monohydroxyeicosanoids with very low concentrations of TFA (24). Increasing the concentration of TFA results in a reduction in the retention times of peptido-leukotrienes without affecting those of other eicosanoids (*Figure 9*). Thus, the retention times of peptido-leukotrienes can be manipulated, relative to those of other eicosanoids, by altering the concentration of TFA in the mobile phase. Using this approach, peptido-leukotrienes can be analysed with a gradient between 0.0008% and 0.02% TFA in 70% acetonitrile (*Figure 10*).

One problem with the use of TFA for preparative applications is that it becomes con-

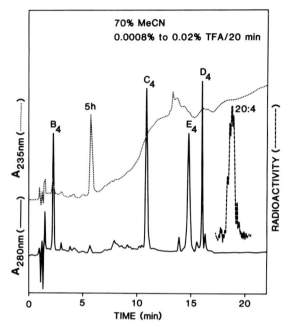

Figure 10. Reversed phase-high-pressure liquid chromatography of peptido-leukotrienes using a trifluoroacetic acid (TFA) gradient on a 5 μm Ultrasphere ODS column. A gradient between 0.0008% TFA in 70% acetonitrile and 0.02% TFA in 70% acetonitrile over 20 min was used to separate leukotrienes B_4, C_4, D_4 and E_4, as well as 5-HETE and [1-14C]arachidonic acid. The flow-rate was 2 ml/min. Solid line, absorbance at 280 nm; dotted line, absorbance at 235 nm; dashed line, radioactivity. Taken from ref. 24.

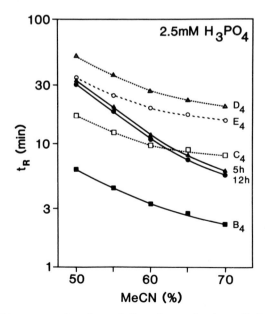

Figure 11. Effects of the concentration of acetonitrile on the retention times of leukotrienes B_4, C_4, D_4 and E_4, and 5-HETE and 12-HETE in the presence of 2.5 mM phosphoric acid. The flow-rate was 2 ml/min and the stationary phase, 5 μm Ultrasphere ODS. Taken from ref. 24.

91

centrated when column fractions are evaporated down. This results in a very low pH just prior to complete removal of the solvent, which can cause decomposition of peptido-leukotrienes. This problem can be alleviated to some extent by addition of a small amount of trimethylamine to the column fractions before evaporation.

7.2.3 *Effects of acetonitrile concentration on retention times*

The degree of ionization of TFA and phosphoric acid is partially suppressed as the concentration of water in the mobile phase is reduced. Raising the concentration of acetonitrile in the mobile phase might therefore be expected to affect the retention times of peptido-leukotrienes differently from those of other eicosanoids. The retention times of leukotrienes C_4, D_4 and E_4, as well as LTB_4, 5-HETE and 12-HETE, as a function of the concentration of acetonitrile in 2.5 mM phosphoric acid are shown in *Figure 11*. As the acetonitrile concentration is raised, the retention times of peptido-leukotrienes drop much more slowly than those of the other arachidonic acid metabolites (24).

7.3 **Gradients for reversed-phase-h.p.l.c. of arachidonic acid metabolites**

Some of the major problems which must be confronted when separating mixtures containing many different types of arachidonic acid metabolites are:

(i)   prostaglandins and TXB_2 should be separated from one another;
(ii)   dihydroxy products should be as well separated as possible; and
(iii) peptido-leukotrienes should preferably be eluted as a group with retention times clearly different from those of other products.

Cyclo-oxygenase products can best be separated by constructing a gradient which initially consists primarily of water and acetonitrile. This is not suitable for the separation of dihydroxy products, which can be optimally separated with a mixture of water, methanol and acetonitrile (*Table 3*). Therefore the concentration of methanol should be increased in the intermediate part of the gradient. Finally, peptido-leukotrienes can be eluted after all of the other arachidonic acid metabolites by using either phosphoric acid or a very low concentration of TFA in the initial stages, and then raising the concentration of TFA at the end of the gradient. Since the retention times of peptido-leukotrienes are shorter relative to those of other eicosanoids at low compared with high concentrations of acetonitrile (*Figure 11*), the gradient should be fairly rapid. If the gradient is too long, the retention times of peptido-leukotrienes on a Beckman Ultrasphere ODS column can overlap with those of monohydroxy metabolites.

A system that we have developed (24) for the separation of arachidonic acid metabolites on a 5 μm Beckman Ultrasphere ODS column is illustrated by *Figure 12*. The sample consisted of a mixture of extracts obtained after incubation of a suspension of human polymorphonuclear leukocytes and a bovine lung homogenate with [1-^{14}C]arachidonic acid, together with 15-HETE, 12-HETE, LTC_4, LTD_4 and LTE_4. The mobile phase was a linear gradient between: (i) 95% solvent G [water/acetonitrile/phosphoric acid (76:25:0.025)] and 5% solvent H [methanol/acetonitrile/water/TFA (60:40:0.08: 0.0016)] and (ii) 20% solvent G and 80% solvent H over 32 min. Prepare the two solvents by adding appropriate amounts of stock solutions of 250 mM phosphoric acid and 2% TFA to water/acetonitrile (75:25) and methanol/acetonitrile (60:40), respectively; use a flow-rate of 2 ml/min. This system separates all of the major cyclo-oxy-

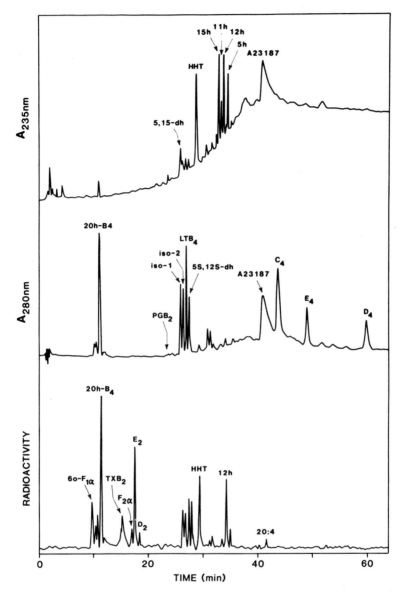

Figure 12. Reversed-phase-high pressure liquid chromatography of a mixture of arachidonic acid metabolites similar to that described in the legend to *Figure 3* on a column of 5 μm Ultrasphere ODS. A linear gradient between (i) 95% solvent G (water:acetonitrile:phosphoric acid, 76:25:0.01) and 5% solvent H (methanol: acetonitrile:water:trifluoroacetic acid, 60:40:0.08:0.0016) and (ii) 80% solvent H and 20% solvent G over 32 min was used. The solvents were prepared by mixing appropriate amounts of 0.25 M phosphoric acid or 2% TFA with either 25% acetonitrile in water or 40% acetonitrile in methanol, respectively. The flow-rate was 2 ml/min. Although the sample did not contain PGB_2, its elution position with identical conditions is indicated by an arrow. 5,15-dh, 5,15-dihydroxy-6,8,11,13-eicosatetraenoic acid. Taken from ref. 24.

genase products and 5,12-dihydroxy isomers of arachidonic acid. Leukotrienes C_4, D_4 and E_4 are eluted at the end of the gradient, after arachidonic acid and the calcium ionophore, A23187 (which had been added to the leukocytes).

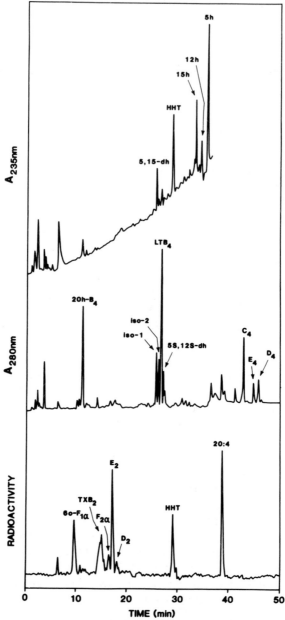

Figure 13. Reversed-phase-high pressure liquid chromatography of a mixture of arachidonic acid metabolites on a Spherisorb ODS-2 column. The sample was a mixture of extracts from incubations of (**i**) [1-^{14}C]arachidonic acid with a bovine lung homogenate and (**ii**) unlabelled arachidonic acid with a suspension of porcine polymorphonuclear leukocytes. It should be noted that the leukocyte products were not labelled as was the case for *Figure 12*. The mobile phase consisted of a ternary gradient between solvent J [water/acetonitrile/TFA (75.05:25:0.001)], solvent K [methanol/acetonitrile/water/TFA (60:40:0.05:0.001)] and solvent L [methanol/acetonitrile/water/TFA (60:40:0.5:0.01)] as follows: 0 min, 100% J; 35 min, 10% J and 90% K; 50 min, 10% J, 90% L. Both gradients were linear, and the flow-rate was 2 ml/min. The solvents were prepared as described in the legend to *Figure 12*.

The system described above has been designed specifically for an Ultrasphere ODS column, in which the stationary phase has been end-capped with trimethylsilyl groups, and will not give satisfactory results with ODS columns which are not end-capped. Spherisorb ODS-2 columns, which are not end-capped, retain peptido-leukotrienes much more than Ultrasphere columns, and they are not eluted using the above gradient. They can be eluted by using a higher concentration of TFA, however. Using this strategy, a mixture similar to that described above (monohydroxy and dihydroxy products were not labelled with ^{14}C in this case) can be separated with a gradient between 100% solvent J [water/acetonitrile/TFA (75.05:25:0.001)] and 90% solvent K [methanol/acetonitrile/water/TFA (60:40:0.05:0.001)] in solvent J for 35 min, followed by a second gradient to 90% solvent L [methanol/acetonitrile/water/TFA (60:40:0.5:0.01)] in solvent J over an additional 15 min (*Figure 13*). Prepare the solvents as described above, by adding appropriate amounts of 2% TFA to water/acetonitrile (75:25) and methanol/acetonitrile (60:40). Peptido-leukotrienes are not eluted during the first part of the chromatography, due to the low concentration of TFA, but only when the concentration of TFA is increased during the second gradient. The chromatographic behaviour of other eicosanoids on the Spherisorb column is almost identical to that on the Ultrasphere column. The baseline at 235 nm increases rapidly shortly after 5-HETE is eluted from the column using these conditions. This problem could have been avoided by maintaining the mobile phase at 90% solvent K (0.001% TFA) for a few minutes before starting the second gradient to 0.01% TFA.

With stationary phases such as Spherisorb ODS-2, which interact strongly with peptido-leukotrienes, another possibility would be to use a pH gradient rather than a TFA gradient for the second phase of the h.p.l.c. This approach has been used by Borgeat and co-workers, who have used a Waters Radial-Pak C_{18} cartridge to separate mixtures containing various lipoxygenase products, including mono- and di-hydroxy products and leukotrienes (5). The mobile phase consisted of an initial gradient in the presence of phosphoric acid (pH ~ 3), followed by a second gradient, in which the pH is increased to 5.5 by the addition of ammonium hydroxide (5).

One disadvantage of the methods described above, utilizing Spherisorb ODS and Radial Pak ODS columns, is that three pumps are required. On the other hand, the system shown in *Figure 12* is simpler, consisting of a linear gradient between only two solvents. The peaks for peptide-leukotrienes are not as sharp with the latter system, however, since they are eluted after the gradient, using isocratic conditions. Mixtures not containing peptido-leukotrienes can be separated using gradients similar to those described in *Figures 12* and *13*. In this case, TFA (0.001%), phosphoric acid (0.025%) and acetic acid (0.02%) give nearly identical results. In the absence of peptido-leukotrienes, it is therefore not necessary to use a third solvent with a Spherisorb ODS column.

8. QUANTITATION OF EICOSANOIDS BY HIGH-PRESSURE LIQUID CHROMATOGRAPHY

8.1 Quantitation by u.v.-absorbance or fluorescence

High-pressure liquid chromatography can be used to quantitate arachidonic acid metabolites, using either a u.v.- or a radioactivity-detector. Most lipoxygenase products can be quantitated on the basis of u.v. absorbance, whereas prostaglandins and

Table 4. Ultraviolet absorption characteristics of some arachidonic acid metabolites.

Compound	λmax (nm)[a]	Molar extinction coefficient	Reference
LTB$_4$	281	39 500	35
6-*trans*-LTB$_4$	280	44 000	36
6-*trans*-12-*epi*-LTB$_4$	280	44 000	36
6-*trans*-8-*cis*-12-*epi*-LTB$_4$ (5S,12S-dh-20:4)	278		16
5,15-dihydroxy-20:4	243	30 000	37
LTC$_4$	280	40 000	25
LTD$_4$	280	40 000	25
LTE$_4$	280	40 000	38
PGB$_2$	278	28 680	25
5-HETE	235	30 500	39
12-HETE	237	30 500	40
HHT	232	33 400	40

[a]LTB$_4$ and other 5,12-dihydroxy metabolites exhibit maximal absorbance at about 270 nm, and have a third λ$_{max}$ at 260 nm. Peptido-leukotrienes also have absorption maxima at 270 nm and 290 nm.

other cyclo-oxygenase products can be measured in experiments where radioactive arachidonic acid has been used as the substrate. The conversion of endogenous arachidonic acid by cyclo-oxygenase can also be investigated by quantitating 12-*L*-hydroxyheptadecatrienoic acid (HHT) on the basis of u.v. absorbance. We have found HHT to be a very good index of cyclo-oxygenase activity in rat pleural leukocytes; the amount formed under various conditions, as estimated by u.v. absorbance, closely paralleled the amounts of TXB$_2$, PGE$_2$ and PGF$_{2\alpha}$, which were quantitated either by gas chromatography-mass spectrometry, or by radioactivity measurements (30).

In order to quantitate arachidonic acid metabolites by h.p.l.c., it is important to add an internal standard to correct for differences in recoveries between samples. Prostaglandin B$_2$ (λ$_{max}$, 278 nm; molar extinction coefficient, 28 650) is often used as an internal standard for quantitation of leukotrienes and monohydroxy metabolites of arachidonic acid by RP-h.p.l.c. (31); add the PGB$_2$ [~50−250 ng (150−740 pmol)] to the medium or biological fluid prior to extraction. The column eluate can be monitored for u.v. absorbance at 235 nm for monohydroxy products and 280 nm for leukotrienes and PGB$_2$. This can either be done simultaneously, or the wavelength of the detector can be changed during the run. The extinction coefficients of various arachidonic acid metabolites are listed in *Table 4*. The amounts of leukotrienes and monohydroxy products can be determined by comparison of their peak areas with that of PGB$_2$, after correction for the difference in extinction coefficients, as shown below. The sensitivity of this method is about 1 ng.

$$\text{Amount of X (pmol)} = \frac{[\text{peak area (X)}] \times [28\ 650] \times [\text{amount of PGB}_2 \text{ added (pmol)}]}{[\text{peak area (PGB}_2)] \times [\text{molar extinction coefficient (X)}]}$$

Eicosanoids which do not have conjugated double bonds can be measured, in some cases, on the basis of their absorbance at 195 nm (8). This requires prior removal of contaminants by open column chromatography, however. Sensitivity can be improved by using a microbore column (internal diameter, 2 mm) (8). Alternatively, prostaglandins can be quantitated using either u.v. or fluorescence detectors after conversion to suitable derivatives as discussed in Section 4.1 (11 − 14). Cyclo-oxygenase products from rat pleural cells were derivatized by treatment with 9-anthryldiazomethane and quantitated using a fluorescence detector (13). The sensitivity of this assay was about 0.5 ng. A very sensitive method (sensitivity, 30 pg/3 ml plasma) has recently been reported for quantitating 15-methylPGE$_2$ as its panacyl ester (14). This method requires several chromatographic steps that can be automated (14). One of the disadvantages of detection after derivatization or detection at very low wavelengths is a reduction in specificity, which must be compensated for by preliminary purification steps prior to analysis.

8.2 Other methods of quantitation by h.p.l.c.

In order to increase specificity, h.p.l.c. can be coupled with radioimmunoassay. Although this can be rather time-consuming, it is a very sensitive and specific method, which has been used for both cyclo-oxygenase products (32) and leukotrienes (33).

Radioactive arachidonic acid metabolites can be quantitated by using either a liquid scintillation counter or a radioactivity monitor. In this case, we normally incubate tissues with ^{14}C-labelled substrate and add either [9β-^{3}H]PGF$_{1\alpha}$ or [9α-^{3}H]PGF$_{1\beta}$ as an internal standard (18). These tritium-labelled standards can be synthesized inexpensively by reducing unlabelled PGE$_1$ with sodium boro[^{3}H]hydride (34).

9. ACKNOWLEDGEMENTS

The author is grateful to Ms Francine Gravelle for expert technical assistance. This work was supported by the Medical Research Council of Canada and the Quebec Heart Foundation. The author holds a Scientist award from the Medical Research Council of Canada.

10. REFERENCES

1. Powell,W.S. (1980) *Prostaglandins*, **20**, 947.
2. Powell,W.S. (1982) In *Methods in Enzymology*. Lands,W.E.M. and Smith,W.L. (eds), Academic Press, New York, Vol. 86, p. 467.
3. Powell,W.S. (1987) *Anal. Biochem.*, in press.
4. Pickett,W.C. and Douglas,M.B. (1985) *Prostaglandins*, **29**, 83.
5. Borgeat,P., Fruteau de Laclos,B., Rabinovitch,H., Picard,S., Braquet,P., Hebert,J. and Laviolette,M. (1984) *J. Allergy Clin. Immunol.*, **74**, 310.
6. Serhan,C.N., Hamberg,M. and Samuelsson,B. (1984) *Proc. Natl. Acad. Sci. USA*, **81**, 5335.
7. Van Rollins,M., Aveldano,M.I., Sprecher,H.W. and Horrocks,L.A. (1982) In *Methods in Enzymology*. Lands,W.E.M. and Smith,W.L. (eds), Academic Press, New York, Vol. 86, p. 518.
8. Rydzik,R., Terragno,A. and Tackett,R. (1984) *J. Chromatogr.*, **308**, 31.
9. Morozowich,W. and Douglas,S.L. (1975) *Prostaglandins*, **10**, 19.
10. Fitzpatrick,F. (1976) *Anal. Chem.*, **48**, 499.
11. Turk,J., Weiss,S.J., Davis,J.E. and Needleman,P. (1978) *Prostaglandins*, **16**, 291.
12. Hatsumi,M., Kimata,S.I. and Hirosawa,K. (1982) *J. Chromatogr.*, **253**, 271.
13. Kiyomiya,K., Yamaki,K., Nimura,N., Kinoshita,T. and Oh-ishi,S. (1986) *Prostaglandins*, **31**, 71.
14. Pullen,R.H. and Cox,J.W. (1985) *J. Chromatogr.*, **343**, 271.
15. Porter,N.A., Logan,J. and Kontoyiannidou,V. (1979) *J. Org. Chem.*, **44**, 3177.

16. Borgeat,P., Picard,S., Vallerand,P. and Sirois,P. (1981) *Prostaglandins Med.*, **6**, 557.
17. Powell,W.S. (1985) In *Biochemistry of Arachidonic Acid Metabolism*. Lands,W.E.M. (ed.), Martinus Nijhoff Publishing, Boston, p. 375.
18. Powell,W.S. (1982) *J. Biol. Chem.*, **257**, 9465.
19. Maclouf,J., Fruteau de Laclos, B. and Borgeat,P. (1982) *Proc. Natl. Acad. Sci. USA*, **79**, 6042.
20. Powell,W.S. (1981) *Anal. Biochem.*, **115**, 267.
21. Merritt,M.V. and Bronson,G.E. (1977) *Anal. Biochem.*, **80**, 392.
22. Powell,W.S. and Funk,C.D. (1983) In *Advances in Prostaglandin, Thromboxane, and Leukotriene Research*. Samuelsson,B., Paoletti,R. and Ramwell,P. (eds), Raven Press, New York, Vol. 11, p. 111.
23. Powell,W.S. (1983) *Anal. Biochem.*, **128**, 93.
24. Powell,W.S. (1985) *Anal. Biochem.*, **148**, 59.
25. Mathews,W.R., Rokach,J. and Murphy,R.C. (1981) *Anal. Biochem.*, **118**, 96.
26. Metz,S.A., Hall,M.E., Harper,T.W. and Murphy,R.C. (1982) *J. Chromatogr.*, **233**, 193.
27. Metz,S.A., Hall,M.E., Harper,T.W. and Murphy,R.C. (1983) *J. Chromatogr.*, **275**, 468.
28. Muller,M. and Sorrell,T.C. (1985) *J. Chromatogr.*, **343**, 213.
29. Bennett,H.P.J., Browne,C.A.B. and Solomon,S. (1981) *Biochemistry*, **20**, 4530.
30. Yue,T.L., Varma,D.R. and Powell,W.S. (1983) *Biochim. Biophys. Acta*, **751**, 332.
31. Borgeat,P. and Samuelsson,B. (1979) *Proc. Natl. Acad. Sci. USA*, **76**, 2148.
32. Alam,I., Ohuchi,K. and Levine,L. (1979) *Anal. Biochem.*, **93**, 339.
33. Beaubien,B.C., Tippins,J.R. and Morris,H.R. (1984) *Biochem. Biophys. Res. Commun.*, **125**, 97.
34. Powell,W.S. (1982) In *Methods in Enzymology*. Lands,W.E.M. and Smith,W.L. (eds), Academic Press, New York, Vol. 86, p. 168.
35. Borgeat,P. and Samuelsson,B. (1979) *J. Biol. Chem.*, **254**, 2643.
36. Borgeat,P. and Samuelsson,B. (1979) *J. Biol. Chem.*, **254**, 7865.
37. Maas,R.L., Turk,J., Oates,J.A. and Brash,A.R. (1982) *J. Biol. Chem.*, **257**, 7056.
38. Lewis,R.A., Drazen,J.M., Austen,K.F., Clark,D.A. and Corey,E.J. (1980) *Biochem. Biophys. Res. Commun.*, **96**, 271.
39. Borgeat,P. and Samuelsson,B. (1976) *J. Biol. Chem.*, **251**, 7816.
40. Hamberg,M. and Samuelsson,B. (1974) *Proc. Natl. Acad. Sci. USA*, **71**, 3400.

CHAPTER 7

Gas chromatography and mass spectrometry of eicosanoids

SUSAN E.BARROW and GRAHAM W.TAYLOR

1. INTRODUCTION

Mass spectrometry (m.s.) provides the most sensitive and specific physicochemical method for the analysis of eicosanoid derivatives. This technique has been used widely for both structure elucidation and for quantification of extremely low concentrations of eicosanoids derived from many biological sources.

Specificity is enhanced by using gas chromatography coupled to mass spectrometry (g.c. −m.s.) where two independent parameters are used to characterize the compound of interest − g.c. retention time and detection of characteristic fragment ions by mass spectrometry. G.c. −m.s. is highly versatile and can be used to perform simultaneous analyses of a number of different arachidonic acid metabolites in a single sample.

Structure elucidation of eicosanoids can also be performed by alternative analytical methods such as nuclear magnetic resonance (n.m.r.), u.v. and i.r. spectroscopy but require concentrations in excess of those generally available from biological sources. Such methods tend to be of greater use to the synthetic organic chemist. The most common quantitative methods for the analysis of eicosanoids are bioassay, radioimmunoassay (RIA), g.c. with electron capture detection and g.c. −m.s. Sensitivities of the order of 10^{-12} g have been reported using g.c. −m.s. with selected ion monitoring (s.i.m.) techniques. Of these, only RIA compares with g.c. −m.s. for sensitivity but has limited specificity because of potential cross-reactivity of antibodies with biologically related compounds which may carry through even quite complex purification procedures.

Although g.c. −m.s. is the method of choice for acquisition of definitive results, it requires costly apparatus, highly skilled personnel and, compared with RIA, relatively few samples can be analysed. In our laboratories we process and assay approximately 25 samples over a period of 3−4 days depending upon the biological fluid and the degree of purification required. For larger sample numbers, it is feasible to employ an RIA technique provided that it is preceded by adequate purification and the method is validated for a given biological system using g.c. −m.s.

2. PRINCIPLES OF GAS CHROMATOGRAPHY

It is now a relatively simple matter to interface a gas chromatograph to a mass spectrometer. There is clearly an absolute requirement for sample volatility and many polar species, including the prostaglandins (PGs), are not amenable to g.c. without conversion to suitable derivatives (see Section 4.6). This not only confers volatility but also

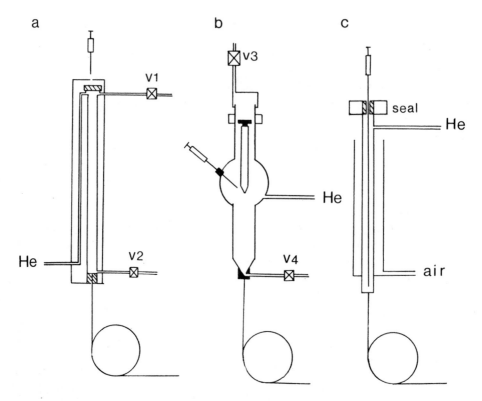

Figure 1. Schematic of the three basic types of gas chromatography injector. **(a)** Grob split-splitless injector. The sample is injected in 1−2 µl of a suitable solvent (e.g. dodecane) through a septum into a heated injector port. The sweep valve (V1) is closed on injection, but open during the g.c. run to minimize septum bleed. The split valve V1 is opened 30 sec after injection in the splitless mode to remove excess solvent. **(b)** Dropping needle injector. The sample in any solvent is loaded onto a helium cooled needle; solvent is vented through valve V3. This valve is closed and the needle is dropped into the heated injector port. After 30 sec valve V4 is opened to eliminate peak tailing. **(c)** On-column injector. The sample in solution is loaded into a syringe fitted with a long, thin needle. The needle is passed through an air-operated elastomer seal, through the air-cooled injector port and into the g.c. column.

a degree of thermal stability. Even as derivatives, high temperatures (>240°C) are required to volatilize these species. The derivatized samples are loaded onto the g.c. via one of three basic types of injector (*Figure 1a, b,* and *c*).

Once on the g.c. column, chromatography occurs via partition of the solute between a non-volatile stationary phase and a mobile phase. The rate at which samples are eluted from the column is dependent upon the temperature and flow-rate of the column. Samples can be chromatographed isothermally, but for optimal resolution, a temperature gradient is often used (e.g. 100−250°C at 5°C/min). The most common mobile phase is helium although nitrogen and other inert (and inexpensive) gases may be used. The optimum velocity of the carrier gas is proportional to the square root of the molecular weight of the gas, and thus chromatography is much slower with nitrogen compared with helium or hydrogen. The attendant risks of fire and explosion with hydrogen have limited its use.

As with h.p.l.c., which is covered elsewhere (Chapter 6), the composition (polarity) of the stationary phase may be chosen to give high selectivity and good resolution for many different classes of compounds. In general, stationary phases are based on silicon polymers which were originally adsorbed onto finely powdered inert supports and packed into open columns (internal diameter ~4 mm). High carrier gas flow-rates were required which presented some problems for mass spectrometric analysis and excess carrier gas was removed either by stream splitting (with consequent loss of sensitivity) or by inserting a jet separator between the g.c. outlet and the mass spectrometer. Packed columns provide poor resolution, and sensitivity is limited by adsorption of sample material onto the stationary phase. Most investigators now routinely work exclusively with fused silica capillary columns of about 0.2 mm internal diameter. These columns are robust; they provide high resolution and have very low adsorption characteristics. The stationary phase is bonded as a thin film to the silica surface of the column and the low flow-rates of $1-2$ ml/min are easily handled by the mass spectrometer without the need for stream splitting. These columns can be operated at temperatures of up to 325°C and are ideal for high molecular weight derivatives.

3. GENERAL PRINCIPLES OF MASS SPECTROMETRY

Mass spectrometry is based on the formation of ions and their separation in a magnetic or electrostatic field. Charge is a prerequisite for analysis; neutral molecules are not mass analysed. Mass spectrometers are normally operated at low pressure ($10^{-6}-10^{-8}$ Torr) to lessen ion-molecule interactions which would lead to reduced sensitivity and resolution.

There are two principal types of mass spectrometers commercially available — magnetic sector and quadrupole (electrostatic) instruments. Each possesses advantages and drawbacks peculiar to their design. Both types may be interfaced with gas or liquid chromatographs allowing complex biological systems to be analysed directly.

3.1 **Magnetic sector instruments**

The main features of a magnetic sector instrument are shown in *Figure 2a* and consist of an ion source, electrostatic and magnetic analysers and an ion detector. The sample is introduced to the ion source, either directly on a solid probe, via g.c. or h.p.l.c. and is ionized (see Section 3.3). The ions, which carry either positive or negative charge, are ejected from the source by the influence of an electrostatic field. In high performance instruments, this is usually achieved by floating the ion source at 8000 V (8 kV) and earthing the exit slit. Ions are thus generated with a Gaussian distribution of energies (centred on 8 keV) and accelerate towards and through the slit into the body of the mass spectrometer. The ions, of slightly differing energies, pass through the electrostatic analyser and are brought to a focus. This step is essential to obtain high resolution. The ions then pass into the magnetic analyser (i.e. the region experienced by the magnetic field) and are deflected in an arc in this field according to their charge (ze), mass (m) and certain instrument parameters [i.e. the magnetic field strength (B), the accelerating voltage (V) and the radius of the magnet (r)]. By considering the force acting on a charged species travelling at velocity (v) in a magnetic field ($= Bzev$), and that acting on a particle travelling in an arc ($= mv^2/r$), the fundamental equation governing

101

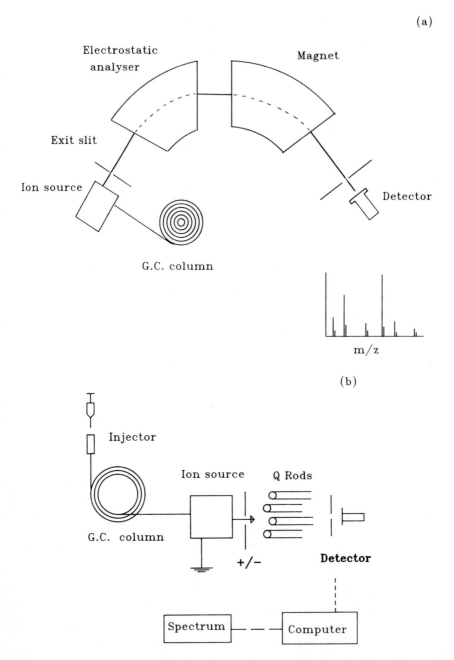

Figure 2. (a) Schematic of a magnetic sector mass spectrometer, consisting of the ion source, electrostatic analyser, magnetic analyser and ion detector. Separation of ions is carried out by scanning the magnetic field, focussing ions at the detector according to their mass to charge (m/z) ratio. **(b)** Schematic of a quadrupole mass spectrometer. The mass analyser consists of four rods, which carry a d.c. voltage and a varying radiofrequency field. The mass spectrum is generated by scanning the r.f. field. At any r.f. field value, ions of one fixed m/z value will pass through the mass analyser to the detector; other ions are unstable and are lost to the instrument walls.

behaviour of charged species in a magnetic field is:

$$\frac{m}{ze} = \frac{B^2.r^2}{2V}$$

Here z is the integral electronic charge on e. For a singly charged ion (z = 1) the equation reduces to:

$$m = k\,B^2 \quad (V,\ r \text{ and } k \text{ are constants})$$

Thus the mass of the ion is proportional to the applied magnetic field. As the magnetic field is scanned, ions of different mass are brought to a focus at the detector slit, generating an electric current, related to the intensity of the ion beam. This is the mass spectrum. Top-of-the-range magnetic sector instruments can now analyse samples with masses in excess of 10 000 daltons. More importantly for eicosanoid analysis, they are high resolution instruments which can separate ions differing in mass by only 6 p.p.m. This is of great value in structure elucidation as it allows accurate masses to be determined from which the molecular formulae may be derived.

3.2 Quadrupole mass spectrometers

The main difference between magnetic sector and quadrupole mass spectrometers lies in the principles governing the separation of ions. In a quadrupole mass spectrometer, ions are generated in the source with low energy (typically a few electron volts). They are ejected into the mass analyser, which consists of four symmetrically positioned rods (hence the term 'quadrupole'). These rods carry a low voltage d.c. potential, overlayed with a varying radiofrequency (r.f.) signal (*Figure 2b*). Ions pass into this region (down the axis of the rods) and experience an electrostatic field, deflecting their flight path. At particular d.c. and r.f. potential, ions of one particular mass to charge (m/z) ratio will pass through the analyser to the detector; ions with other m/z values possess unstable trajectories and are deflected towards the sides of the analyser (and are thus not detected). As the r.f. value is scanned, the paths of ions of different m/z become stable. Ions pass into the detector generating the mass spectrum. Quadrupole mass spectrometers operate at low voltages, with none of the requirements for high quality insulation necessary with magnetic sector instruments. There are two major limitations of quadrupoles. They have maximum resolution of approximately 1000−2000 and the mass range is normally less than 1800 u. They are however, ideally suited to g.c. −m.s. operation, and other operations when high ion source pressures are generated.

3.3 Ionization

As only ions may be mass analysed, the question arises as to how mass spectrometry can be of use for the analysis of neutral molecules, which make up the vast majority of substances of interest in the biological sciences. Various ionization techniques have been developed which impart greater or lesser amounts of energy to the molecule, and these will be briefly considered below.

3.3.1 *Electron impact (e.i.) ionization*

The sample is introduced into the ion source as a vapour which is bombarded by high energy (70 eV) electrons (e^*) forming a radical cation ($M^{\cdot+}$), termed the molecular ion and a low energy thermal electron (e_{th}).

$$M + e^* \rightarrow M^{\cdot} + e_{th} + e^*$$

This is a high energy process, and the molecular ion normally breaks down into a series of fragment ions from which structural information may be obtained. The molecular ion is generally of low intensity, and, in many cases, may not be observed. Clearly, electron impact ionization is only applicable to volatile and thermally stable compounds, and, as with g.c., derivatization is necessary in many cases. This will be considered in detail in other sections.

3.3.2 *Chemical ionization (c.i.)*

This is a softer form of ionization than occurs with e.i., with less energy imparted to the molecule and less fragmentation observed. The sample is volatilized into the ion source which contains a reagent gas such as methane, isobutane or ammonia. The reagent gas R is bombarded with electrons and ionizes to the molecular ion $R^{\cdot\,+}$ (cf. electron impact). In the presence of excess reagent gas, intermolecular collisions occur, with transfer of a proton to form the active ionizing species RH^+ — the c.i. plasma. RH^+ protonates the sample molecules M to form the protonated molecular ion $M+H^+$. This is of lower energy than the corresponding $M^{\cdot\,+}$, and undergoes less fragmentation. Chemical ionization mass spectra therefore contain intense protonated molecular ions, with some fragmentation — interestingly the fragmentation pathway differs from that obtained by e.i.m.s. and can be useful in structure elucidation. As with e.i.m.s., there is an absolute requirement for sample volatility, either as the free material or a suitable derivative.

$$CH_4 + e^* \rightarrow CH_4^{\cdot\,+} + e_{th} + e^*$$
$$CH_4^{\cdot\,+} + CH_4 \rightarrow CH_3^{\cdot} + CH_5^{+}$$
$$M + CH_5^{+} \rightarrow M+H^+ + CH_4$$

Adduct ions corresponding to MRH^+ (e.g. $M+CH_5^+$) are also observed in c.i. spectra.

Negative ion chemical ionization mass spectra may also be generated. Reagent gases such as nitric oxide and oxygen are employed. Molecular ion species are again generated by collision of sample molecules with the ionizing species such as O_2^-, NO^-. The technique has not been widely employed.

3.3.3 *Electron capture negative ion chemical ionization (n.i.c.i.)*

Under chemical ionization conditions, a large number of low-energy thermal electrons are generated from the reagent gas as a consequence of $R^{\cdot\,+}$ formation. These electrons may be captured by certain compounds to generate negative molecular ions $(M^{\cdot\,-})$. As with c.i., this is a low-energy process, and little fragmentation occurs, making it suitable for quantification (see Section 6.4). Most molecules however have a low cross-sectional capture area for e_{th}, and to all intents and purposes, are not ionized under these conditions and it may be necessary to convert them to electron capturing species by suitable derivatization. Fluorinated aromatics (e.g. pentafluorobenzyl, bis-trifluoromethylbenzoyl) have been found to be most suitable for this purpose as they possess low lying anti-bonding molecular orbitals (π^*) and can readily accept these thermal electrons. Other fluorinated derivatives may also be used (notably trifluoroacetyl, heptafluorobutyryl). However, on ionization, these derivatives fragment to generate the acid anion (e.g. CF_3COO^-) almost exclusively, and are of little value for mass spectrometric studies. These derivatives are most suitable for use with g.c. electron capture detectors.

3.3.4 *Soft ionization*

Both e.i. and c.i. require samples to be volatile for analysis. This can be a problem for many substances, which either derivatize incompletely, or form involatile or high mass derivatives. Mass spectrometric data can readily be obtained by softer methods such as desorption chemical ionization (d.c.i.) and fast atom bombardment (f.a.b.) ionization. These are suitable for underivatized polar, involatile or thermally labile materials. For d.c.i., the sample is loaded onto a rhenium wire and inserted into a c.i. plasma. The wire is rapidly heated, resulting in desorption (not volatilization) and ionization of the material with little thermal degradation. Both positive ion ($M+H^+$) and negative ion ($M^{\cdot-}$, $M-H^-$) spectra can be obtained with little fragmentation. Desorption electron impact (d.e.i.) spectra may be obtained in the same way. Again volatility is not essential. D.c.i. (and d.e.i.) are most suitable for less polar species; highly polar materials give superior data with f.a.b. ionization. Here the sample is loaded in solution onto a stainless steel platform, covered in glycerol ($1-2$ μl). It is bombarded with high energy (6 keV) xenon ions. The sample ionizes to give $M+H^+$ and $M-H^-$ ions with limited fragmentation. Fast atom bombardment and d.c.i. can be carried out on sub-microgram quantitites, provided samples are of high purity (although the limits of detection are well above those for g.c. $-$m.s.) and yield molecular weight information.

4. SAMPLE PREPARATION

The extraction and purification of eicosanoids from biological fluids and tissue homogenates has been discussed in Chapters 4 and 6. Here, we shall describe methods which are routinely used in combination with g.c. $-$m.s. and some general considerations when adapting other sample preparations for g.c. $-$m.s. analysis.

4.1 **General precautions**

Because of the low concentrations of eicosanoids often present in biological samples, extensive purification procedures may be required before g.c. $-$m.s. analysis. It is very important to avoid exacerbating the situation by introducing contaminants from solvents, reagents and apparatus during sample processing. Such contaminants may cause assay problems by interfering with the efficiency of one or more of the required derivatization steps (see Section 4.6) or they may prevent measurement by appearing as artefactual peaks during analysis. Contaminants may blank out the signal by suppressing ionization within the source of the mass spectrometer. Some of the most important basic considerations are detailed in *Table 1*.

Eicosanoids are chemically labile compounds and are susceptible to degradation. As a general rule, the pH of samples should not exceed the limits of $3-10$. For the E and D series of prostaglandins, the limits should be $4-8$ since they readily undergo isomerization and dehydration. The majority of mammalian A-series prostaglandins identified during the early years of research are in fact artefacts derived from the degradation of the E series of prostaglandins.

Table 1. Prevention of sample contamination during processing.

1.	Solvents and reagents must be of analytical grade.
2.	Re-distill all solvents before use.
3.	Distilled water may contain organic contaminants. Water which has been purified using a Milli-Q type system, which incorporates a carbon filter, is preferable.
4.	Use disposable vials, syringes, pipettes, etc. wherever possible to avoid cross-contamination of samples.
5.	Do not expose organic solutions to plastic surfaces. Plasticizers may leach out and interfere with the efficiency of subsequent derivatization steps and may produce interfering peaks on g.c. – m.s. analysis.

High temperatures can have a marked effect on eicosanoid recovery and samples should not be heated to greater than 30°C. There is always a temptation to speed up solvent evaporation by heating samples but caution should be exercised. In our laboratories, we have found that solvents can be removed in a water bath set at 30°C under a stream of nitrogen in a relatively short time. However, once dry, samples should not be allowed to stand at this temperature. Our experiences with vortex evaporators which remove solvents under reduced pressure are not favourable. Bumping tends to cause sample losses and cross-contamination.

4.2 Sample extraction

Sub-nanogram quantities of various eicosanoids can be extracted from most biological systems. Samples are acidified to pH 3 – 4 to suppress ionization of the carboxyl group and increase lipophilicity. For conventional organic extraction, the solvent of choice is usually ethyl acetate but this method has been replaced in many laboratories by liquid chromatography using proprietary products such as μBondapak C_{18} Sep-Paks (Waters Associates, Harrow, UK) and Bond-Elut columns (Jones Chromatography Ltd., Llanbradach, UK). These are disposable mini columns containing a bonded reverse phase silica sorbent. The biological fluid is applied to these columns after acidification to pH 3. The columns are washed with water, water/methanol (90/10) or other suitable solvent mixtures to remove salts and polar components. Eicosanoids can then be eluted with an organic solvent such as ethyl acetate. By varying the polarity of the washing solvent, some separation can be achieved between eicosanoids of differing polarity (e.g. the HETEs and peptidoleukotrienes).

Occasionally, it is possible to exploit a unique property of a given eicosanoid during extraction to obtain a pure sample. A good example of this is the method described by Oates and colleagues for the quantitative analysis of 2,3-dinor-6-oxo-PGF$_{1\alpha}$, a urinary metabolite of prostacyclin (1). Selective purification of this metabolite takes advantage of the fact that this PG can exist in several isomeric forms depending upon pH conditions. The ketone form of the free acid is in equilibrium with a hemiketal where the hydroxyl and carbonyl groups are in a configuration favourable for the formation of a γ-lactone (*Figure 3*). 2,3-Dinor-6-oxo-PGF$_{1\alpha}$ exists as the lactone at acid pH and can be extracted with organic solvents. However, it is sufficiently stable to resist hydrolysis to the free acid during extraction of the organic solvent with mild aqueous base. This property allows inclusion of an extraction step, which can remove many fatty acid contaminants. If the lactone is dissolved and allowed to stand in base, hydrolysis to the free acid will occur and the dinor compound will behave as a conven-

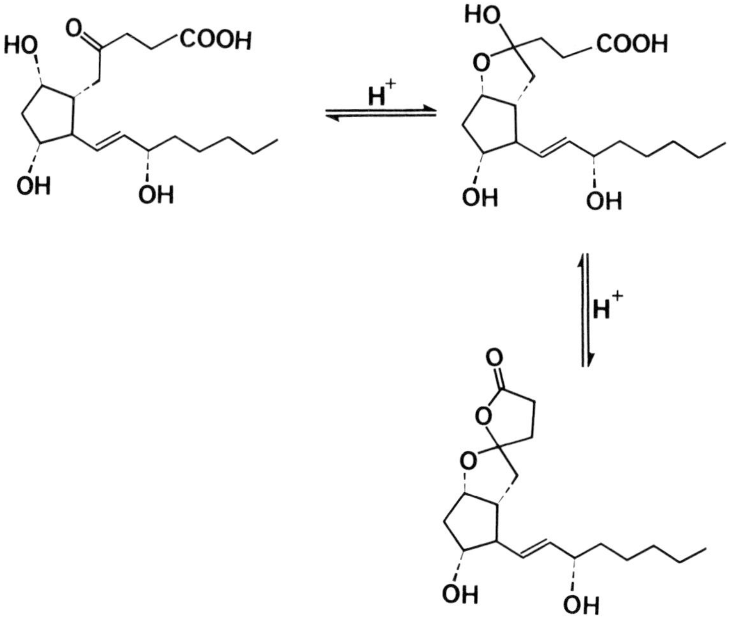

HO · COOH

H⁺

HO · COOH

H⁺

Figure 3. Equilibrium between the ketone form and γ lactone of 2,3-dinor-6-oxo-PGF$_{1\alpha}$. The lactone is favoured at acid pH.

Table 2. Selective extraction of 2,3-dinor-6-oxo-PGF$_{1\alpha}$.

1.	Add internal standard to a 5 ml sample of urine.
2.	Adjust to pH >8 and stand at ambient temperature for 15 min.
3.	Acidify to pH 3.
4.	Apply to a Clin Elut column and elute with 2 × 20 ml of dichloromethane.
5.	Wash organic extract with 0.05 M sodium borate buffer at pH 8.
6.	Evaporate the organic phase to dryness under a stream of nitrogen.
7.	Add 50 μl of pyridine and then 1 ml of 0.05 M sodium borate buffer at pH 8 to the residue. Stand at ambient temperature for 15 min.
8.	Wash with 2 × 10 ml of ethyl acetate.
9.	Acidify the aqueous layer to pH 3 and extract with 2 × 4 ml of dichloromethane.
10.	Wash organic extract with 1 ml of water and evaporate to dryness under a stream of N$_2$.
11.	Add 40 μl of pyridine/water/triethylamine (10/10/1; by vol.) to the residue and stand at ambient temperature for 1 h.
12.	Evaporate to dryness under a stream of N$_2$.
13.	Purify by t.l.c. and derivatize as the methyloxime, pentafluorobenzyl ester, trimethylsilyl ether derivative as described in Section 4.6 and *Table 4*.

tional acid. These steps can be combined to give a highly selective purification of 2,3-dinor-6-oxo-PGF$_{1\alpha}$ from urine (*Table 2*).

4.3 Sample purification

Some form of chromatographic separation is usually required before most biological extracts can be assayed by g.c. −m.s. Relatively clean biological extracts derived from

Gas chromatography and mass spectrometry of eicosanoids

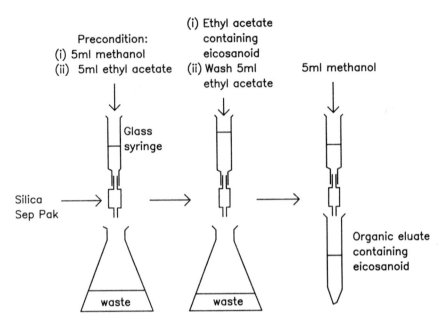

Figure 4. Clean up of organic solutions containing prostaglandins and thromboxanes (not suitable for leukotrienes or HETES). Eicosanoids contained in ethyl acetate or other relatively non-polar solvent are applied to a silica Sep-Pak. They are washed with the same solvent and eicosanoids are eluted with a more polar solvent such as methanol (5 ml).

sources *in vitro* (e.g. cell incubation medium or buffer solutions which have been used to perfuse isolated organs) can be purified using silica Sep-Paks (*Figure 4*). Otherwise, the most common chromatographic procedures in current use are t.l.c. and h.p.l.c. Other open column chromatographic procedures such as silicic acid, Sephadex gel and ion-exchange resins are used less frequently but can be successfully used in combination with g.c. −m.s.

H.p.l.c. provides the greatest degree of resolution but is time consuming when assaying large numbers of samples. Details of h.p.l.c. procedures have been described in Chapter 6. These methods can be incorporated into any work-up procedure for g.c. −m.s. analysis provided that salt-free buffers or non-buffered solvent systems are employed. Salt residues can interfere with analysis either by physical exclusion or by interference with derivatization.

T.l.c. is a popular method of purification primarily because of its wide range of applicability, ease of operation and suitability to handling large numbers of samples (*Figure 5*). ^{3}H-Labelled eicosanoids can be used to locate bands on t.l.c. plates either by direct radiochromatogram scanning or by scraping bands and counting the silica directly by liquid scintillation counting. Purification of some eicosanoids by t.l.c. is complicated by rearrangements taking place on the silica. For example, 6-oxo-PGF$_{1\alpha}$, a stable hydrolysis product of PGI$_2$, can exist in the form of a hemi-ketal (*Figure 6*). Partial conversion to the isomeric form on silica results in chromatography as a poorly defined wide band (2). To prevent isomerization, we routinely convert 6-oxo-PGF$_{1\alpha}$ to an O-methyloxime derivative (Section 4.6) before t.l.c. It is advisable to chromatograph

Silica multi—channel
t.l.c. plate

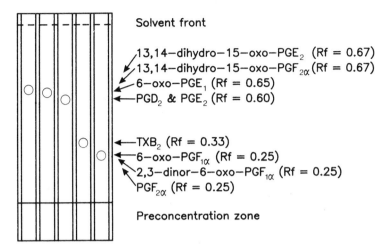

Solvent front

13,14—dihydro—15—oxo—PGE$_2$ (Rf = 0.67)
13,14—dihydro—15—oxo—PGF$_{2\alpha}$(Rf = 0.67)
6—oxo—PGE$_1$ (Rf = 0.65)
PGD$_2$ & PGE$_2$ (Rf = 0.60)

TXB$_2$ (Rf = 0.33)
6—oxo—PGF$_{1\alpha}$ (Rf = 0.25)
2,3—dinor—6—oxo—PGF$_{1\alpha}$ (Rf = 0.25)
PGF$_{2\alpha}$ (Rf = 0.25)

Preconcentration zone

Figure 5. Thin-layer chromatography of prostaglandin and thromboxane methyloxime derivatives. Samples are applied to the pre-concentration zone of a silica t.l.c. plate and are developed in the organic phase separated from a mixture of ethyl acetate:acetic acid:hexane:water (54:12:25:60). Radiolabelled eicosanoids are run as chromatographic markers in a separate channel on the plate. Eicosanoids can be eluted from the silica with methanol.

Figure 6. Hemiketal-ketone isomerization of 6-oxo-PGF$_{1\alpha}$. Formation of the methoxylamine derivative drives the reaction over to the ketone form.

all D- and E-series PGs as O-methyloxime derivatives to prevent isomerization of the 13,14-double bond into more favourable conjugated positions.

Selective purification of many eicosanoid extracts can be achieved by t.l.c. as esters in addition to the free acids (see Section 4.6 on derivatization). Leukotriene (LT) B$_4$, isolated from ionophore-stimulated serum, is purified firstly by t.l.c. of the free acid and then by further t.l.c. of the pentafluorobenzyl ester to remove other interfering eicosatetraenoic acids (3).

4.4 Use of stable isotope internal standards

For quantitative analysis, stable isotope analogue internal standards are added to bio-logical samples immediately following collection. Such compounds have physical pro-

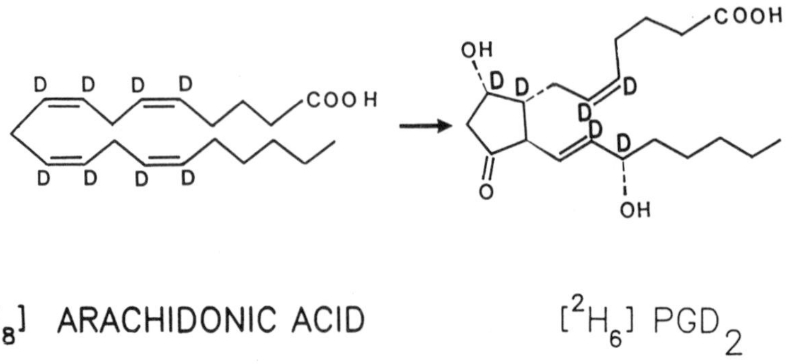

[^{2}H$_8$] ARACHIDONIC ACID [^{2}H$_6$] PGD$_2$

Figure 7. Conversion of [^{2}H$_8$]arachidonic acid to [^{2}H$_6$]PGD$_2$.

perties almost identical to the natural isomers and recovery through extraction, purification and derivatization procedures are the same for both standard and eicosanoid to be measured. The ratio between the internal standard and the eicosanoid of interest can be measured by m.s. By knowing the amount of standard added initially, one can calculate the amount of unlabelled compound present. The isotopic compounds are added in excess of the eicosanoids to be measured and act as carriers through often extensive purification procedures. They compete for active sites which would otherwise completely adsorb very small quantitites of eicosanoids to be measured. This method was poineered by Axen at the Upjohn Company (Kalamazoo, USA) and Hamberg and Samuelsson at the Karolinska Institute (Sweden).

The most commonly used stable isotope is deuterium but ^{18}O has been used on some occasions. The isotope must be incorporated into the eicosanoid in non-labile positions. Many deuterium-labelled 3,3,4,4-[^{2}H$_4$]PGs and thromboxanes (TXs) have been synthesized by the Upjohn Company and have been generously supplied to many laboratories involved in g.c.−m.s. analysis. At the present time, these deuterated standards are not commercially available but [^{2}H$_8$]arachidonic acid can be readily synthesized by catalytic reduction of eicosatetraynoic acid with deuterium gas (4). This provides a starting material for the synthesis and biosynthesis of many deuterated metabolites. Many of these procedures have been documented in the literature (5−7).

The deuterated arachidonic acid synthesized by catalytic addition of deuterium across the alkyne bonds does not yield exclusively [5,6,8,9,11,12,14,15 ^{2}H$_8$]arachidonic acid. The product will always consist of a polytopic mixture where deuteration is incomplete and where a certain degree of isotopic scrambling has taken place during preparation. Complete deuteration at all eight positions is not critical for use as a precursor provided that no [^{2}H]arachidonic acid is present.

We have prepared deuterated PGD$_2$ by incubation of rat peritoneal mast cells with deuterated arachidonic acid (*Figure 7*) (8). In our study the starting material consisted of a mixture of 1% [^{2}H$_{11}$], 3% [^{2}H$_{10}$], 6% [^{2}H$_9$], 65% [^{2}H$_8$], 22% [^{2}H$_7$] and 3% [^{2}H$_6$]. Deuterated PGD$_2$ was prepared from this mixture with a conversion of approximately 20% (equivalent to ~4 µg per 10^6 cells). After removal of labile deuteriums at C-12 by acid-catalysed enolization, the PGD$_2$ consisted of a mixture of 1% [^{2}H$_9$], 3% [^{2}H$_8$], 35% [^{2}H$_7$], 48% [^{2}H$_6$], 11% [^{2}H$_5$] and 2% [^{2}H$_4$]. The major isotope, [^{2}H$_6$]PGD$_2$, was

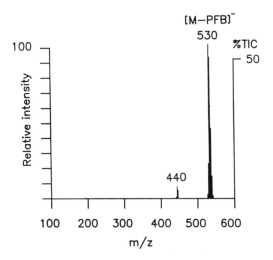

Figure 8. The electron capture mass spectrum of the methyloxime-methyl ester, bis-trimethylsilyl ether derivative of deuterated PGD_2.

used as internal standard without any need for separation from the mxiture. No ($<0.1\%$) non-deuterated PGD_2 was present in the standard (*Figure 8*).

It is critically important to have deuterated standards of high purity where the amount of non-deuterated material is very low ($<0.1\%$). Methods based on h.p.l.c. have been described for the separation of deuterated and non-deuterated PGs and TXs (9). The limitation on the amount of deuterated standard to be used in any given assay is determined by the contribution of non-deuterated material from the internal standard. We have found in practice that a minimum of 2 ng per sample is required as an effective carrier. If this standard contains 0.1% non-deuterated material, a detection limit for this assay must be at least twice this contribution (i.e. 2 pg).

The internal standard must be added in excess of the amount of compound to be measured to minimize the contribution of natural isotope peaks at $M+1$, $M+2$ and $M+3$, etc. into the measurement. If the internal standard has a mass of 4 or more greater than the natural isomer, this contribution will be negligible.

4.5 Estimation of efficiency of extraction and purification

During assay development, recovery can be monitored using ^{3}H-labelled eicosanoids. Many of these compounds are available commercially (NEN Research Products, Stevenage, UK; Amersham International plc, Amersham, UK). In instances where they are not, the methods outlined in Section 4.4 for the preparation of stable isotopes are equally applicable to ^{3}H-labelling.

Each step of an extraction and subsequent purification can be checked quickly for recovery using liquid scintillation counting, but it is important to remember that the ^{3}H label may be carried by degraded products of the eicosanoid in addition to the parent compound. Any ^{3}H-labelled recovery study should be confirmed by g.c. — m.s. when the full work-up procedure has been finalized. This is done by extracting and purifying a known amount of an eicosanoid standard and by adding an equal amount

Table 3. Conditions for the preparation of suitable derivatives for g.c. and m.s. analysis.

Functional group	Derivative	Conditions
α-Amino	N-acetyl	1. Add one drop of water to the sample followed by 0.5 ml of methanol:acetic anhydride (3:1 v/v). After 5 min, remove the reagent under vacuum. If the reaction is continued for 1 h, lactone formation may occur with the peptidoleukotrienes.
		2. Dissolve the sample in 100 μl of pyridine:acetic anhydride (1:10 v/v) and leave to stand for 1–3 h at room temperature. Remove the reagent under vacuum. This reagent will also acetylate hydroxyl functions.
Hydroxyl	Trimethylsilyl ether	1. Dissolve the sample in 100 μl of BSTFA. Leave to stand overnight at room temperature. Remove excess reagent under a stream of nitrogen.
		2. Silylation may also be carried out at 60°C for 1 h. There is some danger of poor yield with low levels of material.
		3. Dissolve the sample in 100 μl of BSTFA:TMCS:pyridine (6:1:1 by vol.). Leave to stand for 30 min at room temperature and remove the reagents under vacuum. This results in more powerful silylation than with BSTFA alone.
	Butyldimethylsilyl ether	1. Add 100 μl of N-methyl-N-(t-butyldimethylsilyl)trifluoroacetamide. Leave to stand at room temperature for 18 h and remove the reagent under nitrogen.
	O-acetyl	1. Carry out with pyridine:acetic anhydride as for amino groups.
	Butyl boronate	1. Add 30 μl of a solution of n-butyl boronic acid in dry 2,2-dimethoxypropane (5 mg/ml). Stand at room temperature for 3 h and then at −20°C overnight. The derivative is highly sensitive to moisture. Assay without removal of solvent or reagent, or immediately following silylation of any remaining hydroxyl groups.

Carboxylic acid	Methyl ester	1. Dissolve the sample in 100 μl of methanol and add 0.5 ml of ethereal diazomethane solution (*Table 7*). After 30 min, remove the solvent and reagents with a stream of nitrogen. **CARE:** diazomethane is a potential explosive.
		2. Bubble dry hydrogen chloride gas through methanol for 30 sec. Allow the solution to cool to room temperature and add 100 μl to the dry sample. Leave to stand for 1 h at room temperature and remove the reagent under vacuum.
		3. Add one drop of Aristar grade hydrochloric acid to 30 drops of methanol. Add 100 μl of reagent to the dry sample and leave to stand for 20 min at room temperature. Remove the reagent under vacuum.
	Pentafluorobenzyl ester	1. Dissolve the sample in 30 μl of dry acetonitrile, add 5 μl of di-isopropylethylamine and 10 μl of a solution of pentafluorobenzyl chloride in acetonitrile (35% v/v). Leave to stand at room temperature for 40 min and remove reagents under nitrogen.
	3,5-Bis-(trifluoromethyl)benzyl	1. Carry out the reaction with 3,5-bis(trifluoromethyl)benzyl bromide under the same conditions for the PFB derivative (above).
Ketone, aldehyde	Methyloxime	1. Add 100 μl of a solution of methoxyamine hydrochloride in pyridine (5 mg/ml). Leave to stand overnight at room temperature and remove the solvent with nitrogen. Note that methoxyl-amine hydrochloride is not volatile but can be removed using Sephadex LH-20 (see *Table 6*).
		2. Methoxymation may also be undertaken at 60°C for 1 h. The *syn-anti* isomer ratio may be different.
		3. For samples in simple biological matrices, methoxymation may be carried out in aqueous solution. An equal volume of aqueous methoxylamine hydrochloride (5 mg/ml) in acetate buffer at pH 5 is added to the biological fluid and heated at 60°C for 10 min. The solution is then acidified to pH 3 and extracted using a μBondapak C_{18} Sep-Pak.

Unless otherwise stated, all the reagents are volatile.

of deuterated material immediately before derivatization and g.c. −m.s. analysis. The ratio between the protium and deuterium forms provides a measure of percentage recovery.

[3]H-Labelled eicosanoids can be added to samples as chromatographic markers in routine assays provided that they are of sufficiently high specific activity and do not contribute significantly to the measurement of the endogenous eicosanoids of interest.

4.6 **Derivatization**

Before eicosanoids can be successfully subjected to g.c., or analysed by m.s., the polar functional groups within the molecule (amino, carboxylic acid, hydroxyl and any ketone) must be converted to less polar derivatives. This reduces intermolecular hydrogen bonding and results in more volatile species. Different derivatives will also affect the direction of mass spectrometric fragmentation (see later). By using isotopically labelled derivatizing reagents, stable isotopes can be incorporated into the molecule which facilitate identification and structural analysis. This is considered in detail in Section 6. The different derivatives used for g.c. −m.s. of eicosanoids are described in detail in the following sections. Reaction conditions are summarized in *Table 3*.

4.6.1 *Amino groups*

The N-acetyl derivative can be prepared by a short acetylation method of Morris and colleagues (10) using a mixture of methanol:acetic anhydride (3:1; v/v) for 5 min. This reagent, widely used for peptide studies, only acetylates primary amino groups; hydroxyl functions are not affected (cf. pyridine:acetic anhydride mixtures which will derivatize most nucleophilic functional groups). Only the primary α-amino function of amino acids are fully acetylated in this time, whereas other amino groups (the ξ-NH$_2$ of lysine for example) are only fully blocked after 3 h.

4.6.2 *Carboxylic acids — methyl esters*

These are easily prepared in high yield using diazomethane. The product is relatively stable. The disadvantages of this method are that the reagent is highly toxic, potential-

Table 4. Preparation of diazomethane.

1.	Prepare diazomethane only in specially designed[a] smooth glass joint apparatus available from companies such as Aldrich Chemical Co., Gillingham, UK.
2.	Carry out the reaction in a fume cupboard behind a protective screen[a].
3.	Dissolve 5 g of KOH in 8 ml of water and 25 ml of ethanol. Place in a flask equipped with a dropping funnel and distillation apparatus.
4.	Heat the solution to 65°C in a water bath.
5.	Add 21.5 g (0.1 mol) of Diazald (N-methyl-N-nitroso-p-toluenesulphonamide; Aldrich) in 200 ml diethyl ether from the dropping funnel over a period of about 25 min.
6.	Distill the ethereal diazomethane at a rate approximately equal to the rate of reagent addition.
7.	Cool the collection flask in an ice/KCl bath.
8.	After addition of the Diazald solution, add 40 ml of diethyl ether dropwise to the reaction flask and continue distillation until the condensate is colourless.
9.	The ethereal/alcoholic distillate usually contains about 3 g of diazomethane.
10.	Use approximately 0.5 ml of this solution for esterification of eicosanoid samples (see Section 4.6 and *Table 4*).

[a]**IMPORTANT!** These reactions are potentially hazardous.

ly explosive and has to be freshly prepared and distilled before use (*Table 4*). Aldrich Chemical Company (Gillingham, UK) provide a kit to be used exclusively for the preparation of diazomethane which minimizes the hazards associated with this preparation. Diazomethane will only attack acid functional groups. Hydroxyl groups are normally unaffected. However, in the presence of boron trifluoride as a catalyst, phenolic hydroxyl groups will undergo *O*-methylation. Side reactions (including insertion of CH_2 and ring expansion) are common with this reagent. This can lead to reduced yield in some cases, and problems with the interpretation of mass spectra. Other diazoalkanes may be prepared to generate higher esters. Esterification may also be undertaken with an alcoholic solution of hydrogen chloride or hydrochloric acid.

4.6.3 *Carboxylic acids — polyfluorinated benzyl esters*

These esters are prepared for electron capture n.i.c.i.m.s. where there is a need to incorporate an electron capturing substituent into the molecule (see Section 6.4.1). These derivatives can be prepared under mild conditions but the esterifying reagents are lachrymators and should be handled only in an efficient fume cupboard. The most commonly used reagent is pentafluorobenzyl bromide (Fluorochem, Glossop, UK) but recently, we have changed to using 3,5-bis(trifluoromethyl)benzyl bromide (Fluka AG, Buchs, Switzerland) because of difficulty in obtaining consistently pure batches of the former. These esters have good g.c. characteristics and are relatively stable.

4.6.4 *Ketones*

Ketones, present in a variety of PGs are generally converted to *O*-alkyl oxime derivatives, the most common one being *O*-methyl oxime. The disadvantage with this is that *syn* and *anti* isomers are produced which are often not fully resolved even using capillary g.c. columns. Either full separation must be achieved or column programming conditions should be adjusted so that the signal is contained in a single well-defined Gaussian peak. For PGs E_2 and D_2, the *syn* and *anti* isomers are fully resolved under normal g.c. operating conditions and we have noted that the ratio of isomers produced varies with the derivatization reaction conditions. When samples are allowed to stand overnight at ambient temperature, the major proportion of the signal is concentrated in the isomer eluting second. The reverse is the case when samples are heated. The first methyloxime isomers of PGs D_2 and E_2 co-chromatograph on capillary g.c. It is advisable to prepare derivatives overnight at ambient temperature and monitor the more specific second eluting isomer of each PG (see *Figure 24*). Other alkyl oximes have been used to derivatize PGs and thromboxanes (TXs) in an attempt to modify the separation of *syn* and *anti* isomers or for detection of alternative fragment ions when there are problems with peak interference from contaminants. Excess methoximating reagent, present in samples, causes rapid deterioration of capillary g.c. columns. It is necessary to remove this reagent before analysis and we have found that the most appropriate method is to chromatograph the derivative (after esterification) on a short column of Sephadex LH-20 (*Table 5*).

4.6.5 *Hydroxyl groups*

(i) *Silylation*. Hydroxyl functions are normally converted to *O*-silyl ether derivatives. The trimethylsilyl (TMS) ether and the higher homologue, tert-butyl bis-(dimethylsilyl)

Table 5. Sample clean-up using Sephadex LH-20.

1.	Swell Sephadex LH-20 in dichloromethane.
2.	Dissolve the methyloxime, ester derivative in approximately 500 μl of dichloromethane.
3.	Prepare the Sephadex column by placing a small plug of cotton wool at the bottom of a short Pasteur pipette. Add about 2 ml of Sephadex slurry and wash down the sides of column with a few drops of dichloromethane.
4.	Add the solution containing the eicosanoids and washings. Elute with 2 ml of dichloromethane. Collect all the eluate.
5.	Evaporate to dryness under a N_2 stream.
6.	Complete derivatization by adding silylating reagent (see Section 4.6 and *Table 3*).

(BDMS) ether are used most frequently. Bis-(trimethylsilyl) trifluoroacetamide [BSTFA; Pierce & Warriner (UK) Ltd., Chester, UK] is normally employed for trimethylsilylation, either on its own, or in the presence of a non-hydroxylic solvent such as acetonitrile of pyridine. BSTFA generates volatile by-products, and is sufficiently powerful to silylate most hydroxyl functions present in the eicosanoids without the need for an acid catalyst. BSTFA has superceded earlier reagents such as bis-(trimethylsilyl)acetamide and hexamethyldisilazane-trimethylchlorosilane mixtures. Powerful trimethylsilylating reagents such as TMS-imidazole, are not normally required for eicosanoid derivatization, and indeed, suffer the drawback of involatility. They are immensely useful for hindered hydroxyl groups as are found in steroids. The trimethylsilylation reaction is normally carried out at 60°C for 1 h, or at room temperature overnight. It is good practice to carry out these reactions under nitrogen, to minimize oxidation which will reduce yield. The most useful reagent for preparation of BDMS derivatives is *N*-methyl-*N*-(tert butyl-dimethylsilyl) trifluoroacetamide [MTBSTFA; Pierce & Warriner (UK) Ltd.]. This is a relatively new derivatization reagent. It is volatile and as such, should be used in preference to the Corey and Venkateswarlu formulation known as tert-butyl dimethylsilyl chloride/dimethyl formamide/imidazole.

Alkylsilyl ether derivatives have good g.c. properties. They shield the oxygen atom and have poor electron donating properties which means that they do not readily adsorb onto g.c. stationary phases. TMS ethers must be stored under anhydrous conditions as they are readily hydrolysed whereas BDMS ethers are stable and can be stored without any special precautions.

BDMS derivatives are sometimes chosen in preference to TMS derivatives because they provide more intense high molecular weight fragment ions using e.i.m.s. which are useful both for quantification and for structure elucidation. One disadvantage of the higher homologues is that they are bulky, and derivatization of sterically hindered hydroxyl groups may be difficult. Also, they may have unacceptably long g.c. retention times and assays of large sample numbers may be very time consuming.

The eicosanoid carboxylic acid can be converted to a TMS or BDMS ester at the same time as silylation of hydroxyl functions. This saves time and eliminates one derivatization step but the TMS ester derivative is extremely water labile (much more so than the *O*-TMS ether) and is used infrequently. BDMS esters are however stable to hydrolysis.

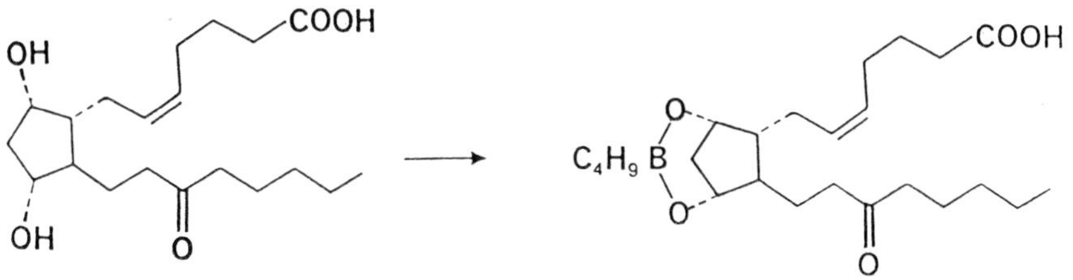

Figure 9. The butylboronate derivative of $PGF_{2\alpha}$. The *trans* epimer cannot form this derivative.

(ii) *O-Acetylation.* Hydroxyl groups may also be converted to their *O*-acetyl derivatives using pyridine-acetic anhydride. The derivatives possess poorer g.c. characteristics compared with alkylsilyl derivatives and are generally not used for eicosanoids.

(iii) *Alkylboronation.* For the F series prostaglandins, where the ring hydroxyl groups are in the *cis* position, cyclic bornate derivatives can be used as alternatives for g.c. −m.s. These derivatives provide a means of determining the stereochemistry of the ring hydroxyls and have been used recently (11) to show that PGD_2 is reduced to a biologically active PGF metabolite with an $9\alpha,11\beta$ hydroxyl-configuration (*Figure 9*). The most commonly used alkyl boronate derivative is the *n*-butyl boronate. This is prepared by reaction with *n*-butyl boronic acid under anhydrous conditions.

4.6.6 *Order of reaction*

Derivatization is normally carried out in the following order: N-acetylation, methyloxime formation, esterification, alkylboronation and finally *O*-silyl ether formation. This order minimizes side reactions.

5. GAS CHROMATOGRAPHY OF EICOSANOIDS

For the purposes of mass spectrometric analysis, the eicosanoids fall into two categories, depending whether or not they are amenable (as suitable derivatives) to gas chromatography. Derivatized PGs, mono- and di-hydroxy eicosatetraenoic acids (HETEs and di-HETES) can be introduced into the mass spectrometer via g.c., but the peptidoleukotrienes (LTs C_4, D_4 and E_4) can only be analysed by direct probe analysis. However, these compounds have been analysed by g.c. −m.s. following cleavage of the peptide side-chain by Raney nickel hydrogenation, and analysis of the derivatized fatty acid residue generated (12).

Most investigators now routinely undertake g.c. with robust and inert fused silica capillary columns. Those suitable for eicosanoid analysis include SE-30, SE-54, SP2100, OV-1, OV-101 and Sil 5 which can be obtained from Chrompack UK Ltd. (London, UK), Jones Chromatography Ltd. (Llanbradach, UK), and from Phase Separations (Queensferry, UK). These columns can be operated at temperatures up to 325°C and are ideal for high molecular weight derivatives. Optimum resolution is generally achieved by temperature programming from between 100 and 200°C up to 325°C at a rate suitable for resolution of the compounds of interest.

In our laboratories, samples, once derivatized, are usually stored in a high boiling solvent such as *n*-dodecane (usually 10 μl). Samples (up to 3 μl) are injected onto the column using a Grob-type splitless injector. The high boiling solvent allows temperature programming to begin at 200°C at a rate of up to 20°C min^{-1}.

5.1 Identification by comparison of retention times

Great reliance is placed on the reproducibility of chromatographic separations. This is important for comparison of standard authentic eicosanoids with those of biological origin. However, the chromatography of an eicosanoid in a biological extract may differ slightly from the chromatography of a clean standard of the same compound. When a deuterated analogue has been incorporated with the sample of interest there is no problem in identification. Deuterated compounds have retention times $1-2$ sec shorter (in an approximately 10 min g.c. capillary run) than the natural analogues and this relative retention time will be constant and independent of sample origin. When a deuterated analogue is not available, a structurally similar compound [but not one which cannot be synthesized by the biological system studied (i.e. preferably another deuterated eicosanoid)] should be used as an internal standard to determine a relative retention time. For absolute confirmation of peak identity under these circumstances, it is essential that an injection of the sample of interest is made in combination with an appropriate amount of authentic standard to confirm co-chromatography. In addition, when an eicosanoid has been provisionally characterized, the retention time of one or more alternative derivatives should be compared with authentic standards.

6. MASS SPECTROMETRY OF EICOSANOIDS

The use of a mass spectrometer as a method of detecting derivatives as they are eluted from a gas chromatograph has proved to be a flexible, sensitive and a selective technique for the analysis of eicosanoids. Despite its relatively high cost and complexity, many laboratories use this method for routine measurements. The mass spectrometer provides a greater degree of specificity when compared with its closest rival the electron capture detector. In m.s., detection is based upon the fragmentation of molecules into characteristic ions which can be used for identification or for quantification.

Sensitivity is based upon the efficacy of ionization. At present, this efficiency is relatively poor and there is a great deal of scope for improvement in instrumentation in the future.

6.1 Preliminary structural studies

Mass spectrometric analysis is rarely undertaken on complete unknowns. Biochemical and/or pharmacological data on the impure sample will often be available. For example, the early work on the peptido-leukotrienes (or slow-reacting substances as they were known) indicated that they were lipoxygenase products of arachidonic acid. Biosynthesis of the biologically active material was potentiated by arachidonic acid, blocked by lipoxygenase inhibitors, but unaffected by aspirin. Further data pertinent to the structure were obtained by careful design of the purification procedure; (e.g. the approximate molecular weight was determined by gel filtration).

Table 6. Chemical inactivation experiments.

Inactivation of biological activity:	Structural inference: functional group(s) present:
1. Acetylation (methanol:acetic anhydride, 3:1 v/v, 5 min).	Primary α-amino.
2. Acetylation (pyridine:acetic anhydride, 1:10 v/v, 1 h).	Amino, hydroxyl.
3. Diazomethane treatment (30 min).	Carboxylic acid, activated hydroxyl.
4. Methanol:HCl treatment (1 h).	Carboxylic acid (reaction is slow with aromatic acids).
5. Catalytic hydrogenation (PtO_2/H_2).	Unsaturation (double, triple bonds). Aromatics are unaffected. Possible loss of sample on the catalyst.
6. Cyanogen bromide.	Thioether linkage.
7. Borohydride reduction.	Ketone, aldehyde, hydroperoxide.
8. Lithium aluminium hydride reduction.	Ester, carboxylic acid, lactone, amide.
9. Acid/base hydrolysis.	Ester, lactone, amide.
10. Enzyme treatment:	
Protease (e.g. trypsin, elastase).	Peptide.
Esterase, sulphatase, phosphatase.	Ester, sulphate, phosphate.
Glycosidase.	Carbohydrate.
Lipoxidase.	*Cis* 1,4 pentadiene.
11. Purification:	
Gel filtration.	Approximate mass.
Electrophoresis, ion-exchange chromatography.	Charge — anionic, cationic groups.
Solvent extraction from acid/base.	Polarity, charged groups (e.g. ether extraction at pH 3 shows the presence of a carboxylic acid).
H.p.l.c., u.v. detection at two wavelengths.	Polarity. Type of u.v. chromophore.

The action of specific chemical reagents on biological activity (or immuno activity) can be used to determine the presence of functional groups within a molecule. Only small amounts of impure material are required for these tests.

119

The use of chemical inactivation studies is also invaluable in the structural elucidation of unknowns. These may give an insight into which derivatives may be suitable for mass spectrometric examination. Here, the effect of various chemical reagents on the biological/immunological activity of an unknown are determined (*Table 6*). If a reagent, known to be specific for certain functional groups, leads to a marked reduction in biological activity, then it is likely, although not certain, that the unknown contains that functional group. For example, the presence of a carboxylic acid may be inferred if biological activity is destroyed by diazomethane treatment; similarly, borohydride inactivation indicates the presence of a ketone or hydroperoxide. Chemical inactivation may be applied to small quantitites of impure material, but suffers the drawback that unexpected side reactions may occur and result in inactivation.

6.2 Electron impact mass spectrometry

6.2.1 *Structure elucidation by e.i.m.s.*

The structural elucidation of many PGs, TXs and LTs has been dominated by the use of e.i.m.s. Structural features can be identified from the characteristic ions generated in this process and additional information can be obtained by using deuterated derivatizing reagents. The mass spectra of most compounds are unique in the combination and relative intensities of ions produced.

Methyl ester, TMS-ether derivatives were used to elucidate the structure of the mono-HETEs and many of the di-HETEs including LTB_4, a potent chemotactic agent (13 – 15). These derivatives elute from the g.c. column with invariant retention times

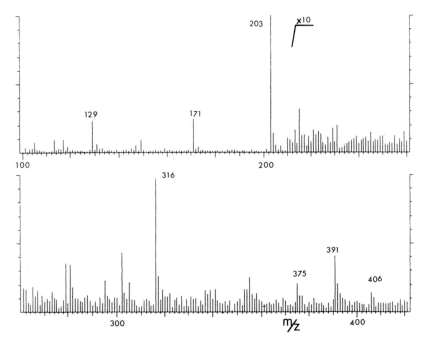

Figure 10. E.i. mass spectrum of 5-HETE as the methyl ester, *O*-trimethylsilyl ether. The ion at m/z 203 is characteristic of 5-hydroxy species.

as single peaks and generate mass spectra. The e.i. mass spectrum of the methyl ester-TMS ether of 5-HETE (*Figure 10*) shows a weak molecular ion ($M^{\cdot +}$) at m/z 406 with ions at m/z 391 ($M^{\cdot +} - CH_3^{\cdot}$) and 375 ($M^{\cdot +} - OCH_3^{\cdot}$) indicating the presence of a methyl ester; some of the ion current associated with m/z 391 also arises by loss of $CH_3^{\cdot}$ from the O-TMS moiety. Other structurally significant ions include m/z 316 (loss of TMSOH) and 203 cleavage at C5 to form TMSO $=$ $CH.CH_2.CH_2.CH_2.$ $COOCH_3^{+}$). Further structural information may be obtained by using isotopically labelled reagents. For example, if the $[^{2}H_3]$methyl ester were used, then the losses of 18 u and 34 u would be observed. Similarly, the $[^{2}H_9]$trimethylsilation would cause 9 u mass shifts for those ions containing the derivatized hydroxyl group. Non-enzymic hydrolysis of LTA_4 generates two pairs of diastereoisomers: 5-(S),6-(S),5-(R),6-(R) and 5-(S),12-(S),5-(S),12-(R) dihydroxyeicosatetraenoic acids with E,E,E,Z stereochemistry. The 5,6 and 5,12 pairs are separated by g.c., although the individual stereoisomers co-elute. LTB_4 [5-(S),12-(R)-dihydroxy (Z,E,E,Z) eicosatetraenoic acid] is only form-ed enzymically. LTB_4 separates from both the 5,6 and 5,12 isomers by g.c. The elec-tron impact mass spectrum of the methyl ester-TMS ether derivatives of 5-(S), 12-(R) (E,E,E,Z) di-HETE is shown in *Figure 11*. A molecular ion ($M^{\cdot +}$) at m/z 494 is pre-sent, with associated fragments at m/z 479 ($M^{\cdot +} - CH_3^{\cdot}$), 463 ($M^{\cdot +} - OCH_3^{\cdot}$), 404 ($M^{\cdot +} - TMSOH$), 383 ($M^{\cdot +} - CH_2(CH_2)_4CH_3$), 314 ($M^{\cdot +} - 2\times TMSOH$) and 203 (TMSO $= CH.CH_2.CH_2.CH_2.COOCH_3^{+}$). If LTA_4 is hydrolysed in the presence of methanol, the 12-O-methyl derivative is also produced. The g.c. profile of the diastereoisomeric mixture (as the methyl-TMS derivative) is shown in *Figure 12*. The

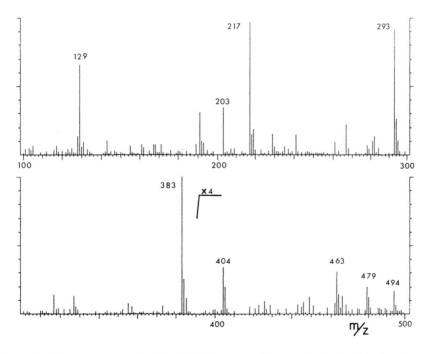

Figure 11. E.i. mass spectrum of a 5,12,di-HETE as the methyl ester, *O*-trimethylsilyl ether. The ion at m/z 203 is characteristic of 5-hydroxy species.

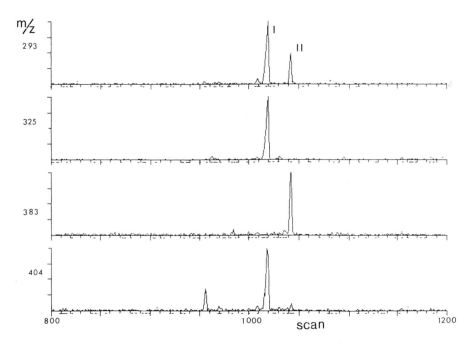

Figure 12. Gas chromatography – mass spectrometric profile of the methyl ester, TMS ether derivatives of 5,12-di-HETE (I) and 12-*O*-methyl-di-HETE (II) generated by treatment of leukotriene A_4 with aqueous methanol. Ions at m/z 293, 325, 383 and 404 were monitored, allowing ready differentiation of the two major species. Other species, including 5,6 di-HETEs are present in low amounts.

e.i. mass spectrum of 12-*O*-methyl di-HETE is shown in *Figure 13*. Ions are observed at m/z 436 ($M^{\cdot+}$), 421 (($M^{\cdot+}$ − $CH_3^{\cdot}$), 404 ($M^{\cdot+}$ − CH_3OH), 325 ($M^{\cdot+}$ − $CH_3(CH_2)_4CH = CHCH_2^{\cdot}$), 293 (325 − CH_3OH), 235 (325 − TMSOH), 203 (TMSO = $CH.CH_2.CH_2.CH_2.COOCH_3^{+}$) and 159 (TMS derived signal). The formation of this species allowed Samuelsson and Corey to deduce the structure of LTA_4. The 5,6 di-HETEs are readily differentiated from the 5,12 isomers by their e.i. mass spectra — the ion at m/z 291 is characteristic for these species (cleavage between C5 and C6). It can be seen that with molecular weight and fragmentation data available, structure can be readily determined. These data were obtained post-g.c., with any impurities (including those derived from the reagents) separated from the eicosanoid of interest. The equivalent probe spectrum of this derivative of, for example, a di-HETE is more complex, with reagent-derived by-products and impurities from the solvents used during purification. These impurities suppress the sample spectrum and account for an appreciable proportion of the ion current. This poses problems only for low microgram amounts of material.

The structure of LTD_4 was determined by direct probe mass spectrometric analysis (10). Only 5 μg of purified material was available. Chemical inactivation experiments, and other biochemical data indicated the presence of amino, hydroxyl and carboxylic acid functions (but no ketones). The sample was acetylated with equimolar acetic and [$^2H_3$]acetic anhydrides in methanol, esterified with diazomethane and trimethylsilylated with a mixture of BSTFA:TMCS:pyridine (6:1:1; by vol; *Table 3*). At the time of the

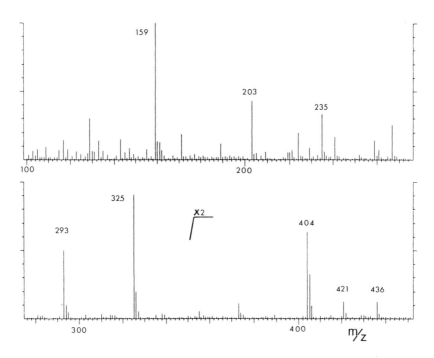

Figure 13. E.i. mass spectrum of 12-O-methyl di-HETE, generated by methanolysis of leukotriene A_4.

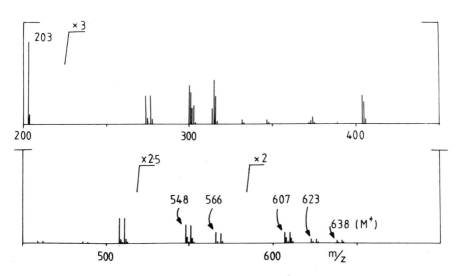

Figure 14. The pure mass spectrum of LTD_4 as the N-(1:1 acetyl:$^2H_3$-acetyl)-methyl ester, O-trimethylsilyl ether derivative. This may be obtained by subtracting background impurities or by analysis of larger amounts of synthetic material.

study, the structure of LTD_4 was unknown, so a powerful trimethylsilylating mixture was used to react with any hindered or unreactive groups present. The use of the isotope label was an important factor in identifying LT-derived ions since any amino group

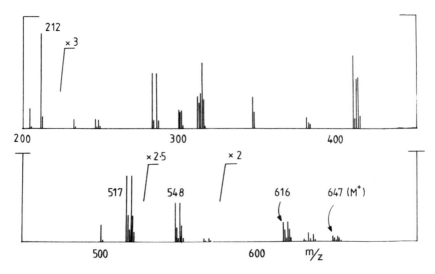

Figure 15. The e.i. mass spectrum of LTD_4 as the N-(1:1 acetyl:[$^2H_3$]acetyl)-methyl ester, *O* [$^2H_9$]trimethylsilyl ether derivative. Ions containing a trimethylsilyl moiety are shifted in mass by 9 u (i.e. the molecular ion is now m/z 647).

present will carry this label. For example, ions containing one acetylated amino group will appear as 1:1 doublets, 3 mass units apart and two such groups will form 1:3:1 triplets. The derivative was examined by probe e.i.m.s. using a temperature gradient approach. At 150°C, many of the reagent-derived impurities vapourized; it was not until 240°C that LT-derived signals were observed. These were clearly visible above the still intense background as 1:1 doublets, 3 mass units apart. By examining the mass spectra generated at each temperature, ions corresponding to impurities could be eliminated and the spectrum of the unknown obtained (*Figure 14*). Isotopic labelling clearly aids identification. The molecular ion of the derivative was identified as the 1:1 doublet at m/z 638/641 by the presence of ions at m/z 623/626 and 607/610 (corresponding to loss of CH_3^- and OCH_3^-, respectively from a methyl ester). Loss of TMSOH to form 548/551 indicated the presence of a derivatized hydroxyl group. The doublet at ion at m/z 566/569 arises from incomplete derivatization of the hydroxyl group. These are all doublets, showing that they contain the acetylated N terminus. Intense singlets were also observed at 203 and 405/404. These do not contain the N terminus. M/z 203 is an ion common to 5-hydroxy acids (e.g. 5-HETE), of structure $TMSO = CH.CH_2.CH_2.CH_2.COOCH_3^+$; 404/405 arise by loss of the peptide part of the molecule. When trimethylsilylation was carried out with [$^2H_9$]BSTFA, the mass spectrum shown in *Figure 15* is obtained. Ions containing the TMS moiety shift by 9 u (*Table 7*), facilitating structural analysis. There is one set of doublets at m/z 508/511 that do not arise by an obvious fragmentation pathway; the ion shifts to 517/520 on [$^2H_9$]trimethylsilylation. This fragment contains the N terminus (i.e. the peptide portion) and one derivatized hydroxyl group. High resolution mass spectrometric analysis (carried out on a magnetic sector instrument) gave a molecular formula of the ion as 508.279 allowing a plausible ion structure to be determined as $M^{\cdot+}$ − $HCO(CH_2)_3COOCH_3$, that is cleavage between C_5 and C_6, with transfer of a TMS

Table 7. Ions generated from the N-(1,1-acetyl-$^2H_3$-acetyl)-methyl ester-O-trimethylsilyl ether and the N-(1,1-acetyl-$^2H_3$-acetyl)-methyl ester-O-$^2H_9$-trimethylsilyl ether of leukotriene D_4.

Ion (m/z)		No. of TMS groups	N terminus	
[$^1H_9$]TMS	[$^2H_9$]TMS			
638 (d)	647	1	+	$M^{\cdot+}$
623 (d)	632	1	+	$M^{\cdot+} - CH_3^\cdot$
607 (d)	616	1	+	$M^{\cdot+} - OCH_3^\cdot$
566 (d)	566	0	+	$M - OH^{\cdot+}$
548 (d)	548	0	+	$M^{\cdot+} - TMSOH$
508 (d)	517	1	+	$M^{\cdot+} - HCO(CH_2)_3COOCH_3$
405 (s)	414	1	–	$M^{\cdot+} - SCH_2CHNHCOCH_3$
404 (s)	413	1	–	$(H)\ CONHCH_2COOCH_3$
315 (s)	315	0	–	$405 - TMSOH$
314 (s)	314	0	–	$404 - TMSOH$
203 (s)	212	1	–	$TMSO = CH(CH_2)_3COOCH_3^+$

Doublets (d) appear for ions containing the N terminus (labelled +); ions containing a trimethylsilyl group are shifted by 9 units.

group. This ion is characteristic for the peptidoleukotrienes, with the analogous fragment at m/z 451/454 observed in the mass spectrum of LTE$_4$.

6.2.2 *Quantification by e.i.m.s.*

Many studies have focussed on the development of g.c. −e.i.m.s. methods for the quantitative analysis of PGs, TXs, mono- and di-HETES (16). This is performed by monitoring selected ions unique to the mass spectrum of a given eicosanoid. The signal of this ion relative to that of an internal standard is a measure of the amount of eicosanoid present. It is not always possible to choose a unique ion as many compounds, including related eicosanoids, may produce potentially interfering ions. The majority of such ions can be effectively removed by rigorous purification, high resolution capillary column g.c. and by choice of high molecular weight ions. However, quantification using e.i.m.s. suffers from being relatively insensitive due to multiple fragmentation. For example, *Figure 16* illustrates the e.i. mass spectrum of the *O*-methyloxime, methyl ester, tris-TMS derivative of 6-oxo-PGF$_{1\alpha}$. The molecular ion (M$^{\cdot+}$) is present, but weak at m/z

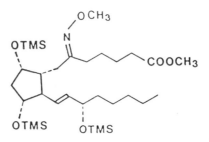

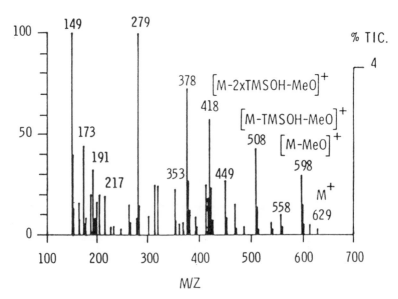

Figure 16. The e.i. mass spectrum of the *O*-methyloxime, methyl ester, tris-trimethylsilyl derivative of 6-oxo-PGF$_{1\alpha}$. The molecular ion is weak, and extensive fragmentation occurs.

629. The major ions correspond to fragments at m/z 598 ($M^{\cdot +}$ − OCH_3), 508 ($M^{\cdot +}$ − OCH_3 − TMSOH) and 418 ($M^{\cdot +}$ − OCH_3 − 2 × TMSOH). The intensity of any ion signal represents a relatively small proportion of the total ion current which limits the applicability of this method. Using s.i.m. techniques, the detection limit for this derivative of 6-oxo-$PGF_{1\alpha}$ is approximately 200 pg injected on column (signal:noise ratio of 3:1). Poor sensitivity can be overcome by extracting large volumes of biological fluid but this puts severe constraints on projects undertaken and has encouraged many investigators to resort to less specific but more sensitive methods such as RIA. Nevertheless, for laboratories which are not equipped for n.i.c.i.m.s. (the optimal method for quantification which will be discussed in the following section) g.c. −e.i.m.s. can be used for assays where relatively high eicosanoid concentrations are to be measured and when derivatives such as benzyl oximes and butyldimethylsilyl ethers are used to maximize the intensity of higher molecular weight fragment ions.

6.3 Chemical ionization mass spectrometry

C.i.m.s. is a softer ionization method than electron impact, resulting in minimal fragmentation. Positive ion chemical ionization (p.i.c.i.) is a relatively inefficient technique but can be used to obtain molecular weight data. For example, *Figure 17* shows the ammonia p.i.c.i. mass spectrum of the methyloxime, methyl ester, tris-TMS ether derivative of 6-oxo-$PGF_{1\alpha}$. The major fragment ion at m/z 540 corresponds to the protonated $[M+H]^+$ molecular ion from which the molecular weight of the derivative may be determined. Although the vast majority of the total ion current is contained in the protonated molecular ion, the efficiency of ionization is poor and the detection limit for this compound using s.i.m. procedures is 1.2 ng injected on column (eight times higher than obtained using e.i.m.s.).

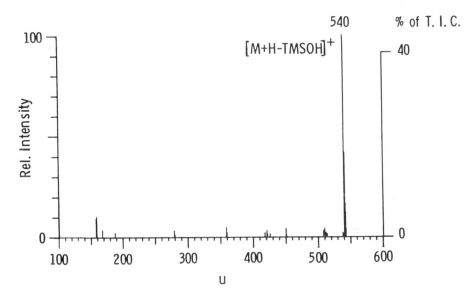

Figure 17. The positive ion chemical ionization mass spectrum of the methyloxime, methyl ester, tris-trimethylsilyl derivative of 6-oxo-$PGE_{1\alpha}$. There is little fragmentation but efficiency of ionization is poor.

6.4 Electron capture ionization

Eicosanoids are not naturally electron capturing substances, but all possess at least one terminal carboxyl group which can be esterified with a suitable electron capturing group. Thermal electron capture by the polyfluorinated benzyl esters is a highly efficient process. After initial electron capture to form the molecular anion $M^{\cdot -}$, a cleavage occurs in the gas phase with loss of the fluorinated benzyl radical leaving a stabilized carboxylate anion corresponding to the intact eicosanoid (*Figure 18*). This can be monitored by electron capture negative ion chemical ionization mass spectrometry (n.i.c.i.m.s.).

6.4.1 *Structural elucidation by electron capture n.i.c.i.m.s.*

In many cases, there is insufficient material to obtain definitive electron impact mass spectra for structure elucidation. The sensitivity of the electron capture method means that molecular weight information can readily be obtained on nanogram amounts of material. By using isotopically labelled derivatives, the number of functional groups present can be determined. This is illustrated by the identification of 6-oxo-PGE$_1$, a

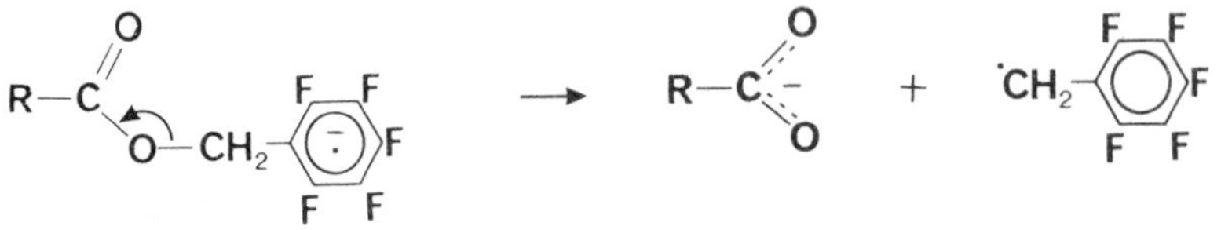

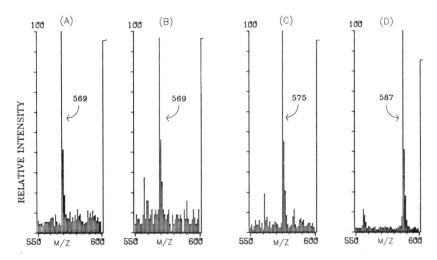

Figure 18. Formation of the eicosanoid anion $(M-PFB)^-$ from the pentafluorobenzyl ester under electron capture ionization.

Figure 19. Partial electron capture mass spectra (post-g.c.) of: **(a)** Rat lung 6-oxo-PGE$_1$ as the methyl oxime, pentafluorobenzyl ester, *O*-trimethylsilyl ether. The ion at m/z 569 corresponds to $(M-PFB)^-$. **(b)** Authentic 6-oxo-PGE$_1$ as the same derivative. **(c)** The ion at m/z 569 shifts to m/z 575 with the [$^2H_3$]methoxyamine derivative, showing the presence of two carbonyl functions. **(d)** The ion at m/z 569 shifts to m/z 587 with the [$^2H_9$]BSTFA derivative, showing the presence of two hydroxyl functions.

biologically active metabolite of PGI_2, in rat lung perfusates (18). The unknown was purified, and converted to the methyloxime PFB ester, bis-TMS ether (*Table 3*). The electron capture spectrum was obtained post-g.c., and showed an intense ion at m/z 569. This shifted to m/z 587 with deuterated silylating reagent, and to m/z 575 with deuterated methyloxime (*Figure 19*). This showed that the mass of the derivatized anion was 569, and it possessed two hydroxyl and two carbonyl functions. The g.c. retention times of the isomers were indistinguishable from those derived from authentic 6-oxo-PGE_1.

6.4.2 *Quantification by electron capture n.i.c.i.m.s.*

The sensitivity of quantitative analysis of eicosanoids can be improved by the use of electron capture mass spectrometry. This a highly efficient ionization process. For many eicosanoids, the carboxylate anion carries greater than 50% of the total ion current and limits of detection using s.i.m. techniques are in the range 200 fg−5 pg injected on column. Such detection limits are two orders of magnitude lower than possible using e.i.m.s. and it is not surprising that during the last 4 years g.c.−n.i.c.i.m.s. has been adopted as the method of choice for quantitative analysis by every leading laboratory involved in eicosanoid research.

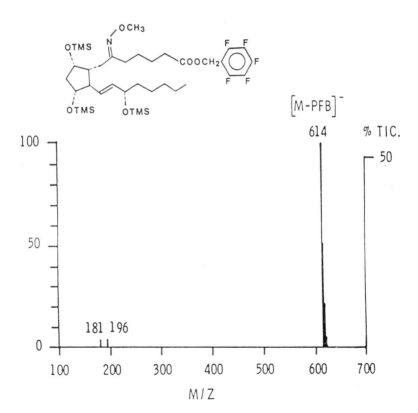

Figure 20. The electron capture mass spectrum of *O*-methyloxime, pentafluorobenzyl ester, tris-trimethylsilyl derivative of 6-oxo-$PGF_{1\alpha}$ showing the presence of an intense $(M-PFB)^-$ at m/z 618.

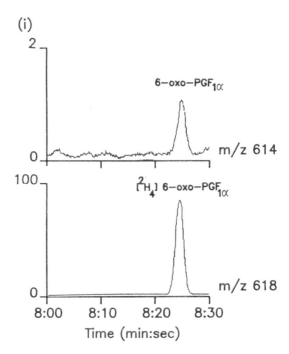

Figure 21. Representative selected ion monitoring chromatograms of the methyloxime, pentafluorobenzyl ester, tris-trimethylsilyl derivative of 6-oxo-PGF$_{1\alpha}$. The deuterated ion at m/z 618 represents addition of 2 ng of internal standard before extraction. The concentration of endogenous 6-oxo-PGF$_{1\alpha}$ is 2.4 pg/ml.

We used this method originally to quantify 6-oxo-PGF$_{1\alpha}$ in human plasma (18) to clarify the diverse range of values (up to 1 ng/ml) quoted in the literature. The n.i.c.i. mass spectrum of the methyl oxime, PFB ester, tris-TMS derivative of 6-oxo-PGF$_{1\alpha}$ is illustrated in *Figure 20*. This derivative elutes as a single peak on fused silica capillary columns (*Figure 21*). The mass spectrum consists of a single major fragment ion at m/z -614 corresponding to the $(M-PFB)^-$ ion. The structural integrity of the PG molecule is retained in this fragment providing optimum specificity. The internal standard, 3,3,4,4[^{2}H$_4$] derivative of 6-oxo-PGF$_{1\alpha}$ has an n.i.c.i. mass spectrum identical to the natural isomer but with the $(M-PFB)^-$ ion is four mass units higher. Endogenous concentrations of 6-oxo-PGF$_{1\alpha}$ can be quantified in plasma and in urine as well as in other biological fluids using this method. The concentration of 6-oxo-PGF$_{1\alpha}$ in the sample illustrated in *Figure 21* is 2.4 pg/ml. The normal range for human plasma 6-oxo-PGF$_{1\alpha}$ is <500 fg/ml-3 pg/ml which is considerably lower than had been previously estimated by bioassay and RIA.

The n.i.c.i.m.s. of the PFB ester, bis-TMS derivative of LTB$_4$ is illustrated in *Figure 22*. Two major fragment ions are produced which correspond to $(M-PFB)^-$ at m/z 479 and $(M-PFB - TMSOH)^-$ at m/z 389. Both these ions can be used to quantify LTB$_4$ but sensitivity is reduced compared with the PGs since the signal is divided between the two ions. However, specificity is significantly improved by the availability of two fragment ions and there is a trade off between specific and sensitivity. Under these circumstances, not only should the ratios of 479 and 389 to their deuterated

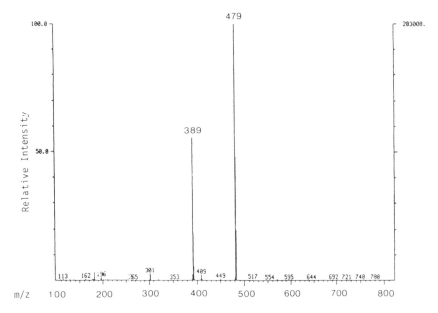

Figure 22. The electron capture mass spectrum of the pentafluorobenzyl ester, tris-trimethylsilyl derivative of LTB_4 showing the presence of an intense $(M-PFB)^-$ ion at m/z 479 and a fragment at m/z 389 $(M-TMSOH)^-$.

analogue ions be identical, the ratios of 479 and 389 and the equivalent deuterated ratio should remain constant. Any deviation from these parameters indicates the presence of an interfering contaminant. A further problem with di-HETE analysis arises from the large number of structural isomers. There are a number of possible isomers of LTB_4, including the naturally occurring 5,6 and 5,12 di-HETEs. They each form the same derivative (of identical mass) and specificity must therefore rely on chromatographic separation. This may cause problems, as the 5,6 di-HETEs, generated by non-enzymic hydrolysis of LTA_4 chromatographs on g.c. in the same region as LTB_4, leading to erroneous results. They can however be separated by h.p.l.c.

Many different eicosanoids can be assayed in a single sample and we have used this technique to measure 6-oxo-$PGF_{1\alpha}$ and 2,3-dinor-6-oxo-$PGF_{1\alpha}$ in human urine (*Figure 23*), to profile PG and TX production by activated platelets, to profile PG and LTB_4 production by human pulmonary macrophages, rat peritoneal mast cells, rat aortic rings and perfused sensitized guinea-pig lungs during anaphylaxis among many other systems (18−23). Many of these *in vitro* systems do not require extensive purification. A typical s.i.m. profile of primary PGs and TXB_2 derived from a single sample is illustrated in *Figure 24*. Each PG has a characteristic $(M-PFB)^-$ which has been exploited for s.i.m. The pairs 6-oxo-$PGF_{1\alpha}$ and TXB_2 and PGs E_2 and D_2 have common fragment ions but can be separated by the high resolution of the capillary column. Note that PGs E_2 and D_2 are separated into *syn* and *anti* oxime isomers. The first eluting isomer of each co-chromatograph but the second eluting isomers are resolved and can be used for quantification. In each case, deuterated internal standards are used; all standards carry four deuterium atoms with the exception of $[^2H_6]PGD_2$ prepared as described earlier.

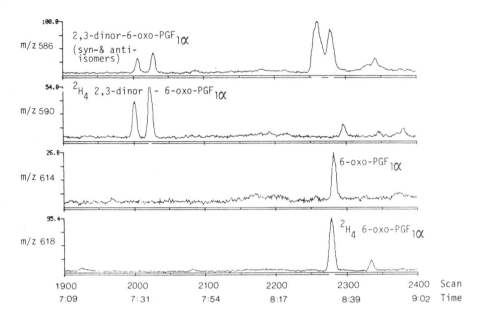

Figure 23. Representative selected ion chromatograms showing the simultaneous analysis of 2,3-dinor-6-oxo-PGF$_{1\alpha}$ and 6-oxo-PGF$_{1\alpha}$ derived from human urine.

(i) *Preparation of standard curves for quantification.* Standards should be prepared in a concentration range appropriate to the samples to be measured with a constant amount of internal standard identical to that in the samples to be measured. The lowest standard should be at the limit of detection of the assay (usually with a signal:noise ratio of at least 3:1) and the highest standard at a value greater than anticipated for the highest concentration to be assayed. Although calibration curves are linear over a wide range of values, it is not advisable to extrapolate beyond the upper limit of the curve prepared. Typical extracted calibration curves are illustrated in *Figure 25a* and *b* where the peak area ratio of protium- to deuterium-labelled PG is plotted against known weights of the PG. The curves are generated using a least squares linear regression analysis which provide gradient and intercept parameters which allow unknown levels of 6-oxo-PGF$_{1\alpha}$ to be determined.

A standard curve that has been extracted and purified through the same work-up procedure as unknown samples should be prepared with every assay.

(ii) *Precision and accuracy.* Accuracy and precision measurements must be checked before eicosanoid assays are set up on a routine basis. These should be performed by measuring known amounts of standards at the lowest end of the concentration range. They should be extracted and purified through a full work-up procedure. A minimum of five samples should be assayed together to provide intra-assay coefficient of variation. A minimum of five samples should be prepared on five separate occasions with five different calibration curves to provide an inter-assay coefficient of variation.

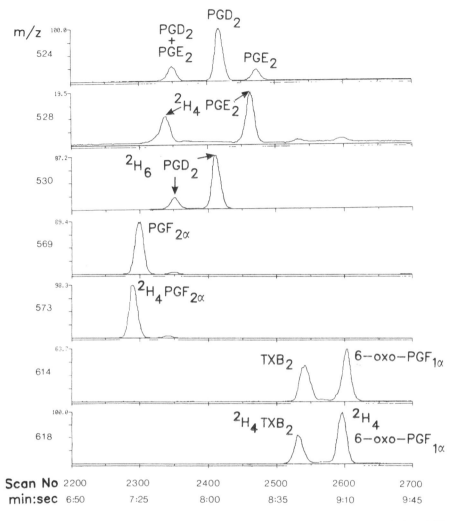

Figure 24. Representative selected ion chromatograms showing the simultaneous analysis of PGD_2, PGE_2, $PGF_{2\alpha}$, 6-oxo-$PGF_{1\alpha}$ and TXB_2.

6.5 Soft ionization

Soft ionization techniques such as d.c.i. and f.a.b. have been employed to determine the molecular weights of both underivatized PGs and LTs. The value of such techniques are best outlined by reference to the peptido-leukotrienes. During the structure elucidation of LTD_4, its molecular weight was inferred from the e.i. mass spectrum but this could not be considered definitive. Molecular ions are often not observed in e.i. mass spectra, and the ions at m/z 607/610, 623/626 and 638/641 may have arisen from breakdown of a much heavier species. However, under f.a.b. ionization, LTD_4

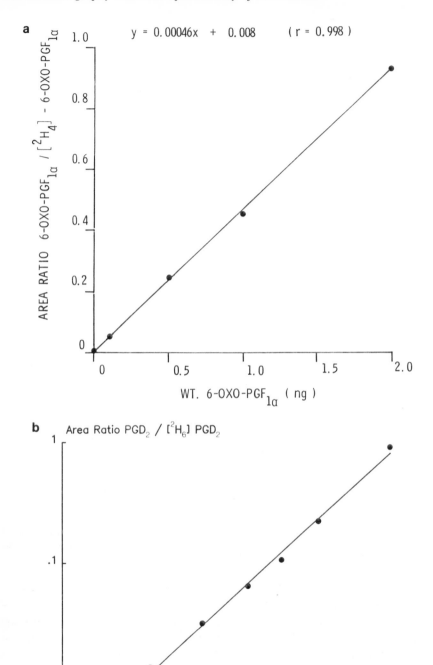

Figure 25. (a) A typical extracted calibration curve for the quantification of 6-oxo-PGF$_{1\alpha}$. **(b)** A typical extracted calibration curve for the quantification of PGD$_2$. When a wide range of values are to be measured, a better fit of the data is obtained using a log/linear plot.

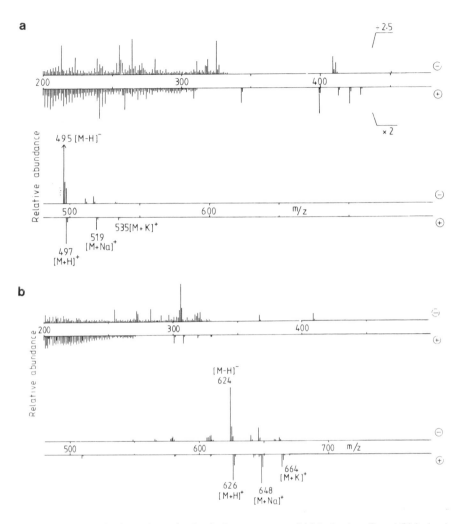

Figure 26. The positive ion and negative ion f.a.b. mass spectra of **(a)** leukotriene C_4 and **(b)** leukotriene D_4. Intense molecular ion species $(M+H^+, M-H^-)$ are observed with little fragmentation. Cationized species $(M+Na^+, R.COONa^-)$ are also observed.

and the other peptido-leukotrienes generate molecular ion species (e.g. $M+H^+$, $M-H^-$ at m/z 497, 495 for LTD_4 and 626, 624 for LTC_4) with little fragmentation (*Figure 26*) (25,26). Only $0.5-5$ µg are required to obtain convincing spectra. Although derivatization is not required, short acetylation in methanol (*Table 3*), especially with an equimolar mixture of acetic and [$^2H_3$]acetic anhydrides (see Section 6.2.1), can be valuable in defining the presence of a free N terminus in the molecule. Under these conditions LTs C_4 and D_4 acetylate to yield 1:1 doublet protonated molecular ion species $(M+H^+)$ at m/z 668/671 and 539/542 and deprotonated negative ions $(M-H^-)$ at 666/669 and 537/540, respectively. Interestingly, if the acetylation is allowed to continue for 30 min the *N*-acetyl lactone becomes the major product, with a small amount of the *N*-acetyl-monomethyl ester (*Figure 27a* and *b*). This behaviour

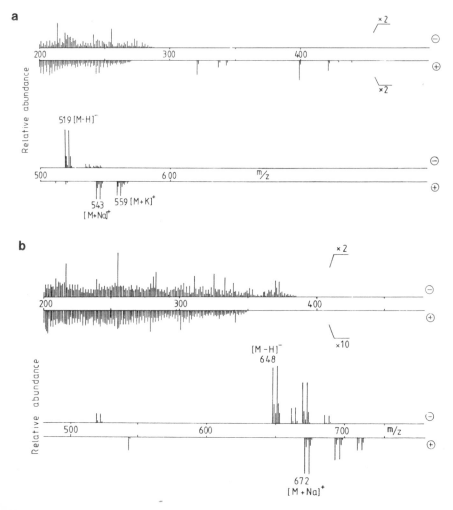

Figure 27. The f.a.b. mass spectra of **(a)** LTC_4 and **(b)** LTD_4 following acetylation in methanol:acetic anhydride:$[^2H_3]$acetic anhydride (6:1:1 by vol.) for 30 min showing the formation of a lactone. The lactone is not generated by short acetylation (5 min). Note also the use of isotopic labelling to facilitate identification.

was rationalized as occurring through a mixed anhydride between the reagent (acetic anhydride) and the lipid carboxylic acid. Once formed, internal nucleophilic attack of the 5-hydroxyl group eliminates acetate (a good leaving group) forming a stable 6-membered cyclic lactone. Methanol can also attack the mixed anhydride to generate the mono-methyl ester; this is less favoured on entropy grounds and the yield is consequently lower.

Interestingly, the prostaglandins generate only weak molecular ion species by both positive ion f.a.b. and d.c.i.; the major ions in the spectra correspond to loss of one or two molecules of water, which could lead to confusion during structural studies; deprotonated molecular ions are however observed in the negative ion spectra (*Figure 28*). Isotopic labelling can also be used to assist structural analysis (*Figure 29*). Fast

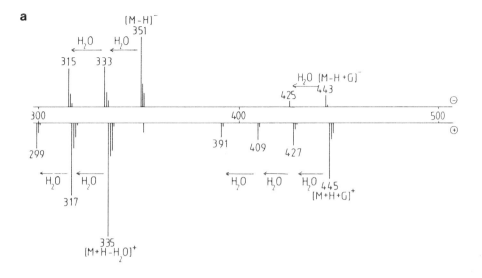

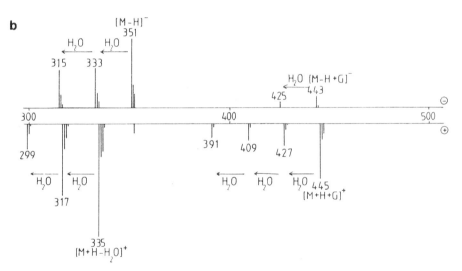

Figure 28. F.a.b. mass spectra for **(a)** PGD$_2$ and **(b)** PGE$_2$. Water loss is common with these species in the positive ion mode and the protonated molecular ion is not observed. The deprotonated molecular ion (M−H$^-$) is observed in the negative spectra. D.c.i. spectra of the prostanoids give similar results. Glycerol adducts (+G), 92 u higher than the molecular ion species, are common with f.a.b.m.s.

atom bombardment and d.c.i. mass spectra may be generated on approximately 1 μg of sample but the sample must however be of high purity (i.e. post-h.p.l.c.).

7. FUTURE TRENDS

Mass spectrometry is constantly evolving, such that analyses considered impossible 5 years ago are now commonplace. There are many developments in the pipeline that should prove extremely useful for eicosanoid analysis. Two such developments are the

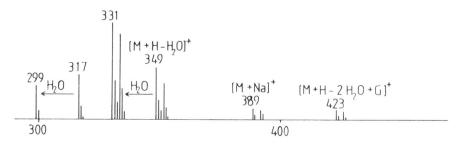

Figure 29. Isotopic labelling facilitates the identification of prostanoids by f.a.b.m.s. PGE_2 was esterified with methanol:$[^2H_3]$methanol:hydrogen chloride (0.4 M) for 30 min leading to the characteristic 1:1 doublets in the positive ion mass spectra. The 1:1 doublet at m/z 349/352 corresponds to $(M+H-H_2O)^+$. The lower energy cation $(M+Na)^+$ is present, together with a glycerol adduct of the dehydrated species.

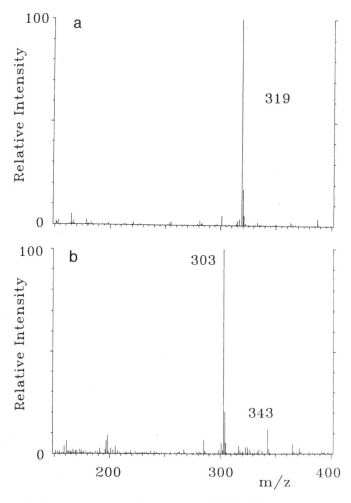

Figure 30. (a) Positive ion thermospray mass spectra of 5-HETE. The protonated molecular ion species readily loses water to generate the base peak at m/z 303. **(b)** Negative ion thermospray mass spectra of 5-HETE, with the deprotonated molecular ion species at m/z 319 as the base peak.

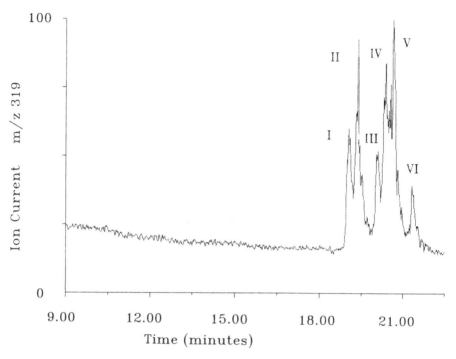

Figure 31. Thermospray l.c. – m.s. profile of six synthetic HETEs. HETEs were chromatographed on Nova Pak ODS, eluting with acetonitrile:water:trifluoroacetic acid system. The h.p.l.c. chromatogram was monitored in the negative mode at m/z 319. I: 14/15 HETEs, II: 11-HETE, III: 8-HETE, IV: 9-HETE, V: 12-HETE, VI: 5-HETE. All isomers are resolved, except 14/15 HETEs which co-elute on this h.p.l.c. system.

thermospray liquid chromatography – mass spectrometry interface and the ion trap g.c. detector.

7.1 Liquid chromatography – mass spectrometry

There is a large body of information on the high resolution h.p.l.c. purification of eicosanoids. Clearly, by coupling the h.p.l.c. with a mass spectrometer, spectra can be obtained on polar and thermally labile species without the need for prior purification or derivatization. One such method — thermospray l.c. – m.s. — has recently become commercially available. Thermospray m.s. is a soft ionization technique (cf. f.a.b., c.i.) generating molecular ion species ($M+H^+$, $M-H^-$) post-h.p.l.c. with little fragmentation (24). The technique has been applied to analyse HETEs generated from human inflammatory cells (*Figures 30 and 31*) (27). Thermospray mass spectra have also been generated from the peptido-leukotrienes (28), species which are not amenable to g.c. analysis even as derivatives. The technique at present lacks the sensitivity of g.c.-based assays, with limits of detection in the low nanogram range. However, as the interface is refined, sensitivity limits should improve, making thermospray l.c. – m.s. a viable alternative to h.p.l.c. – RIA for the assay of the peptido-leukotrienes.

7.2 Ion trap g.c. detector

Many laboratories undertake a large amount of g.c. work, but do not possess mass spectrometric facilities. Recently an inexpensive bench top mass spectrometer has been developed by Finnigan MAT, primarily for use as a g.c. detector. The 'ion trap' is a development of the quadrupole mass spectrometer, and although of limited mass range (650 u), full electron impact mass spectra may be generated post-g.c. Further developments should extend the range of ionization modes available. The ion trap should prove of great value to those already working with g.c., who require structural information, but lack the available funds to purchase a conventional mass spectrometer.

8. ACKNOWLEDGEMENTS

Many of the examples described in this chapter result from experiments performed at the Royal Postgraduate Medical School and Imperial College, London. This work was supported by the Medical Research Council, The British Heart Foundation and The Wellcome Trust.

9. REFERENCES

1. Fallardeau,P., Oates,J.A. and Brash,A.R. (1981) *Anal. Biochem.*, **115**, 359.
2. Barrow,S.E., Waddell,K.A., Ennis,M., Dollery,C.T. and Blair,I.A. (1982) *J. Chromatogr.*, **239**, 71.
3. Blair,I.A., Brash,A.R., Daugherty,J. and Fitzgerald,G.A. (1985) In *Advances in Prostaglandin, Thromboxane and Leukotriene Research.* Hayaishi,O. and Yamamaoto,S. (eds), Raven Press, London, Vol. 15, p. 61.
4. Hamberg,M., Nihaus,W. and Samuelsson,B. (1968) *Anal. Biochem.*, **22**, 145.
5. Green,K., Hamberg,M., Samuelsson,B., Smigel,M. and Frolich,J.C. (1978) In *Advances in Prostaglandin and Thromboxane Research.* Frolich,J.C. (ed.), Raven Press, London, Vol. 5, p. 39.
6. Lands,W.E. and Smith,W.L. (1982) *Methods in Enzymology.* Vol. 86, Academic Press, London.
7. Axen,U., Green,K., Horlin,D. and Samuelsson,B. (1971) *Biochem. Biophys. Res. Commun.*, **45**, 519.
8. Barrow,S.E., Heavey,D.J., Ennis,M., Chappell,C.G., Blair,I.A. and Dollery,C.T. (1984) *Prostaglandins*, **28**, 743.
9. Powell,W.S. (1983) In *Advances in Prostaglandin, Thromboxane and Leukotriene Research.* Samuelsson, B., Paoletti,R. and Ramwell,P. (eds), Raven Press, London, Vol. 11, p. 207.
10. Morris,H.R., Taylor,G.W., Piper,P.J. and Tippins,J.R. (1980) *Nature*, **285**, 104.
11. Liston,T.E. and Roberts,L.J.,II (1985) *Proc. Natl. Acad. Sci. USA*, **82**, 6030.
12. Murphy,R.C., Hammarstrom,S. and Samuelsson,B. (1979) *Proc. Natl. Acad. Sci. USA*, **76**, 4275.
13. Nugteren,D.H. (1975) *Biochim. Biophys. Acta*, **380**, 299.
14. Borgeat,P., Hamberg,M. and Samuelsson,B. (1976) *J. Biol. Chem.*, **251**, 7816.
15. Borgeat,P. and Samuelsson,B. (1979) *J. Biol. Chem.*, **254**, 2643.
16. Green,K., Granstrom,E. and Samuelsson,B. (1973) *Anal. Biochem.*, **54**, 434.
17. Berry,C.N., Griffiths,R.J., Hoult,J.R.S., Moore,P.K. and Taylor,G.W. (1986) *Br. J. Pharmacol.*, **87**, 327.
18. Blair,I.A., Barrow,S.E., Waddell,K.A., Lewis,P.J. and Dollery,C.T. (1982) *Prostaglandins*, **23**, 579.
19. Waddell,K.A., Wellby,J. and Blair,I.A. (1983) *Biomed. Mass Spectrom.*, **10**, 83.
20. Waddell,K.A., Barrow,S.E., Robinson,C., Orchard,M.A., Dollery,C.T. and Blair,I.A. (1984) *Biomed. Mass Spectrom.*, **11**, 68.
21. MacDermot,J., Kelsey,C.R., Waddell,K.A., Richmond,R., Knight,R.K., Cole,P.J., Dollery,C.T. and Blair,I.A. (1984) *Prostaglandins*, **27**, 163.
22. Ennis,M., Barrow,S.E. and Blair,I.A. (1984) *Agents and Actions*, **14**, 397.
23. Ritter,J.M., Ongari,M.-A., Barrow,S.E., Orchard,M.A., Blair,I.A. and Lewis,P.J. (1982) *Prostaglandins*, **24**, 881.
24 Vestal,M. (1984) *Science*, **226**, 275.
25. Morris,H.R., Taylor,G.W., Panico,M., Dell,A., Etienne,A.T., McDowell,R.A. and Judkins,M.B. (1981) In *Methods in Protein Sequence Analysis.* Elzinga,M. (ed.), Humana Press, Clifton, New Jersey, p. 243.
26. Taylor,G.W., Morris,H.R., Beaubien,B. and Clinton,P.M. (1983) In *Leukotrienes and Other Lipoxygenase Products.* Piper,P.J. (ed.), John Wiley, Chichester, UK, p. 277.
27. Richmond,R., Clarke,S.R., Watson,D., Chappell,C.G., Dollery,C.T. and Taylor,G.W. (1986) *Biochim. Biophys. Acta*, **881**, 159.
28. Taylor,G.W., Chappell,G.C., Clarke,S.R., Heavey,D.J., Richmond,R., Turner,N.C., Watson,D. and Dollery,C.T. (1986) In *Leukotrienes: Their Biological Significance.* Piper,P.J. (ed.), Raven Press, p. 67.

10. GENERAL BIBLIOGRAPHY

10.1 Gas chromatography

1. *Gas Chromatography with Glass Capillary Columns.* (1980) Jennings,W. (ed.), Academic Press, London, UK.
2. *Recent Advances in Capillary G.C.* (1978, 1981) Bertsch,W., Jennings,W. and Kaiser,R.E. (eds), Vol. I−III. Huthig.

10.2 Mass spectrometry

1. *Soft Ionisation Biological Mass Spectrometry.* (1981) Morris,H.R. (ed.), Heyden, London, UK.
2. *Spectroscopic Methods in Organic Chemistry.* (1980) Williams,D.H. and Fleming,I., McGraw-Hill, Maidenhead, UK.
3. *Mass spectrometry* (biennial review, 1980, 1982, 1984, 1986) Burlingame,A.L. (ed.), Analytical Chemistry.
4. *Mass spectrometry: Specialist Periodical Reports.* (annual), Chemical Society, London, UK.
5. *Quantitative Mass Spectrometry.* (1978) Millard,B.J. (ed.), Heyden, London, UK.

10.3 Derivatization

1. *Handbook of Derivatives For Chromatography.* (1979) Blau,K. and King,G. (eds.), Heyden, London, UK.
2. *Pierce Handbook and Catalogue.* (annual) Pierce Chemical Co., Rockford, Illinois, USA.

10.4 Stable isotopes

1. *Stable Isotopes: Applications in Pharmacology, Toxicology and Clinical Research.* (1978) Baillie,T.A. (ed.), Macmillan Press, London, UK.
2. *Syntheses with Stable Isotopes.* (1981) Ott,D.G. (ed.), J.Wiley and Son, New York, USA.

10.5 Eicosanoids: general methods

1. *Methods in Enzymology.* (1982) Lands,W.E. and Smith,W.L. (eds), Vol. 86, Academic Press.
2. *Advances in Prostaglandin, Thromboxane and Leukotriene Research.* (1976−1985) Vol. 1−15, Raven Press, London, UK.

CHAPTER 8

Measurement of prostaglandins, thromboxanes and leukotrienes by smooth muscle bioassay

PRISCILLA J. PIPER

1. INTRODUCTION

Many of the numerous metabolites of arachidonic acid possess very potent actions on various types of smooth muscle. Indeed, the prostaglandins, thromboxane A_2 and leukotrienes (LTs), originally known as slow-reacting substance of anaphylaxis (SRS-A), were initially detected by their contraction of strips of human uterus (1), rabbit aorta (2) and rabbit jejunum (3), respectively. Bioassay is the determination of the active power of a biologically active substance by noting its effect on a live animal or an isolated organ, as compared with the effect of a standard preparation (4). The technique of bioassay is extremely versatile and, in addition to being used for quantitation of numerous materials, bioassay techniques have played crucial roles in discovering not only naturally-occurring substances but also the metabolic function of the lung (5) and the activity of enzymes such as angiotensin-converting enzyme (6). Measurement of the tone of a strip of smooth muscle suspended in an organ bath was described by Magnus in 1903 (7). The technique of bioassay was used and developed by Dale (8), Finkleman (9) and Gaddum (10). The use of superfusion, the bathing of an assay tissue with a continuous stream of fluid, was introduced by Gaddum (10), developed and extended for use with either buffer solutions or blood by Vane (11). In his Nobel Lecture of 1982, Sir John Vane stated 'with extraordinary simplicity and convenience, by its very nature, bioassay distinguishes between the important biologically active compounds and their closely related but biologically unimportant metabolites' (12).

This chapter will describe bioassay techniques used for the measurement of prostaglandins, thromboxane A_2 and leukotrienes. Only methods involving the use of smooth muscle preparations will be described and, in most cases, methods using superfusion will be used. Ideally, the smooth muscle chosen to assay a given substance should be very sensitive and specific for that substance. Sensitivity may be improved by limiting the amount of fluid bathing the tissue. Specificity may be increased by the use of more than one tissue so that the combination of tissues shows a characteristic response to the test substance (see *Figure 1*). This is based on the use of parallel pharmacological assay described by Gaddum (13). The specificity of a smooth muscle bioassay may be further increased by constantly bathing the tissue(s) with antagonists. For example, rat stomach strip is relaxed by catecholamines but, if this is blocked by a β-receptor antagonist, the tissue is more specifically contracted by prostaglandins (14).

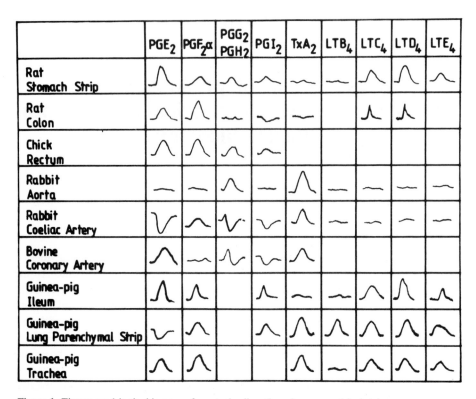

	PGE$_2$	PGF$_{2}\alpha$	PGG$_2$ PGH$_2$	PGI$_2$	TxA$_2$	LTB$_4$	LTC$_4$	LTD$_4$	LTE$_4$
Rat Stomach Strip									
Rat Colon									
Chick Rectum									
Rabbit Aorta									
Rabbit Coeliac Artery									
Bovine Coronary Artery									
Guinea-pig Ileum									
Guinea-pig Lung Parenchymal Strip									
Guinea-pig Trachea									

Figure 1. Tissues used in the bioassay of prostaglandins, thromboxanes and leukotrienes.

2. SUPERFUSION

Assay tissues are suspended in organ baths as shown in *Figure 2* and continuously bathed with either Krebs' or Tyrode's solution, depending on the tissues used. The Krebs' or Tyrode's solutions are gassed with oxygen (95%) and carbon dioxide (5%) or pure oxygen, respectively and heated so that the fluid reaches the tissues at 37°C. Changes in length or tension of the smooth muscles are recorded with transducers. Any antagonists used to increase the specificity of the assay may be either added to the buffer solution or infused over some or all of the tissues.

This technique may be used to detect or quantitate substances released into the effluent of isolated, perfused organs such as the lung (2). Since the perfusate reaches the assay tissues within seconds, this technique can be used to detect chemically unstable materials with a short half-life. Another advantage is that the continuous superfusion of the tissues allows the complete profile and time-course of a response to be recorded.

Vane used the method of superfusion to develop the blood-bathed organ technique (11) in which heparinized blood is taken from an anaesthetized animal and superfused over a series of assay tissues and returned to a suitable vein. When tissues are bathed in blood, antagonists are administered intraluminally to tissues such as chick rectum and rat colon so that they do not enter the circulation of the donor animal.

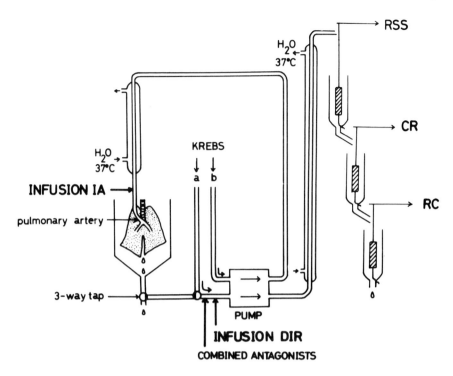

Figure 2. Superfusion of isolated assay tissues. Three to six strips of smooth muscle are superfused in series either with buffer solution or the effluent from an isolated perfused organ. Combined antagonists are either added to the buffer or continuously infused into the superfusing fluid.

3. PROSTAGLANDINS

Classical prostaglandins PGE_2, $PGF_{2\alpha}$ are assayed on a combination of rat stomach strip, rat proximal colon and chick rectum (15). These tissues are blocked with a combination of hyoscine (3.4×10^{-7} M), mepyramine (3.5×10^{-7} M), methysergide (5.5×10^{-7} M), phenoxybenzamine (4.4×10^{-7} M) and propranolol (8.8×10^{-6} M). Under these conditions, a simultaneous contraction of all three tissues indicates the presence of a prostaglandin-like material. These tissues show a differential sensitivity to prostaglandins: rat stomach strip is more sensitive to PGE_2 than to $PGF_{2\alpha}$ and rat colon is more sensitive to $PGF_{2\alpha}$. The fundic portion of the rat stomach strip is cut in a zig-zag manner as described by Vane (16) and suspended under a tension of 4 g. Both the chick rectum and rat colon are tied at the proximal end but have the suspending thread passed through the wall so that perfusing fluid does not pass through the lumen. They require a tension of 2 g. These tissues will respond to doses of PGs in the picomole range.

In order to detect the prostaglandin endoperoxides PGG_2 and H_2, it is necessary to use spirally cut strips of vascular tissue such as rabbit coeliac or mesenteric arteries (17) in addition to the rat and chick tissues. Prostacyclin relaxes spirally cut strips of bovine coronary artery (18) and may be distinguished from PGE_2 which contracts this tissue (see *Figure 1*). Prostacyclin is unstable and therefore should be generated and assayed immediately.

4. THROMBOXANE A_2

Thromboxane A_2 has a half-life of 30 sec in buffer and was initially detected by contraction of spirally cut strips of rabbit aorta (2). Strips of rabbit aorta should be suspended as previously described under a tension of 4 g. Thromboxane A_2 is a powerful vasoconstrictor and will contract strips of various types of arterial tissue such as rabbit coeliac or mesenteric arteries or guinea-pig or rat aorta. These tissues will require less tension than rabbit aorta.

Since thromboxane A_2 is very unstable it either has to be generated from a perfused organ and the effluent superfused over the assay tissues as described or prepared by aggregation of platelets in close proximity to the assay tissues (19).

5. LEUKOTRIENES

The cysteinyl-containing LTs LTC_4, LTD_4, LTE_4 and LTF_4 have potent actions on smooth muscle of the gastrointestinal tract and airways. On the other hand, LTB_4, which has no amino acid residues in its side chain, possesses much less smooth muscle stimulating activity. Accordingly, the smooth muscle bioassays for the two types of LT are different.

5.1 Cysteinyl-containing LTs

Since their original detection, the slow-reacting substances have been identified by their characteristic slow responses on isolated smooth muscle, usually from the gastrointestinal tract. The classical assay tissue for SRS-A, now known to contain LTC_4, LTD_4 and LTE_4, is guinea-pig ileum used in the presence of anti-histaminic and anti-cholinergic drugs (20). Use of this tissue allows distinction to be made between the fast contractions of histamine and the slower, longer-lasting contractions of the cysteinyl-containing LTs. Leukotrienes C_4, D_4, E_4 and F_4 contract guinea-pig ileum but their relative potencies (in terms of height of contraction) and their durations of action vary. The relative potencies are $LTD_4 > LTC_4 > LTE_4 > LTF_4$ and leukotrienes C_4 and F_4 cause contractions which last longer than LTD_4 or LTE_4 (21) (*Figure 3*). In meaningful doses, LTB_4 does not contract guinea-pig ileum.

The terminal part of the guinea-pig ileum is most sensitive to LTs. This section of the ileum is removed from the animal, placed in Tyrode's solution and cut into segments (3–4 cm) as required. Areas containing Peyers' patches should be avoided as they tend to show a high degree of spontaneous activity. Basically, guinea-pig ileum may be used in two different ways to quantitate leukotrienes. Firstly,

(i) Suspend tubular segments containing both longitudinal and circular smooth muscle in conventional organ baths in Tyrode's solution containing anti-cholinergic and anti-histaminic drugs, for example hyoscine and mepyramine, gassed with oxygen.

(ii) Record the changes in length of the tissue with an appropriate transducer.

(iii) Inject agonists into the bathing fluid at regular time intervals, and allow the

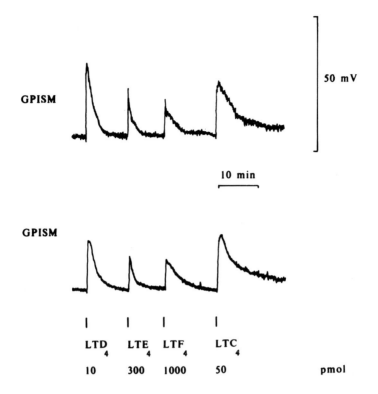

Figure 3. Contractions of guinea-pig ileum smooth muscle induced by LTC_4, LTD_4, LTE_4 and LTF_4. Vertical scale mV. Reproduced from ref. 24 with permission.

responses to reach their maximum before washing out, unless cumulative dose−response curves are being constructed.

This method is suitable for quantitating pure LTs and evaluating antagonists, since it reliably detects very low levels of LTC_4 or LTD_4, around or slightly less than 10^{-10} M but gives only limited information on the profile of LT responses. Secondly,

(i)   Remove strips of longitudinal smooth muscle from the ileum by a modification of the method of Rang (22) and superfuse in series.

(ii) Slide segments of ileum onto a glass pipette (held in a clamp stand) and keep moist.

(iii) Starting from the mesenteric line, divide the longitudinal muscle by firm strokes with the fingers and then strip it free from the deeper circular layer by gentle lateral strokes.

(iv) Suspend the resulting strips in the organ baths under a tension of 1 g and super-fuse with Tyrode's solution (5 ml/min) containing anti-histaminic and anti-cholin-ergic drugs to increase the specificity of the assay.

In addition to providing information about the relative potency and profile of action of LTs, the superfusion method provides information about their stability. For example, LTC_4 is converted to LTD_4 by γ-glutamyl transferase present on guinea-pig ileum. This causes the profile of the contraction of response to LTC_4 to change in the 60 sec

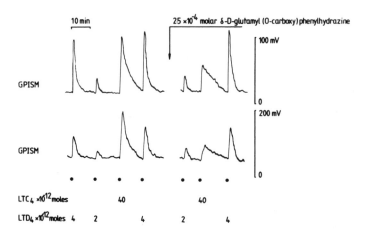

Figure 4. Activation of LTC$_4$ during superfusion over guinea-pig ileum smooth muscle. LTC$_4$ and LTD$_4$ were superfused over six strips; responses of the first and sixth strips are shown, the time between them being 60 sec. **(Left)** In the first strip, 40 pmol of LTC$_4$ caused contraction equivalent in height to that produced by 4 pmol of LTD$_4$. In the last strip, this had increased significantly. **(Right)** In the presence of 0.25 mM 1-D-glutamyl-(*O*-carboxy)phenylhydrazine, the contraction elicited by 40 pmol of LTC$_4$ was reduced to the equivalent of that elicited by approximately 2 pmol of LTD$_4$ and the duration of the response increased. The presence of γ-glutamyltransferase on the surface was confirmed by the method of Szasz (23). Reproduced from ref. 24 with permission.

required to superfuse six strips of guinea-pig ileum smooth muscle in series (*Figure 4*).

When unpurified LTs are being quantitated, either during release from a perfused organ such as the heart or lung or during assay of crude samples, the specificity of the assay may be improved by continuously blocking the last tissue with a leukotriene antagonist such as 4-oxy-8-propyl-4H-1-benzopyran-2-carboxylate (FPL-55712) (25) or 1-L2-hydroxy-3-propyl-4- < 4-(1H-tetrazol-5-yl)butoxy > phenyl > ethanone (LY171883) (26). In the presence of anti-cholinergic and anti-histaminic drugs, a contraction of guinea-pig ileum which is blocked by FPL-55712 is likely to be due to cysteinyl-containing LTs. Assays using guinea-pig ileum will detect picomole amounts of LTC$_4$ or LTD$_4$; this sensitivity is an order of magnitude less than that of radio-immunoassay (RIA).

5.2 Leukotriene B$_4$

Leukotriene B$_4$ is a potent chemotactic agent for polymorphonuclear leukocytes (27) and this property forms the basis of a sensitive assay for LTB$_4$ (28); this technique will not be discussed further here as it does not involve the use of smooth muscle. As mentioned previously, in contrast to the cysteinyl-containing LTs, LTB$_4$ has little smooth muscle-stimulating activity but contracts the guinea-pig ileum parenchymal strip. This action is due to the generation of the powerful bronchoconstrictor agent TxA$_2$ (29,30). Leukotriene B$_4$ has a potent contractile action on guinea-pig parenchyma but does not contract guinea-pig ileum. The responses to LTB$_4$ become tachyphylactic unless the doses are separated by at least 30 min. The LTB$_4$-induced contractions are not antagonized by the LT-antagonist FPL-55712. The differential action of LTB$_4$ on

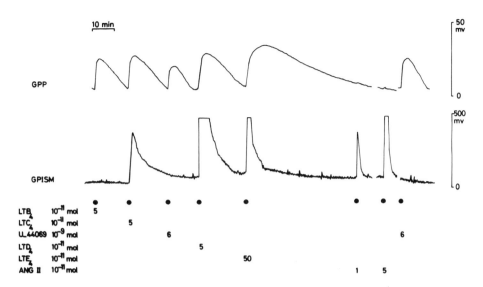

Figure 5. Differential effects of LTB$_4$, LTC$_4$, LTD$_4$, LTE$_4$ and angiotensin II (Ang II) on guinea-pig lung parenchymal strips and guinea-pig ileum smooth muscle. LTB$_4$, LTC$_4$ and LTD$_4$ (5×10^{-11} mol) produced contractions of similar height and duration of action (15, 18 and 20 min, respectively) on guinea-pig lung parenchymal strips. LTE$_4$ (50×10^{-11} mol) was inactive on guinea-pig lung parenchymal strips whereas U-44069 (6×10^{-9} mol) induced stable contractions of this tissue. LTB$_4$ and U-44069 had no effect on guinea-pig ileum smooth muscle unlike the other substances which contracted this tissue, LTD$_4$ being the most active agonist. Vertical scale: mV. Horizontal scale: 10 min. Reproduced from ref. 31 with permission.

guinea-pig ileum and parenchyma has been used in a simple, selective and sensitive bioassay for this LT (31).

(i)   Perfuse guinea-pig lungs with Tyrode's solution until free of blood and cut strips of parenchyma $30 \times 3 \times 3$ mm from the distal parts of the middle or large lobes.

(ii)   Superfuse a strip of parenchyma under a tension of 1 g above one or two strips of guinea-pig ileum smooth muscle.

(iii)   Block the tissues continuously with mepyramine, hysocine, methysergide, propranolol and phenoxybenzamine.

Under these conditions, LTB$_4$ contracts only the parenchyma (*Figure 5*) and is not blocked by FPL-55712. This differential action of LTB$_4$ distinguishes it from its all-*trans* metabolites which are much less active on parenchyma, as well as distinguishing it from a number of mediators, including other arachidonic acid metabolites, which occur in inflammatory fluids and have some action on guinea-pig ileum (31). This assay detects levels of LTB$_4$ of around $0.3-1$ pmol and compares well with the chemotactic assay for LTB$_4$ but is less sensitive than RIA.

6. CONCLUSION

Prostaglandins, TxA$_2$ and LTs can be reliably and reproducibly quantitated by relatively simple bioassay techniques and the results obtained very rapidly. The techniques described here are not quite as sensitive as RIA but can be used as a preliminary method of identifying PGs, TxA$_2$ and LTs in biological fluids whereas, on account of the possibility of unidentified cross-reaction with antisera, RIA should not be used alone for this purpose. Bioassay to detect and quantitate eicosanoids generated from biological sources may be greatly improved by the use of high-performance liquid chromatography to separate, purify and concentrate the active materials.

7. REFERENCES

1. Kurzroc,R. and Lieb,C.C. (1930) *Proc. Soc. Exp. Biol. Med.*, **28**, 268.
2. Piper,P.J. and Vane,J.R. (1969) *Nature*, **223**, 29.
3. Kellaway,C.H. and Trethewie,E.F. (1940) *Q.J. Exp. Physiol.*, **30**, 121.
4. *Dorland's Medical Dictionary*, 25th edition, W.B.Saunders, New York, Philadelphia, Toronto.
5. Bakhle,Y.S. and Vane,J.R., eds (1977) *Metabolic Function of the Lung.* Dekker, New York and Basel.
6. Bakhle,Y.S., Reynard,A.M. and Vane,J.R. (1969) *Nature*, **222**, 956.
7. Magnus,R. (1903) *Ergeb. Physiol.*, **2**, 637.
8. Dale,H.H. (1912) *J. Pharmacol. Exp. Ther.*, **4**, 167.
9. Finkleman,B. (1930) *J. Physiol.*, **70**, 145.
10. Gaddum,J.H. (1953) *Br. J. Pharmacol. Chemother.*, **8**, 321.
11. Vane,J.R. (1964) *Br. J. Pharmacol.*, **23**, 360.
12. Vane,J.R. (1983) *Br. J. Pharmacol.*, **79**, 821.
13. Gaddum,J.H. (1959) *Pharmacol. Rev.*, **11**, 241.
14. Vane,J.R. (1969) *Br. J. Pharmacol.*, **35**, 209.
15. Ferriera,S.H. and Vane,J.R. (1967) *Nature*, **216**, 868.
16. Vane,J.R. (1957) *Br. J. Pharmacol.*, **12**, 344.
17. Bunting,S., Moncada,S. and Vane,J.R. (1976) *Br. J. Pharmacol.*, **57**, 462P.
18. Needleman,P., Bronson,S.D., Wyche,A., Sivakoff,M. and Nicolaou,K.C. (1978) *J. Clin. Invest.*, **61**, 839.
19. Dusting,G.J., Moncada,S. and Vane,J.R. (1977) *Prostaglandins*, **13**, 3.
20. Brocklehurst,W.E. (1960) *J. Physiol.*, **151**, 416.
21. Piper,P.J. (1986) In *The Leukotrienes: Their Biological Significance.* Piper,P.J. (ed.), Raven Press, New York, p. 59.
22. Rang,H.P. (1964) *Br. J. Pharmacol.*, **23**, 356.
23. Szasz,G. (1969) *Clin. Chem.*, **15**, 124.
24. Morris,H.R., Taylor,G.W., Jones,C.M., Piper,P.J., Samhoun,M.N. and Tippins,J.R. (1982) *Proc. Natl. Acad. Sci. USA*, **79**, 4838.
25. Augstein,J., Farmer,J.B., Lee,T.B., Sheard,P. and Tattersall,M.L. (1973) *Nature New Biol.*, **245**, 215.
26. Fleisch,J.H., Rinkema,L.E., Haisch,K.D., Swanson-Bean,D., Goodson,T., Ho,P.P.K. and Marshall, W.S. (1985) *J. Pharmacol. Exp. Ther.*, **233**, 148.
27. Ford-Hutchinson,A.W., Bray,M.A., Doig,M.V., Shipley,M.E. and Smith,M.J.H. (1980) *Nature*, **286**, 264.
28. Ford-Hutchinson,A.W., Bray,M.A., Cunningham,F.M., Davidson,E.M. and Smith,M.J.H. (1980) *Prostaglandins*, **21**, 143.
29. Piper,P.J. and Samhoun,M.N. (1982) *Br. J. Pharmacol.*, **77**, 267.
30. Piper,P.J. and Samhoun,M.N. (1983) In *Advances in Prostaglandin, Thromboxane and Leukotriene Research.* Samuelsson,B., Paoletti,R. and Ramwell,P.W. (eds), Raven Press, New York, p. 127.
31. Samhoun,M.N. and Piper,P.J. (1984) *Prostaglandins*, **27**, 711.

CHAPTER 9

Aggregometry techniques for prostanoid study and evaluation

BRENDAN J.R.WHITTLE

1. INTRODUCTION

Studies on the actions of prostanoids on platelet function have extensively utilized the technique of aggregometry. The potent platelet anti-aggregatory actions of prostaglandin E_1 (PGE$_1$; *Figure 1*), derived from the precursor fatty acid, dihomo-gamma-linoleic acid, were recognized in the early 1970s from studies *in vitro* with platelet-rich plasma from several species (1). However, since only trace levels of PGE$_1$ can be detected under normal dietary conditions *in vivo* (2), the physiological significance of the actions of this prostanoid remain obscure. Later studies with PGD$_2$ (*Figure 1*) derived from the unsaturated fatty acid arachidonic acid, likewise indicated this prostanoid to be a potent inhibitor of platelet aggregation in human platelet-rich plasma *in vitro* (3,4). PGD$_2$ can be generated by human platelets and has been detected in human plasma, while the non-enzymatic conversion of the endoperoxide PGH$_2$ to PGD$_2$ is greatly enhanced by the presence of plasma protein from certain species including man (5,6). Thus, PGD$_2$ formation may play some physiological or pathophysiological role in the local regulation of platelet function in some species.

Prostacyclin is the predominant cyclo-oxygenase product of arachidonic acid in vascular tissue, endothelial cells being a major site of its formation (7,8). Prostacyclin (PGI$_2$) is not only the most potent naturally-occurring prostaglandin which inhibits platelet aggregation, being some 20 times more active than PGD$_2$, but is also the most potent endogenous anti-aggregating agent so far described (9). The role of endogenous prostacyclin in the local regulation of endothelial cell−platelet interaction has been extensively explored. The early characterization of the biosynthesis and activity of prostacyclin has greatly depended on the use of the platelet aggregometer, and this methodology has now become an important tool in the pharmacological study and bioassay of prostacyclin and its derivatives.

2. BASIC PRINCIPLES OF AGGREGOMETRY

2.1 Optical aggregometry

The most widely used technique for the evaluation of platelet anti-aggregating activity is the turbidometric aggregometry system developed originally by Born and colleagues (10,11) which determines the optical density of platelet-rich plasma; as platelets aggregate, the optical density of the plasma decreases and light transmission increases. This change in light transmission is detected by a photo-cell system and the resulting

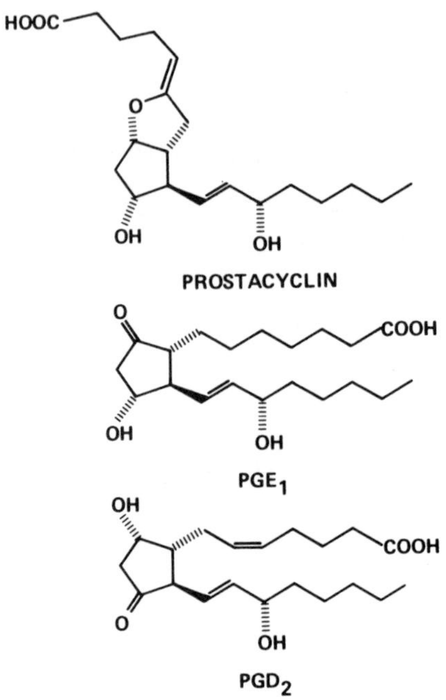

Figure 1. Structure of the endogenous anti-aggregating prostanoids, prostaglandin E$_1$ (PGE$_1$), PGD$_2$ and prostacyclin (PGI$_2$).

chart trace can be accurately quantified (*Figure 2*). Using this system, typical sigmoid dose−response curves can be constructed and subjected to the appropriate analysis.

2.1.1 *Preparation of plasma*

(i)   Collect human blood, following venepuncture in volunteers (the subjects should not have taken any non-steroid anti-inflammatory agent for 1 week before study), into a plastic 150 ml tissue culture flask (Corning) containing trisodium citrate (to give a final concentration of 0.315% w/v).

(ii)   Centrifuge (200 *g* for 15 min) at room temperature using a bench centrifuge to prepare platelet-rich plasma (*Figure 3*).

(iii)   In the same fashion, collect blood into citrate from a cannulated artery or vein or abdominal aorta of various species of laboratory animals including rabbit, dog, rat and guinea-pig (4). For the more rapid preparation of these smaller quantities of platelet-rich plasma (PRP), collect the whole blood in 10 ml plastic neutral tubes (Sarstedt) containing trisodium citrate (to give a final concentration of 0.315%, or in the case of the rat, 0.34%) and centrifuge (3000 r.p.m. for 2 min) at room temperature in a Petalfuge-1 bench centrifuge (12). Remove the PRP carefully, using a plastic syringe, mix and transfer into plastic Universal 30 ml containers (Sterilin) and store closed at room temperature.

(iv)   Determine the platelet count in the PRP using a Coulter Counter (such as Model ZF) or by manual counting (Chapter 3); the values for the various species are shown in *Table 1*. If desired, the platelet count can be adjusted by the addition

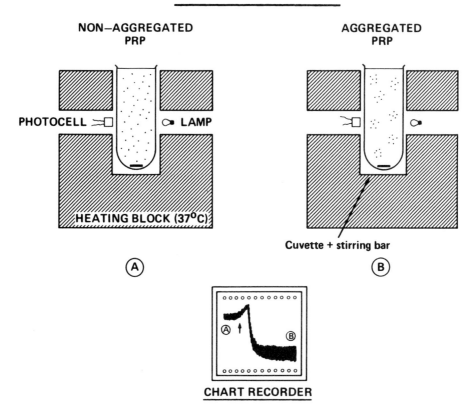

Figure 2. The use of the optical aggregometer for the measurement of platelet aggregation.

of platelet-poor plasma (PPP). This PPP can be prepared by further more-rapid centrifugation of aliquots of the PRP to sediment the platelets, for example by a 1 min centrifugation (9000 *g*) in an Eppendorf bench centrifuge.

2.1.2 *Platelet aggregation*

Measure platelet aggregation in a commercially-available aggregometer such as a Payton dual-channel aggregation module or Chrono-log module connected to a suitable chart recorder such as the 'W + W' recorder 1200. Incubate aliquots (0.5 ml) of PRP for 1 min at 37°C, stir with Teflon-coated magnetic stirrers at 900 r.p.m., prior to the addition of submaximal dose of adenosine diphosphate (ADP) to just cause a non-reversing control aggregation. The concentrations of ADP used for the various species are shown in *Table 1*.

Comparable studies can be conducted where platelet aggregation is induced by other agents including arachidonic acid (using concentrations of $100-400$ μg/ml in human PRP), collagen ($0.5-4$ μg ml), thrombin, and thromboxane mimetics (for example U-46619; $11\alpha,9\alpha$-epoxy methano-PGH$_2$; $0.1-3$ μM). The degree of platelet aggregation can be expressed in terms of percentage change in light transmission, using

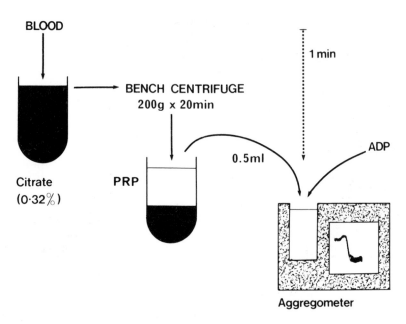

Figure 3. Preparation of PRP from whole blood collected into trisodium citrate for the study of platelet aggregation in an optical aggregometer.

Table 1. The mean platelet count, and the concentration of ADP inducing the non-reversing platelet aggregation in the PRP from different species.

Species	Platelet count ($\times 10^8$ ml)	ADP (μM)
Human	3.2	3.5
Guinea-pig	3.0	3.0
Dog	1.6	10.1
Rat	7.6	3.4
Rabbit	4.9	10.2
Sheep	2.4	1.7
Horse	1.4	1.5

aliquots of PPP to set the value for complete removal of platelets from the light path. Following addition of the aggregating agent (usually in volumes of $< 10\ \mu l$) such as ADP to the PRP, an initial small decrease in light transmission is usually observed, which results from an initial shape change of the platelets from their normal disk shape to a spherical shape. This is followed by a rapid increase in light transmission as the platelets aggregate, accompanied by an increase in trace oscillations reflecting the passage of such platelet clumps across the light path (*Figure 4*). Depending on the species from which the PRP has been prepared, the anti-aggregating agent and the dose employed, the profile of changes observed during aggregation will vary. Thus, ADP can give a biphasic response in human PRP, the initial phase being the primary aggregation following the formation of platelet pseudopods and small aggregates. If low concentrations of ADP ($0.5 - 2\ \mu M$) are employed, this aggregation can reverse, whereas

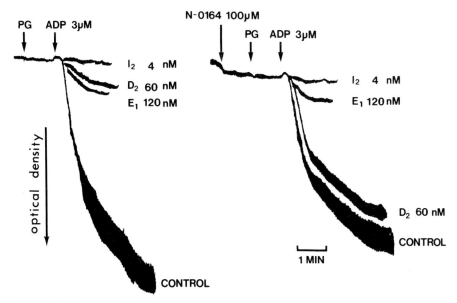

Figure 4. Inhibition of ADP-induced platelet aggregation in human PRP by the prostanoids, PGE_1, PGD_2 and prostacyclin (PGI_2). The figure also shows the selective antagonism by N-0164 on the anti-aggregating actions of PGD_2. The recorder traces from the aggregometer are superimposed.

at higher concentrations of ADP ($2.5-10$ μM), the platelets then release the contents of their dense bodies (including 5-hydroxytryptamine and ADP itself) during the non-reversing secondary aggregation. This secondary phase, in which thromboxane A_2 is also formed and liberated, can be inhibited by pre-incubation with non-steroid anti-inflammatory agents which inhibit platelet cyclo-oxygenase.

2.2 Measurements of aggregation in whole blood

For some pharmacological studies, the effects of eicosanoids on platelet aggregation may be required to be studied in whole blood. Further, it may not be practical in some experimental models to remove adequate volumes of blood to prepare sufficient PRP. Clearly the type of optical aggregometer just described cannot be used in these situations because the density of the whole blood will prevent light transmission. Two systems for the study of platelet aggregation in whole blood have, however, been developed.

2.2.1 Whole-blood aggregometer

Inhibition of platelet aggregation by prostacyclin and other prostanoids in citrated whole-blood *in vitro* can be assessed by use of an impedance electrode system (13,14). In this system, developed by R.J.Flower and colleagues at the Wellcome Research Laboratories, the electrical resistance between two closely-placed platinum electrodes, which initially become coated with a monolayer of platelets, increases when aggregating platelets deposit on these probes. This system which is now commercially available (Chronolog Whole-Blood Aggregometer) gives aggregation traces comparable with those obtained in optical aggregometer (although without shape-change information) and ID_{50} values can be calculated in an analogous fashion.

The experimental details for study of platelet activity using this technique are described in full elsewhere (13). The technique can be adapted further to monitor platelet aggregation in small volumes (100 μl) of citrated whole blood (14), as well as in non-anti-coagulated whole blood (15).

2.2.2 *Platelet counting techniques*

The technique of determining the fall in free platelet count as an index of *in vivo* platelet aggregation was developed by Smith and colleagues, in which blood was continuously removed from a cannulated artery of laboratory animals, mixed with citrate solution and pumped through a Technicon Autocounter (16). Studies in whole blood can likewise be conducted by an *in vitro* platelet counting technique, utilizing an Ultra-Flo Whole Blood Platelet Counter (17,18). Aggregation by ADP (1−5 μM) or collagen (1−4 μg/ml) is induced in samples of whole blood, shaken or stirred at 37°C, and aliquots removed at various time intervals for counting of free platelets. The degree of aggregation is calculated from the fall in free platelet count, and thus inhibition of aggregation can be readily determined.

In our studies (18), human whole blood is collected into trisodium citrate (0.32% final concentration) as described above. Aliquots (0.5 ml) are placed into siliconized glass cuvettes of an aggregation module and after 1 min stirring (900 r.p.m.) at 37°C, collagen (1.6−4 μg/ml), in a dose which produces near maximal aggregation, is added. Blood samples (10 μl) are withdrawn from the cuvette at 0, 1 and 2.5 min intervals and the platelet count recorded using a whole blood platelet counter (Ultra Flo 100, Clay Adams). The platelet count values are expressed as % inhibition using the following calculation:

$$\% \text{ inhibition} = 100 - \left(100 \times \frac{(\text{count at time } 0 - \text{test count at } 2.5 \text{ min})}{(\text{count at time } 0 - \text{control count at } 2.5 \text{ min})}\right)$$

2.3 **Washed platelets**

The study of platelet aggregation in PRP may be complicated by the binding of the various prostanoids to plasma proteins and other constituents. Several techniques for separating and washing platelets free of plasma and its constituents have been described in the literature. These are generally based on the preparation of platelet suspensions by differential centrifugation, gel filtration or centrifugation through an albumin gradient. In an approach to improve viability of these preparations, Shio and Ramwell (19) used the anti-aggregatory prostanoid PGE_1 during preparation and storage, and noted a markedly improved yield of platelets in the final suspension. However, prostacyclin is a more potent inhibitor of platelet aggregation. Thus, in our laboratory we have found that the use of prostacyclin during separation and washing of human platelets from whole blood produces stable platelet suspensions which respond to agonists and inhibitors readily and remain morphologically normal and physiologically active for long periods (20,21).

The platelet suspensions are prepared from whole blood from different species using

Table 2. The simplified method for washing platelets with prostacyclin.

	PGI_2 ($\mu g/ml$)	Tyrode's solution	Centrifu- gation (g)	Time (min)	Tempera- ture (°C)	Citrate (0.32%)
Collect blood	–	–	–	–	22	+
Obtain PRP	–	–	250	20	22	–
Sediment platelets	0.3	–	900	10	22	–
Sediment platelets	0.3	+	800	10	37	–
Final sus- pension	–	+	–	–	37	–

(+) indicates the presence and (−) indicates the absence of the reagents. In some situations the blood can be collected directly into citrate-containing prostacyclin (2 $\mu g/ml$) which can improve the final yield of platelets.

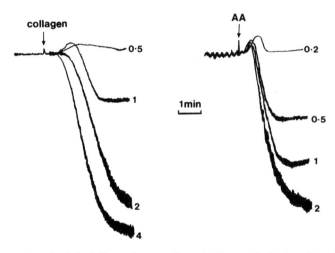

Figure 5. Aggregation of an 0.5 ml aliquot of prostacyclin washed human platelets by collagen (0.5−4 $\mu g/ml$) and by arachidonic acid as the sodium salt (0.2−2 $\mu g/ml$), as determined in an optical aggregometer.

the general procedure described by Vargas *et al.* (20) with the following modifications as detailed elsewhere (21):

(i)   in some experiments prostacyclin (PGI_2) is added at the initial step of blood collection, which can improve the final platelet yield;

(ii)   a slightly higher centrifugal force (250 g) is used during centrifugation of the blood, to remove leukocytes and erythrocytes without the need for further centrifugation of the PRP;

(iii)   platelets are washed only once;

157

(iv) resuspension of the loose upper layer of the platelet pellet is achieved using an Oxford pipette (5 ml) with the tip cut approximately 5 mm from the end, whilst for the bottom more-compact layer, a Precision pipette (0.5 ml) is used.

The details of this modified technique are summarized in *Table 2*. The use of siliconized plastic containers throughout the procedure promotes a higher yield of platelets.

Aggregation studies are carried out in this albumin-free medium in a dual-channel aggregometer such as the Chronolog Lumi aggregometer which can additionally determine ADP release from the platelets. Although no great change in the sensitivity of the platelets is observed during the first $1-2$ h after final resuspension in prostacyclin-free Tyrode's solution, studies are usually commenced 2 h after final resuspension. As shown in *Figure 5*, these platelets respond well to aggregating agents such as ADP and collagen, and the lack of plasma protein binding of arachidonic acid greatly enhances its potency.

2.4 Data analysis

In our studies, the inhibition of ADP-induced aggregation is determined by pre-incubation (1 min at 37°C) with the prostaglandin under investigation prior to the addition of a sub-maximal dose of ADP. Dose−inhibition curves are constructed and the IC_{50} (dose causing 50% inhibition) is calculated as the dose required to reduce the aggregation to 50% of its control amplitude. Comparable studies are conducted using the other aggregating agents.

Others have investigated the anti-aggregating potency of prostanoids at different phases of ADP-induced aggregation, determining both the extent and rate of aggregation (22).

2.5 Materials

(i) Make up the solution of ADP (Sigma Chemical Co.) in distilled water and keep on ice, as with the suspension of collagen in isotonic glucose solution (suspended fibrils, Horman-Chemie, Munchen).

(ii) Store arachidonic acid (Grade I, Sigma Chemical Co.) in *n*-hexane (10 mg/ml) at -20°C and use freshly as the sodium salt. Following evaporation of the *n*-hexane from 1 ml aliquots, add sodium hydroxide (0.5 M in methanol, 0.5 ml) and subsequently evaporate to dryness. Dissolve the residue (10 mg/ml) in 1 M Tris buffer (pH 9.6 at 24°C), and store in a light-proof container on ice.

(iii) Store the endoperoxide analogue $11\alpha,9\alpha$-epoxy methano-PGH_2 (U-46619), supplied by the Upjohn Company, in ethanol at -20°C and dissolve in isotonic saline when required.

(iv) Dissolve prostacyclin (as the sodium salt), obtained from the Wellcome Foundation, freshly in 1 M Tris buffer (pH 9.6 at 4°C) and store on ice; make subsequent dilutions with ice-cold Tris buffer (50 mM, pH 8.6) or with isotonic sodium bicarbonate solution (1.25% w/v; pH 8.6) and use immediately.

(v) Store prostaglandin D_2, PGE_1 (obtained from the Upjohn Company, Kalamazoo)

Table 3. Inhibition of ADP-induced aggregation in citrated platelet-rich plasma obtained from several species by prostacyclin (PGI$_2$), PGE$_1$ and PGD$_2$.

	IC_{50} (ng/ml)		
	PGI$_2$	PGE$_1$	PGD$_2$
Human	0.4 ± 0.1	21 ± 3	11 ± 2
Guinea-pig	0.8 ± 0.2	20 ± 3	200 ± 20[a]
Dog	0.8 ± 0.2	9 ± 3	970 ± 300
Rat	1.7 ± 0.5	8 ± 1	50 000
Rabbit	2.8 ± 0.5	16 ± 3	370 ± 50
Sheep	3.7 ± 0.8	37 < 8	16 ± 5
Horse	3.7 ± 0.5	39 ± 10	27 ± 6

Results expressed as the dose causing 50% inhibition (IC_{50}) are the mean ± S.E. mean of 3−20 experiments for each value.
[a]PGD$_2$ exhibits a bell-shaped dose−response curve in guinea-pig plasma.

or other prostanoids in ethanol (10 mg/ml; −20°C) and dilute with 50 mM Tris buffer (pH 7.5 at 4°C) when required.

3. INHIBITION OF PLATELET AGGREGATION BY PROSTANOIDS

Using the Born-type optical aggregometer, the potency of the naturally-occurring anti-aggregatory prostanoids in PRP of various species has been determined. Prostacyclin is the most potent inhibitor of platelet aggregation in all species investigated (*Table 3*). In our studies in human PRP, prostacyclin is 50 and 20 times more active than PGE$_1$ and PGD$_2$, respectively. In a comparison of the anti-aggregatory potency of these prostanoids at different stages of ADP-induced aggregation, they had comparable relative activities against full aggregation, the first-phase of aggregation and the initial rate of aggregation (22).

3.1 Species sensitivity

The potency of prostacyclin as an inhibitor of platelet aggregation in PRP differs between various species, yet as shown in *Table 3*, the range of IC_{50} values from human plasma (the most sensitive species to prostacyclin) to sheep or horse plasma (the least sensitive species) are within one log unit of concentration. The anti-aggregating potency of PGE$_1$ varies in a comparable fashion between the species investigated, suggesting that both prostacyclin and PGE$_1$ act on the same or very comparable receptor sites on platelets. In marked contrast, the anti-aggregating potency of PGD$_2$ spans 4 log units of concentration from the most sensitive species (human plasma) to the least sensitive species (rat plasma). Thus, it is unlikely that PGD$_2$ is acting at comparable platelet receptor sites to those for prostacyclin or PGE$_1$.

A further difference between PGD$_2$ and prostacyclin was noted in studies on guinea-pig platelets. Whereas prostacyclin and its chemically-stable mimetic, carbacyclin, produce full inhibitory dose−response relationships with IC_{50} values comparable with those in human PRP (*Table 3*), PGD$_2$ acts as a weak inhibitor of guinea-pig platelet aggregation, producing a bell-shaped response (12). Recent studies suggest that this may reflect an interaction of PGD_2 at pro-aggregatory thromboxane-sensitive sites on these platelets (23).

3.2 Studies in whole-blood

The dose−inhibitory activity of both prostacyclin and its chemically-stable analogue, 9β-methyl carbacyclin (24) on ADP-induced platelet aggregation has been compared in whole blood and PRP. In rabbit PRP (determined using optical aggregometry) and in whole blood (determined using the platelet counting technique) these prostanoids had a comparable potency ratio in either system (*Figure 6*). In a similar comparison of the anti-aggregating activity of prostacyclin and 9β-methyl carbacyclin in human

a

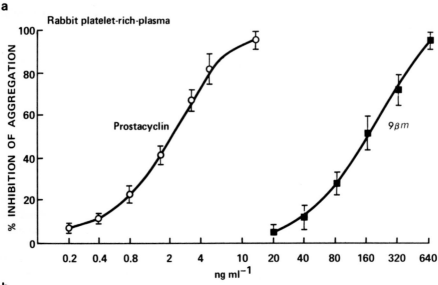

b

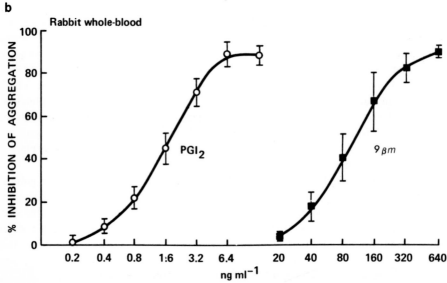

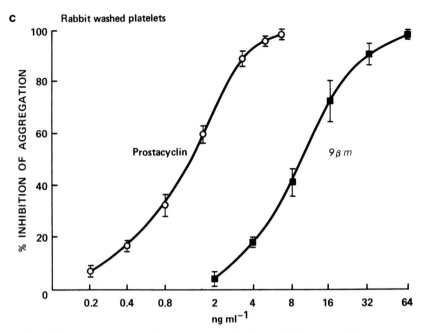

Figure 6. Inhibition by prostacyclin or 9β-methyl carbacyclin (9βm) of ADP-induced rabbit platelet aggregation in (**a**) PRP, (**b**) whole blood and (**c**) washed platelets. In washed platelets, 9βm was significantly ($P < 0.001$) more potent than in PRP using optical aggregometry techniques, or in whole blood using a platelet counting technique.

PRP and in whole blood aggregated with collagen, the IC_{50} concentrations for prostacyclin were 0.91 ± 0.08 and 0.88 ± 0.15 ng/ml and for 9β-methyl carbacyclin were 123 ± 32 and 73 ± 20 ng/ml, respectively (18).

In another study, prostacyclin had comparable anti-aggregating activity in human PRP and in citrated whole blood, as determined by the Impedance Aggregometer (25). The activity of the putative prostacyclin metabolite, 6-oxo-PGE$_1$ (IC_{50} in our studies in human PRP is 6 ± 1 ng/ml) is enhanced in whole blood, as measured by the latter technique. The mechanism of this enhanced activity in whole blood, which is also found with PGE$_1$ is unknown but may reflect the reduction in ADP release from erythrocytes (25).

3.3 Washed platelets

As with whole blood, the anti-aggregating activity of prostacyclin is comparable in PRP and in platelet suspensions washed free of plasma, as shown in *Figure 6* with rabbit platelets. However, the activity of 9β-methyl carbacyclin was enhanced some 10-fold in washed platelets, indicating a significant binding of the analogue to some plasma component compared with prostacyclin itself. Similar differential potency with carbacyclin in human PRP and washed platelet suspensions have also been observed (26).

4. BIOASSAY OF INHIBITORY PROSTANOIDS

The anti-aggregatory activity of prostacyclin has been extensively utilized in its detection, and in the subsequent bioassay of endogenously-synthesized prostacyclin.

PREPARATION OF GASTRIC MUCOSAL EXTRACTS

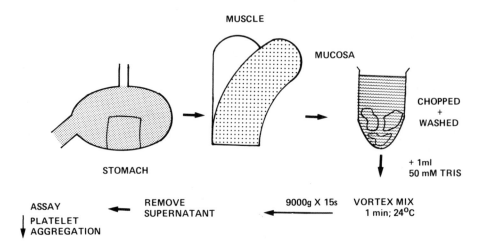

Figure 7. Preparation of a gastric mucosal tissue and subsequent generation of prostacyclin-like anti-aggregating activity using the vortex-mixing procedure.

4.1 Formation of prostacyclin

The generation of prostacyclin from strips or rings of vascular tissue has been determined from various species including man, by incubating such excised tissue *in vitro* in a buffer or physiological salt solution, and subsequent bioassay of the supernatant for prostacyclin-like anti-aggregating activity (7,9,27).

In this laboratory, we use this bioassay technique to measure the formation of prostacyclin-like activity from gastro-intestinal and vascular tissue following a vortex-mixing procedure (27) to stimulate its formation (*Figure 7*). This presumably acts by stimulation of phospholipase-A_2 with subsequent release of substrate, arachidonic acid.

(i)   Remove segments (0.3−0.5 g) of jejunum or upper ileum (3−6 cm from the caecum and freed from adherent mesentery), strips of gastric mucosa (0.3 g), removed from underlying muscle by peeling off with forceps, or the abdominal aorta (1.5 cm in length) cut into rings. Wash in Tris buffer (50 mM; pH 8.4 at 4°C) and weigh.

(ii)   Chop the tissues in 1 ml of buffer, centrifuge in an Eppendorf bench centrifuge (10 sec at 9000 *g*), re-wash in 1 ml buffer, re-centrifuge, and finally incubate in 0.5 ml of buffer by vortex mixing for 1 min at room temperature.

(iii)   After a 15-sec centrifugation (9000 *g*), test aliquots (5−50 μl) of the supernatant immediately for their ability to inhibit ADP-induced aggregation of human platelets (using 0.5 ml of citrated PRP as described above) in a dual-channel aggregometer and assay against authentic prostacyclin (27).

4.2 Characterization of prostacyclin-like activity

Pre-treatment of the animals with a non-steroid anti-inflammatory agent such as indomethacin to inhibit cyclo-oxygenase and reduce prostanoid biosynthesis prior to removal of the tissues should be employed to confirm that the platelet-inhibitory activity is a prostanoid. Incubation *in vitro* with such agents can also be used, but in tissue fragments, relatively high concentrations of these aspirin-like drugs may be required due to poor tissue penetrations.

The identity of platelet-inhibitory activity as prostacyclin can be confirmed by several tests. This activity, like prostacyclin itself, should inhibit platelet aggregation in plasma from several species, and such determination in different PRP can be utilized as a parallel bioassay technique. Thus, the material should exhibit a parallel dose−response relationship to authentic prostacyclin, and should exhibit a similar potency ratio to the standard in the PRP from different species. Prostacyclin-like activity can clearly be distinguished from that of PGD_2 since this latter prostanoid has only weak anti-aggregatory in rabbit PRP, and minimal activity in rat PRP (*Table 3*).

The instability of prostacyclin, especially under acid conditions can additionally be used to characterize any endogenously-formed prostacyclin present in extracts. Thus, the anti-aggregating activity should be destroyed by incubation at 37°C for 15 min at pH 7.4, or by a 30-sec incubation at pH 3 with subsequent neutralization. Such thermal and acid instability is not shared by the other anti-aggregatory prostanoids such as 6-oxo-PGE_1. A further definitive test, but which is less readily available, is to determine whether the anti-aggregating activity is also abolished by a 1-min pre-incubation of the extract with a specific antiserum. This antibody, which is raised in rabbits to a stable prostacyclin analogue such as 6β-PGI_1 or carbacyclin, binds and hence inactivates prostacyclin *in vitro* (27).

5. PLATELET PROSTANOID RECEPTOR CLASSIFICATION

5.1 **Prostanoid receptor antagonists**

The inhibition of platelet aggregation in PRP by PGD_2 can be abolished by simultaneous incubation with the prostaglandin antagonist, N-0164, at concentrations which fail to prevent the inhibition by PGE_1 or prostacyclin, as shown in *Figure 4* (28). Like N-0164, di-4-phloretin phosphate (DPP) can selectively antagonize the actions of PGD_2 on human platelets (29). However, the nature of the inhibition with DPP is complex. In PRP from rabbits, DPP inhibits the responses to PGE_1 and prostacyclin, but not to PGD_2, the converse of the effects in human platelets. The specificity of DPP as a prostanoid receptor antagonist on platelets thus requires carefuly analysis. Furthermore, N-0164 can act as a thromboxane receptor antagonist in guinea-pig platelets (27). However, both N-0164 and DPP could be used to characterize further any prostanoid anti-aggregating activity in biological extracts.

It is clear that potent and selective antagonists for both prostacyclin and PGD_2 receptors would be of great benefit in characterizing the pharmacological profile of these prostanoids. The technique of platelet aggregometry thus offers a rapid and precise model for the development of such agents.

Although PGE_2 can inhibit platelet aggregation (but only at high concentrations, ~20 μm), it can, conversely, potentiate aggregation induced by agents such as ADP. Furthermore, PGE_2 can interfere with the anti-aggregatory actions of PGE_1, prostacyclin and also PGD_2. Although PGE_2 is thus not a selective prostanoid receptor antagonist, such effects can potentially interfere with bioassay of tissue extracts for prostacyclin. However, a 4-fold concentration excess of PGE_2 has only minimal effects on the dose-inhibiting relationship with prostacyclin, although its effects on the responses to PGD_2 are greater (22). Thus, the determination of prostacyclin levels by aggregometry bioassay techniques may lead to an underestimation of the levels present in an extract if a large excess of PGE_2 is concurrently generated. Under these conditions, it may be more appropriate to employ alternative assay techniques.

5.2 Prostanoid receptor agonists

The development of probes for prostanoid receptors will assist in the characterization of the pharmacological actions. With prostacyclin, the identification of appropriate chemically-stable analogues is of importance both for pharmacological studies and for clinical development. Many such analogues have been reported, including 5,6-dihydro analogues, exemplified by 6β-PGI_1, thia-prostacyclins such as (5Z)-6,9-thia prostacyclin, nitrogen-containing analogues such as 9-deoxy-9α-6-nitrilo-PGF_1, ring-expanded 5,9-epoxy derivatives such as 9-deoxy-5,9α-epoxy PGE_1 and interphenylene analogues (24). However, the stable carbocyclin analogues of prostacyclin, in which the enol-ether oxygen is replaced by a methylene group, such as in carbacyclin and 9β-methyl carbacyclin (ciprostene), have proven to be close mimetics.

Less attention has been directed towards agonists at the PGD_2 receptor. However, aggregometry studies on PRP from several species indicate that the hydantoin prosta-glandin, BW245C acts on PGD_2 receptor sites on platelets (30). Indeed, this prostanoid may be more selective than PGD_2 itself, which can also interact with platelet thromboxane receptors (23).

5.3 Thromboxane A_2 mimetics and antagonists

Although TxA_2 and the endoperoxide intermediates, PGG_2 and PGH_2 induce platelet aggregation in PRP and washed platelets from several species, aggregometry techniques are not usually employed for the bioassay of these highly unstable products. However, induction of platelet aggregation with the stable analogues of TXA_2 and the endo-peroxides, such as $11\alpha,9\alpha$ or $9\alpha,11\alpha$-epoxy methano PGH_2 (U-46619 and U-44069, respectively) is used for the investigation of platelet thromboxane receptors (22).

The evaluation of thromboxane receptor competitive antagonists such as 13-aza prostanoic acid and BM 13.177 can thus be conducted in human PRP using U-46619 (0.11$-$2.8 μM) to induce aggregation, and typical rightward shifts of the dose$-$response curve can be achieved, allowing assessment of the nature of the antagonism (for example, 23).

6. LIPOXYGENASE PRODUCTS

The optical aggregometry techniques have been successfully utilized for the study of white cell aggregation, and the stimulant actions of the lipoxygenase product, leukotriene B_4 (LTB_4), have been identified.

Cell suspensions containing greater than 85% polymorphonuclear leukocytes (PMNL) are prepared from rat peritoneal exudates obtained 24 h after the injection of sodium caseinate (31). The cells are suspended in buffered medium to study the aggregation in an aggregometer following addition of LTB_4.

In comparable studies in our laboratories (32), peritoneal exudate cells ($\sim 80\%$ PMNLs) are obtained from male Wistar rats (150−200 g) 17 h after i.p. injection of 0.2% oyster glycogen.

(i)   Harvest the cells immediately following i.p. injection of Hank's balanced salt solution (20 ml) containing 20 U/ml heparin.

(ii)   Wash the cells once in the buffered salt saline without heparin and then resuspend at a concentration of 10^7 cells/ml.

(iii)   Transfer aliquots (490 μl) of the cell suspension to siliconized glass cuvettes, warm the suspensions to 37°C and stir at 800 r.p.m. in a dual-channel aggregometer.

(iv)   After 5 min pre-incubation, add the agonists to the cell suspension in 50 mM Tris buffer (pH 8.0; 10 μl) and monitor the aggregation of the PMNL by changes in light transmission. Aggregation is measured as the maximum height for the change in light transmission induced by buffer alone (32). Aggregation of the rat PMN can be induced by addition of LTB$_4$ ($10^{-9}-10^{-6}$ M).

Studies on aggregation of human blood mononuclear leukocytes by arachidonic acid and LTB$_4$ can likewise be conducted using optical aggregometry on cells prepared on a discontinuous Percoll gradient (33). Aggregation of leukocytes in whole blood using the Impedance whole-blood aggregometer has also been described, where small volumes of blood (100 μl) can be used following dilution with a suitable buffer (14).

7. CONCLUSIONS

The use of the optical platelet aggregometer has clearly played a significant role in the study of the biological profile of endogenous anti-aggregatory prostanoids such as prostacyclin and PGD$_2$, as well as in the early characterization of the pro-aggregatory endoperoxides and TxA$_2$. This relatively simple and reproducible technique, which can use PRP obtained from various species or platelets washed free of plasma, has allowed the pharmacological study of receptor mechanisms for prostanoids in a well-characterized cell system. Such techniques have also provided a sensitive and selective biaossay for the levels of prostacyclin formed by various tissues. The adaptation of the platelet aggregometry techniques for the measurement of leukocyte aggregation has provided a further use of this system. Studies in whole blood on platelet or leukocyte aggregation using either cell-counting techniques or the impedance whole-blood aggregation is a more recent extension to the established methodology. It thus seems likely that aggregometry techniques will remain an important part of pharmacologists equipment for the study and bioassay of eicosanoids and other related mediators.

8. REFERENCES

1. Kloeze,J. (1969) *Biochem. Biophys. Acta*, **187**, 285.
2. Danon,A., Heimberg,M. and Oates,J.A. (1975) *Biochim. Biophys. Acta*, **388**, 318.
3. Smith,J.B., Silver,M.J., Ingerman,C.M. and Kocsis,J.J. (1974) *Thromb. Res.*, **5**, 219.
4. Whittle,B.J.R., Moncada,S. and Vane,J.R. (1978) *Prostaglandins*, **16**, 373.
5. Ali,M., Cerskus,A.L., Zamecnik,J. and McDonald,J.W.D. (1977) *Thromb. Res.*, **11**, 485.
6. Hamberg,M. and Fredholm,B.B. (1976) *Biochim. Biophys. Acta*, **431**, 189.
7. Moncada,S. and Vane,J.R. (1979) *Pharmacol. Rev.*, **30**, 293.
8. Moncada,S. (1982) *Br. J. Pharmacol.*, **76**, 34.

9. Whittle,B.J.R. and Moncada,S. (1984) *Br. Med. Bull.*, **39**, 232.
10. Born,G.V.R. (1962) *Nature*, **194**, 927.
11. Born,G.V.R. and Cross,M.J. (1963) *J. Physiol.*, **18**, 175.
12. Hamid,S. and Whittle,B.J.R. (1985) *Br. J. Pharmacol.*, **85**, 285.
13. Cardinal,D.C. and Flower,R.J. (1980) *J. Pharmacol. Methods*, **3**, 135.
14. Russell-Smith,N.C., Flower,R.J. and Cardinal,D.C. (1981) *J. Pharmacol. Methods*, **6**, 315.
15. Zwierzina,W.D. and King,F. (1985) *Thromb. Res.*, **38**, 91.
16. Holmes,I.B., Smith,G.M. and Freuler,F. (1977) *Thromb. Haemostasis*, **37**, 36.
17. Lumley,P. and Humphrey,P.P.A. (1981) *J. Pharmacol. Methods*, **6**, 153.
18. O'Grady,J., Hedges,A., Whittle,B.J.R., Al-Sinawi,L.A.H., Mekki,Q.A., Burke,C., Moody,S.G., Moti,M.J. and Hassan,S. (1984) *Br. J. Clin. Pharmacol.*, **18**, 921.
19. Shio,H. and Ramwell,P.W. (1972) *Science*, **175**, 536.
20. Vargas,J.R., Radomski,M. and Moncada,S. (1982) *Prostaglandins*, **23**, 939.
21. Radomski,M. and Moncada,S. (1983) *Thromb. Res.*, **30**, 383.
22. Anderson,N.H., Eggerman,T.L., Harker,L.A., Wilson,G.H. and De,B. (1980) *Prostaglandins*, **19**, 711.
23. Hamid-Bloomfield,S. and Whittle,B.J.R. (1985) *Br. J. Pharmacol.*, **88**, 931.
24. Whittle,B.J.R. and Moncada,S. (1984) In *Progress in Medicinal Chemistry*. Ellis,G.P. and West,G.B. (eds), Elsevier Science Publishers, Amsterdam, Vol. 21, p. 237.
25. Wilsoncroft,P.S., Lofts,F.J., Griffiths,R.J. and Moore,P.K. (1985) *J. Pharm. Pharmacol.*, **37**, 139.
26. Moncada,S. and Whittle,B.J.R. (1983) *Br. J. Pharmacol.*, **78**, 160P.
27. Whittle,B.J.R. (1981) *Gastroenterology*, **80**, 94.
28. MacIntyre,D.E. and Gordon,J.L. (1977) *Thromb. Res.*, **11**, 705.
29. Westwick,J. and Webb,H. (1978) *Thromb. Res.*, **123**, 973.
30. Whittle,B.J.R., Moncada,S., Mullane,K. and Vane,J.R. (1983) *Prostaglandins*, **25**, 302.
31. Cunningham,F.M., Shipley,M.E. and Smith,M.J.W. (1980) *J. Pharm. Pharmacol.*, **32**, 377.
32. Terrano,T., Salmon,J.A. and Moncada,S. (1984) *Prostaglandins*, **27**, 217.
33. Villa,S., Colotta,F., de Gaetano,G. and Semeraro,N. (1984) *Br. J. Haematol.*, **58**, 137.

CHAPTER 10

Radioimmunoassay of eicosanoids

ELISABETH GRANSTRÖM, MARIA KUMLIN and HANS KINDAHL

1. INTRODUCTION

Eicosanoids generally occur only in minute amounts in biological material, which necessitates the use of very sensitive and accurate quantification methods. Many immunological methods display satisfactory detection limits for eicosanoid assay, permitting the analysis of even small biological samples, such as sub-millilitre volumes of plasma. Since these methods are also relatively inexpensive and the analyses simple to perform, it is not surprising that they have gained widespread use.

The principle underlying many immunological quantification methods is a competition between unlabelled (standard or sample) and labelled molecules of a certain compound for the binding sites of an antibody directed against the compound in question. The more unlabelled molecules that are present in a sample, the more labelled ones will be displaced from the antibody binding sites. The extent of this displacement is then quantitated − in either the antibody-bound or the free fraction − by the appropriate method, depending on the label, and the absolute amount of the assayed substance is obtained from comparison with a standard curve.

Several different types of label can be employed. In older, less sensitive methods a common marker was red blood cells, whose surface was coated with the compound in question. The quantifiable reaction was agglutination of the erythrocytes, which only occurred when antibodies were bound to the surface ligands. This type of immunological method is still in use, for example in pregnancy tests (determination of human chorionic gonadotropin in urine), although latex beads are now preferred to red blood cells. Each bead or cell is coated with a large number of ligand molecules. This implies that the assay is relatively insensitive, since a large number of unlabelled molecules in the analysed samples are thus also required to inhibit the agglutination.

With the use of other markers, a more favourable situation may be obtained, with a resulting increase in sensitivity. This is obtained by individual labelling of marker molecules, which can be achieved in a number of ways. These include labelling with an easily quantifiable enzyme, a fluorophor, an electron-dense moiety, and so on. An almost classical approach to this problem is the use of radiolabelled markers, the basic principle of radioimmunoassay (RIA). Although some of the more recently introduced methods, such as enzyme immunoassay (EIA, see Chapter 11), may replace RIA in the future because of its far higher sample capacity, the radioimmunological methods will no doubt continue to be widely in use at least for the next decade.

This chapter will describe aspects of the practical performance of eicosanoid RIA: production of an antibody preparation, preparation of labelled ligand(s), incubation procedures, methods for separation of antibody-bound and free fractions, counting of radioactivity and mathematical handling of data. A considerable part of the chapter will also discuss the interpretation of data and various often encountered problems and sources of error.

2. DEVELOPMENT OF AN EICOSANOID RADIOIMMUNOASSAY

2.1 **Preparation of the antigen**

All the eicosanoids, including the prostaglandins, thromboxanes, leukotrienes and lipoxins, are substances of low molecular weight and hence not antigenic in themselves. Thus, in order to obtain antibodies against such compounds, it is necessary to attach them to a larger molecule, for example a protein or a polypeptide. Various methods have been described for coupling an eicosanoid to such a large carrier molecule.

2.1.1 *Choice of carrier*

By far the most commonly used protein in this respect is bovine serum albumin (BSA). Keyhole limpet haemocyanin (KLH) is another protein, often used in this area. γ-Globulins, ovalbumin and thyroglobulin are also sometimes employed. There are different opinions about the importance of the choice of a proper carrier: whether they differ in antigenicity, and whether they can prevent an undesired metabolism *in vivo* of the hapten in the immunized animal. A factor that is likely to be of some importance for the production of many eicosanoid antibodies is the content of lysine residues in the protein, since coupling of the eicosanoid generally takes place between the eicosanoid carboxyl and the ε-amino groups of lysine moieties in the protein. A high molar ratio (eicosanoid:carrier) is supposed to give rise to high titre antibodies. BSA has 59 lysine residues (1); however, many of these may not be accessible to coupling, since reported molar ratios seldom exceed about 20 (2). It should however also be pointed out that efficient immunogens have often been obtained with far lower relative amounts of the eicosanoid: molar ratios can even be as low as $2-3$ and the conjugate still evoke a sufficient antigenic response. A carrier such as polylysine would seem ideal in this respect and has often been employed in prostaglandin RIA. The antigenicity of this polypeptide is however weak, and the conjugate has to be further coupled to, for example, KLH prior to immunization of the animal.

2.1.2 *Coupling methods*

As mentioned, most coupling methods take advantage of the presence of a carboxyl group in the prostanoid which is conjugated to an amino group by formation of a peptide bond. In the case of the cysteinyl-containing leukotrienes (i.e. LTC_4, D_4 and E_4), which have more than one carboxyl $-$ LTC_4 is a tricarboxylic acid $-$ the situation becomes more complicated. Solutions to this problem are discussed more in detail in Section 4.2.

Several different methods can be used to activate a carboxyl group and couple it to an amino group on a peptide or protein. The most widely used reagents for such coupling are water-soluble carbodiimides (CDI) $(2-4)$ and N,N′-carbonyldiimidazole (5,6). The mixed anhydride reaction, for example using isobutylchlorocarbonate as reagent (1,7), has also been used successfully to prepare immunogenic conjugates of eicosanoids. A slightly different approach is to convert the eicosanoid carboxyl into a reactive, water-soluble ester, such as N-hydroxysuccinimide esters (8,9), prior to the conjugation to a carrier protein, which then occurs as a spontaneous process. Coupling to N-hydroxysuccinimide is achieved by for example using carbodiimide (8,9).

When several carboxyls exist in the hapten, as is the case with the cysteinyl-containing leukotrienes, a different approach has been used (10) (see Section 4.2 for a further discussion of this problem). Aehringhaus *et al.* (10) coupled the single free amino group of LTC_4 to amino groups of BSA using glutaraldehyde as cross-linking reagent. Dimethylpimelindiimidate has been used similarly to produce an antigenic conjugate of LTE_4 and BSA (11).

In this chapter, only the first two methods will be described in detail.

(i) *Carbodiimides as the coupling reagent.* Several different carbodiimides can be used for coupling. The most commonly used compound is 1-ethyl-3-(3-dimethylaminopropyl)carbodiimide-HCl (4), but N,N'-dicyclohexylcarbodiimide is also sometimes employed. A general procedure is as follows.

(1) Dissolve the eicosanoid (3−10 mg, about 10−30 μmol) in a small volume of dimethylformamide or ethanol, and add a slight excess of the CDI (5−10 mg).
(2) Add the protein (BSA, 20−40 mg) dropwise in a small volume of water. It is important to keep a slightly acidic pH during this procedure (∼pH 5.5).
(3) Leave the reaction mixture overnight and then dialyse against distilled water to remove any remaining free eicosanoid and also the low molecular weight by-products of the reaction.

To estimate the degree of incorporation of the eicosanoid into the protein, it is recommended to include a small amount of the radiolabelled hapten.

(ii) *N,N'-Carbonyldiimidazole as coupling reagent.*

(1) Dissolve the eicosanoid (e.g. 3−10 mg) in a small volume (0.5−2 ml) of dry dimethylformamide and convert it into a reactive imidazolide by the addition of about equimolar amounts of N,N'-carbonyldiimidazole (2−5 mg).
(2) After about 20 min at room temperature add the solution dropwise to an aqueous solution of the protein (for example, 20−40 mg of BSA in 1−3 ml of water).
(3) After 5 h with stirring at room temperature, dialyse the reaction mixture, first against dimethylformamide:water (2:3, v/v), and then against water.
(4) For convenience, divide the dialysed preparation into several portions (one for each planned injection into the animal) and lyophilize.

2.2 Preparation of the antibody

Most antibody preparations in the prostanoid field have been raised in animals *in vivo*, and are thus polyclonal. In most cases their specificities seem to have been sufficient, and in cases with a too heterogenous population of antibodies, some separation into subpopulations of more specific ones may improve the preparation.

With modern techniques, however, it is possible to prepare monoclonal antibodies (12). Several such antibody preparations have been produced to date against PGE_2

(13,14) and LTB_4 (15), some of these with very high specificity.

It should be pointed out that monoclonal antibodies are not necessarily more specific *per se*. Polyclonal preparations seem less specific because they are a mixture of many different antibodies with varying specificities. The advantage of using a monoclonal preparation is that the clone with the desired properties can be obtained completely pure.

2.2.1 *Preparation of monoclonal eicosanoid antibodies*

The production of a monoclonal antibody preparation involves several steps. First, polyclonal antibodies are raised *in vivo* (see below), generally in mice. The next step consists of hybridization of splenic lymphocytes from the immunized animal with myeloma cells lacking the capacity for antibody production. The heterokaryotic cells from this fusion are then isolated by culture in a special medium. The hybridoma cells are then cloned, and the various clones are tested for antibody production. The clone(s) producing the most specific antibody are selected for the subsequent assay.

For technical details of this rather complex procedure, see for example ref. 16.

2.2.2 *Preparation of polyclonal eicosanoid antibodies*

This technique, which utilizes the immunological response of an intact animal, is still the most common one in this area. The rabbit is the most commonly employed species for antibody production, at least in the eicosanoid field. Other animals sometimes used are the guinea pig, monkey and sheep (for review, 6).

(i)   Dissolve the immunogen in a small volume of water and emulsify with Freund's complete adjuvant (mycobacteria in mineral oil). The adjuvant is necessary to stimulate the immunologic response.

(ii)   Inject the emulsion intradermally, intramuscularly, intraperitoneally or subcutaneously at multiple sites in the animal.

(iii)   Repeat the injections with $1-2$ week intervals until the antibody response is satisfactory. Usually at least $4-5$ injections are necessary.

Samples of the animal's blood are taken regularly to follow the development of the immunologic response. In view of the fact that certain of the arachidonate metabolites are formed in large amounts during sample collection and/or the clotting process, it may be advisable to add an anti-coagulant and thus to obtain the 'antiplasma' rather than the antiserum. If the antibody is raised against a product of the cyclo-oxygenase pathway, an inhibitor of prostanoid biosynthesis, such as indomethacin, may also be included for the same reason.

2.2.3 *Characterization of the antibody*

Data obtained by an immunologic method depend to a great extent on the properties of the employed antibody. One of the most important steps in the development of such an assay is thus the characterization of the antibody preparation, that is the determination of such features as its titre, specificity and avidity. Some of these parameters depend on other factors as well, and will be further discussed below.

(i) *Titre test.* A suitable working dilution (the 'titre') of the antiplasma is one that binds approximately $40-60\%$ of the labelled ligand in the absence of the unlabelled compound.

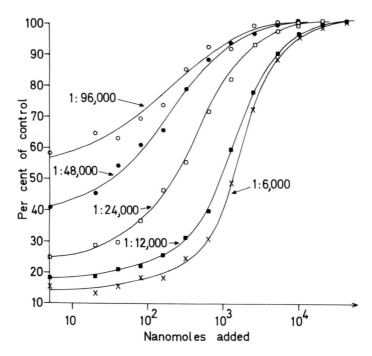

Figure 1. Influence of antibody concentration (in this case an antibody against 15-keto-13,14-dihydro-PGF$_{2\alpha}$) on B$_0$ and the slope and shape of the standard curve. Note increasing sensitivity with increasing antibody dilution. Simultaneously, however, accuracy and precision decrease, since minor differences in measured radioactivity will have correspondingly greater effects on final results.

The use of larger amounts of the antibody will decrease the sensitivity of the assay, since comparatively large amounts of the unlabelled compound will have to be added to saturate the antibody binding sites, before the proper displacement of the labelled compound can begin. In contrast, if smaller amounts of the antibody are used, for example by taking a higher dilution of the plasma, the sensitivity of the assay increases: addition of even small amounts of the unlabelled ligand will affect the binding of the tracer. This may however not be an advantage, since the difference in radioactivity in the 'no displacement' (zero point) tubes and 'total displacement' tubes decreases simultaneously, and thus the uncertainty in the RIA readings increases (the so-called accuracy and precision may decrease, see below).

Figure 1 illustrates the effects of different antibody dilutions on these parameters of a typical RIA standard curve.

(ii) *Sensitivity.* The sensitivity of an assay can be defined in more than one way. Generally in prostaglandin RIA, it is expressed as the minimum amount of the unlabelled ligand that can be distinguished from the 'zero point' tubes (maximum binding tubes, in the absence of added unlabelled substance) with two standard deviations. Usually the amount of substance that causes a 10% displacement of radioactivity from the 'zero point' is regarded as the limit of detection of the assay, and is given as its 'sensitivity'.

The magnitude of this parameter is influenced by several factors. One is the antibody dilution, as was discussed above (see *Figure 1*). Other important factors are the amount

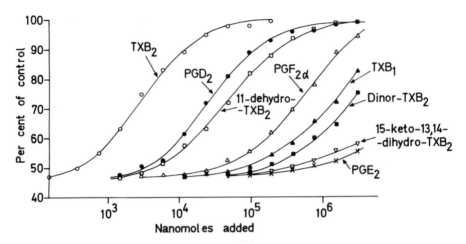

Figure 2. Properties of a relatively non-specific antibody against TXB_2. Cross-reactions were determined by replacing the standard dilutions of unlabelled TXB_2 with other compounds. The antibody recognizes 9,11-dihydroxy compound (TXB_2, $PGF_{2\alpha}$) but also compounds with a keto group at C-11 (PGD_2, 11-dehydro-TXB_2; for a possible explanation, see text). Cross-reaction with compounds structurally altered in the side chain is negligible (such as TXB_1, dinor-TXB_2, 15-keto-13,14-dihydro-TXB_2).

and specific activity of the added tracer, and also the avidity of the antibody (see below).

(iii) *Specificity*. The specificity of an antibody against a certain ligand is expressed in terms of cross-reactions with structurally related compounds. It may seem self-evident that a high specificity is desirable: in many situations, however, it may be preferable to use a low-specificity antibody instead. This is the case, for example, in many leukotriene studies: it is known that the metabolism *in vitro* of the cysteinyl-containing leukotrienes leads to an extensive interconversion between LTC_4, D_4 and E_4, the extent of which may not be known. Assay of only one of these compounds may thus give a false picture of events, and the use of a non-specific antibody that does not differ between these compounds may be preferable. Another situation where a low specificity of the antibody may give more informative results, is in studies aimed at following the total body production of a certain eicosanoid by monitoring a urinary metabolite. Assay of several, major, structurally related compounds together by the use of a non-specific antibody may then give a better picture of events.

The cross-reaction with a compound is usually expressed in percentage terms, calculated from the amount of the compound in question required to displace 50% of the labelled ligand bound to the antibody, in comparison with the proper ligand (the 'cross-reaction' with the proper ligand is thus 100%).

Cross-reactions are determined by replacing the normal standard dilutions by corresponding dilutions of other substances that can be expected to be recognized by the antibody. Usually, however, much larger amounts of these related substances have to be added to achieve displacement of the proper, labelled ligand. *Figure 2* shows the properties of a relatively non-specific antibody against TXB_2. Note the high cross-reactions with 11-dehydro-TXB_2 and PGD_2, indicating that the antibody recognizes an oxo group at C-11, which can be seen in one form of TXB$_2$ (17,18). In contrast, however, the antibody is highly specific for the lengths and structures of the side chains: cross-reactions with TXB$_1$, dinor-TXB$_2$ and 15-keto-13,14-dihydro-TXB$_2$ are low.

(iv) *Avidity.* The avidity of an antibody expresses the energy of binding in the antigen−antibody reaction, and refers to the properties of the antibody. (The corresponding term for the antigen is affinity.) The avidity is essentially the same as the association constant in physical chemistry (K_a), with

$$K_a = \frac{[AbPG]}{[Ab]\,[PG]}$$

where [AbPG], [Ab] and [PG] refer to the molar concentration of the antibody−prostaglandin complex, the free antibody and the free prostaglandin, respectively.

The avidity can be determined by plotting the standard curve as a Scatchard plot (19). The ratio of the antibody-bound to the free antigen is plotted against the concentration of the antibody-bound ligand. K_a is then given by the slope of this line, and the molar concentration of the antibody binding sites by its intercept on the abscissa. The K_a values for prostaglandin antisera are seldom published, but the value is usually in the range of $10^9 - 10^{10}$ M^{-1}, occasionally as high as 10^{12} M^{-1} (2,20). In general, the higher the value, the better the antiserum, since a high figure indicates a strong binding of the ligand: thus, less antibody is required in the assay, and furthermore, influence by disturbing factors is usually minimized.

2.3 Preparation of the tracer (labelled ligand)

A high specific activity and purity of the tracer is essential to obtain a high sensitivity of the RIA. The majority of RIA work today is done with commercially available reagents. Eicosanoids, generally multiply labelled with ^{3}H, can thus be obtained with specific activities over 150 Ci/mmol. These are usually hepta- or octatritiated compounds, prepared biosynthetically from carrier-free [^{3}H$_8$]arachidonic acid.

In some cases, however, this is not possible, and the scientist may have to prepare the tracer him/herself. Several alternatives exist for such preparations (see also below, Section 4.3). The use of ^{14}C-labelled substances is usually not possible in RIA, since the specific activity of such compounds would be far too low. This also holds true for compounds with one or two tritium atoms, such as [9β-^{3}H]PGF$_{2\alpha}$, [17,18-^{3}H]PGF$_{2\alpha}$ and [5,6-^{3}H$_2$]PGF$_{1\alpha}$, which are otherwise easily prepared by chemical reduction of PGE$_2$, PGF$_{3\alpha}$ and PGF$_{2\alpha}$, respectively, using the proper tritium-labelled reducing agent (6).

By far the most common method for tracer preparation in eicosanoid RIA is the enzymatic conversion of a multiple tritium-labelled precursor into the desired compound. To obtain a preparation with high specific radioactivity in good yield, it is recommended to use, if possible, the immediate precursor of the compound in question. The biological system employed for the conversion may be an entire organism, an organ or a tissue preparation or a purified enzyme.

When choosing a biological system for this purpose, the scientist should consider several aspects.

(i)   If possible, the desired compound should be the major metabolite produced by the system, and the amount of by-products that may be difficult to separate from the desired one should be kept at a minimum. This ideal situation may be difficult to attain, particularly at the extremely low substrate concentrations that are employed during tracer preparations. An example of this is given below.

(ii)   Second, dilution with endogenous material must be kept as low as possible. Pre-treatment of the biological system with an appropriate enzyme inhibitor may reduce this problem (for a further discussion, see below, Section 4.3).

(iii)   Third, it is important that the tracer is as pure as possible. In our experience, however, extensive purification with a large number of chromatographic steps is not the best way to achieve this, particularly when working with relatively small amounts of the tracer. The reason is that most chromatographic procedures inevitably concentrate, and even introduce, many interfering substances that will disturb the final RIA. Our recommendation is to prepare a large batch of the compound (if possible, ~ 100 μCi at a time) and purify it by using one extraction step with a Sep-Pak cartridge, and one or two h.p.l.c. steps. The best results are obtained if the final chromatographic fractions containing the compound can simply be diluted directly in the RIA buffer and then used as such.

The preparation of $[^3H_7]$11-dehydro-TXB$_2$ from $[^3H_8]$TXB$_2$ is described here as a typical example. The commonly used tissue preparation for this biosynthesis was earlier the guinea-pig liver supernatant, which is known to have a high capacity for 11-dehydrogenation of TXB$_2$ (21). However, a number of other products are also formed; among them an acyclic compound with alcohol groups at C-11 and C-12: 8-(1,3-dihydroxypropyl)-9,12-dihydroxy-5,10-heptadecadienoic acid (21). This compound was formed in larger amounts at low substrate concentration, together with a number of other, unidentified TXB$_2$ metabolites, resulting in a considerably reduced yield of 11-dehydro-TXB$_2$ (M.Kumlin, unpublished observation). A further difficulty was the fact that this acyclic metabolite co-migrated with one chemical form of 11-dehydro-TXB$_2$ in most tested chromatographic systems.

To solve this problem, other tissues were screened for their TXB$_2$ metabolizing capacity. The best tissue in this respect found so far is rabbit lung (22): the high speed supernatant from this organ converted $[^3H_8]$TXB$_2$ almost exclusively into $[^3H_7]$-11-dehydro-TXB$_2$, even at very low substrate concentration (23). Since the lung also has a high capacity for thromboxane biosynthesis from endogenous arachidonic acid (24), the entire preparation of the subcellular fraction and the incubation were carried out in the presence of indomethacin to prevent dilution with endogenous, unlabelled 11-dehydro-TXB$_2$. Extraction of the desired labelled product was done at pH 2 using ethyl acetate, and the compound was then purified using straight-phase h.p.l.c. (23). The acidification converted the metabolite into one chemical form, a δ-lactone, and the compound was recovered in $1-2$ chromatographic fractions. The yield of the pure compound from 100 μCi of $[^3H_8]$TXB$_2$ (specific activity, 130 Ci/mmol) was about 60 μCi (specific activity, about 100 Ci/mmol) from an incubation with 5 g of rabbit lung (23).

2.4 **Performance of the assay**

2.4.1 *Incubation procedure*

The incubation volume is usually within the range $0.3-0.7$ ml. Glass tubes, approximately 10×80 mm in size, are suitable for this purpose. The different components of the assay are added, for example according to the scheme below. The contents are then mixed by vigorous shaking, and the tubes are left for an incubation time of $1-24$ h, at $+4\,°C$, on ice, or at room temperature, depending on the properties of the antibody.

A common set up of RIA tubes is as given below.

(i)   Tubes $1-3$:   'total radioactivity' tubes, or 'zero binding' tubes; containing only labelled ligand in buffer (no antibody or unlabelled substance present).

(ii)   Tubes $4-6$:   'maximal binding' tubes, or 'zero point' tubes: containing labelled ligand plus antibody but no unlabelled substance.

(iii) Tubes $7-24$:   standard curve, containing labelled ligand, antibody, and increasing amounts of unlabelled ligand; always at least in duplicate and increasing by a factor of two (e.g. 1, 2, 4, 8, 16, 32, ... etc. pg per tube).

(iv)   Tubes $25-n$:   sample tubes: several dilutions of each sample, and duplicates or triplicates of each dilution should preferably be measured.

2.4.2 *Separation of the free and the antibody-bound fraction*

Since RIA is based on an accurate estimation of the extent of tracer displaced from the antibody binding sites, the separation of the free and bound fraction is an extremely important step. Several methods can be employed for this purpose, three of which are particularly common: dextran-coated charcoal (DCC), polyethylene glycol (PEG) and a second antibody.

DCC absorbs the free fraction (low molecular weight substances). Coating of charcoal with dextran is done to prevent the adsorption of large protein molecules, such as the antibodies, to the surface of the charcoal. Dextran only permits the passage of low molecular weight substances; larger molecules are excluded. After the free fraction has thus been absorbed, this heavy complex can be removed by centrifugation. The supernatant, containing the antibody-bound fraction, is then usually counted for radioactivity. The method is simple to perform and has consequently gained widespread use; however, it has one draw-back: the reagent may 'strip' the antibody of bound ligand molecules, leading to falsely high RIA results if not performed with utmost caution.

The other two methods mentioned above lead instead to precipitation of the bound fraction. PEG is an inexpensive, safe and efficient method (6,25); however, it requires a minimum amount of carrier γ-globulin to give complete precipitation. Furthermore, the presence of this compound implies some difficulties in scintillation counting (see below).

Finally, with the second-, or double-, antibody technique, the antibody-bound fraction is precipitated by addition of an antibody directed against the γ-globulin fraction of the species employed for production of the first (anti-eicosanoid) antibody. Such antibodies are commercially available, for example goat or swine anti-rabbit IgG. The use of a second antibody may unfortunately give incomplete precipitation of the antibody-bound fraction, since this step has been shown to be particularly easily disturbed by a number of factors (6,26).

In our laboratory, we prefer to use the PEG technique.

(i)   Add an ice-cold, 25% solution of PEG in water or buffer (w/v) to the pre-cooled incubation tubes in equal volume (to give a final concentration of 12.5%), and vigorously vortex the contents.

(ii)   Collect the formed protein precipitate by centrifugation, and analyse either the pellet (the bound fraction) or the supernatant (free) for radioactivity content, as described below.

An alternate method to achieve separation of free and antibody-bound fractions is to use a solid-phase technique. Two possibilities exist: first, binding of the first antibody to the inner surface of the plastic tubes used in the incubation of the RIA, and second, binding of the first or the second antibody to very fine insoluble dextran particles. These types of methods have gained some interest when it is desirable to simplify the method, for example in kits or in large-scale clinical studies. In general, the methods have somewhat lower sensitivity and reproducibility than the common, liquid phase type of RIA. In the prostaglandin field, solid-phase techniques are uncommon, but a few assays have been developed (e.g. 27).

2.5 Counting of radioactivity

After separation of the antibody-bound and free forms of the eicosanoid, the radioactivity of either fraction is counted. Depending on the choice of emitter (β- or γ-emitters) and the employed separation method, different approaches can be used. γ-Emitters such as ^{125}I are easy to determine in either supernatant or pellet. Most conveniently, the supernatant is discarded and the RIA tubes are allowed to drain upside down on some soft absorbing tissue or filter paper. The whole tube is then counted directly in the γ-counter. This method is preferred in systems utilizing solid phase (see above), or when the separation method yields a firm precipitate. In either case, the tubes should be washed several times with buffer before the final counting.

When β-emitters such as ^{3}H are used, scintillation counting must be done. The choice of scintillation cocktail is very important. The cocktail must have a high capacity for water and in many cases also proteins (e.g. when direct analyses of plasma are done). If PEG is used for separation of the bound and free forms of the ligand, this reagent must be taken into account also. Today several ready-for-use cocktails exist which fulfill these criteria and also give a high efficiency in the counting. The sample and the cocktail can be in one phase or in a gel form. It is, however, extremely important that the system does not separate into two phases, since this can give false radioactivity values.

The following account describes counting of the supernatant after PEG separation (i.e. the free fraction).

(i)   To produce a one-phase system in the scintillation vial, remove 1 ml of the supernatant with an automatic diluter (e.g. LKB Ultrolab System Diluter or Hamilton Microlab 1000 or some comparable equipment).

(ii)   After the aliquot is diluted automatically with, for example, 1 ml of water, transfer it to a scintillation vial.

(iii) Add Instagel (10 ml) and vigorously shake the vials. An emulsion is initially formed, which becomes clear after about 15−20 h at +10°C, or after freezing, thawing and re-shaking.

Correction for quenching is necessary, particularly when large volumes of aqueous samples are assayed directly. In other situations, quench correction is also recommended, due to the possibility of differences in the samples compared with the standards, differences in the plastic vials, and so on. Internal quench correction is the classical method, but for practical reasons when working with large series of vials, an external method must be employed. A simple method is to use the automatic external standard channels ratio. The scintillation counter must then be equipped with a γ-source close to the vial in the counting chamber. Quenched standard vials with known amounts of radioactivity are commercially available and can be used for the calibration curve to show the relationship between the obtained ratio values and the counting efficiency. This relation can be linearized. The obtained counts per minute (c.p.m.) can then easily be converted into disintegrations per minute (d.p.m.) from the following mathematical formula:

$$\text{d.p.m.} = (\text{c.p.m.} \times k)/(\text{ratio} - a)$$

where 'k' is the slope of the calibration curve for the scintillation counter and 'a' is the intercept with the ordinate. The instruments of today are usually equipped with both quench correction facilities and minicomputers for direct calculation of d.p.m. (see also Section 2.6). Our recommendation is to discuss the best method for quench correction with the manufacturer.

2.6 Mathematical handling of data

In the following, only analyses of the free fractions are discussed. The corresponding operations when calculating the bound fractions (supernatant after the use of DCC, or pellet after the use of PEG or double antibody) are in principle the same. However, the slope of the standard curve will then be the opposite to the one obtained when calculating the free fraction.

After the radioactivity contents of the standards have been measured, a standard curve is constructed. This standard curve is then used for calculating the eicosanoid content in the unknown samples. The following variables are used:

T = total radioactivity per tube in the assay (no addition of antibody; radioactivity in 'zero binding' tubes);

B_0 = maximal binding in d.p.m. (antibody present, but no addition of unlabelled eicosanoid; 'zero point' tubes);

B = d.p.m. of the various standard samples;

U = d.p.m. of the unknown samples.

The maximal binding of the labelled ligand is expressed as B_0/T. When selecting the optimal antibody working titre, most scientists prefer to have a maximal binding of around 50% of the radioactive tracer; thus, $B_0/T = 0.5$. The corresponding value for the standards (B/T) then gradually increases from 0.5 until finally total displacement of the bound radiolabelled compound is achieved when $B/T = 1$ or $B = T$.

The standard curve can be plotted in several ways, but the simplest graph is to plot B_0/T and B/T versus the log dose of the concentration of the standard. This graph is a sigmoid curve when drawn on semilogarithmic paper. The amount of eicosanoid in the unknown samples can be calculated from their corresponding U/T values. The construction of this sigmoid curve is always somewhat arbitrary, and the readings of the values for unknowns may be difficult. However, the advantage of the sigmoid curve is the high reliability in the low and high regions of the standard curve, compared with a linearized standard curve.

For automatic, computerized handling of the standards and unknowns — by far the most common method today — linearization of the curve must however be performed. The most convenient procedure for this operation is to make a logit transformation of $(B - B_0)/(T - B_0)$ $(=Y)$ versus $\log_e$ dose (or $\log_{10}$ dose) (28). This gives:

$$\text{logit } (Y) = \log_e Y/(1 - Y)$$

There is a linear correlation between logit (Y) and $\log_e$ dose:

$$\text{logit } (Y) = a_1 + k_1 (\log_e X)$$

where X = the amount of unlabelled eicosanoid in a standard tube, k_1 = slope of the line and a_1 = intercept with the ordinate.

For calculating RIA results, the logit values can conveniently be read from logit—log graph paper, or from tables of logit values. For a computerized handling of the data, a weighted or unweighted least-square regression analysis is done, and k_1 and a_1 are determined. This is the most common curve-fitting model used in the computer programs today (29,30). These programs are commercially available and fit several types of computers. Today several scintillation counters are equipped with microprocessors for calculations of d.p.m. and for automatic handling of this raw data, employing RIA programs to obtain the final results expressed as amounts of eicosanoids in the unknown samples.

3. VALIDATION OF THE EICOSANOID RADIOIMMUNOASSAY

In our opinion, the most important step in the development of an assay is the validation of the results obtained by the method. This is particularly important with RIA, since this type of method may, under certain conditions, be very non-specific. This fact is unfortunately sometimes overlooked, since it is often believed that the use of a highly specific antibody must also result in a highly specific method.

As was mentioned in Section 1, RIA is based on a competition between labelled and unlabelled molecules for antibody binding sites. The quantifiable process is inhibition of the binding of the tracer by the antibody. It must however be kept in mind that this binding may be inhibited by numerous factors or compounds, totally unrelated to the monitored substance. Such non-immunological inhibition will be discussed below

(Section 5). In this section, some methods and experiments will be described that may reveal the presence of such interfering substances.

First, the data obtained must be plausible. A considerable body of data, for example on prostaglandin and thromboxane biosynthesis and metabolism in the intact organism, has accumulated over the years, and the basal concentrations of certain compounds in blood, urine, tissues and other biological material may hence be calculated. If the RIA results obtained deviate from such expected levels, the reason may reside in the method. For example, so-called 'basal' plasma levels of primary prostaglandins, TXB_2 or 6-keto-$PGF_{1\alpha}$, obtained by RIA methods, have often been reported in a range of several hundred pg/ml. If true, such levels would indicate an endogenous prostaglandin or thromboxane biosynthesis associated with severe symptoms. Highly specific mass spectrometric methods have regularly shown that true circulating amounts of all the above mentioned compounds seldom exceed a few pg/ml plasma under normal conditions. Although falsely high values may be caused by other factors (such as uncontrolled biosynthesis of the compound during sample collection, see Chapters 2 and 3), and may thus also be obtained with g.c./m.s. methods, they are far more commonly seen with immunological methods.

Second, the results obtained must not vary with modifications in the method. Analysis of complex biological material frequently necessitates a purification process prior to the RIA step. It is often reported that alterations in the work-up procedure lead to changes in obtained results, which indicates removal (or, unfortunately, sometimes introduction) of interfering material, and necessitates caution in the interpretation of results.

Third, it is important that known, induced variations in the eicosanoid levels are accurately reflected in the final results from the RIA. The simplest experiment, which is a minimum requirement for the validation of an assay, is an addition experiment, where a regression line with a slope around 1.0 between added and measured amounts of the compound must be found. It is important furthermore that the added amounts are of the same order of magnitude as those expected in the biological system for which the RIA is intended. It is not uncommon unfortunately that relatively large amounts of the compound are used for this purpose: highly diluted samples are then analysed, and this dilution may reduce deceptively the deleterious influence of other sample components, which may thus escape detection, but will exert their full effect when the assay is used normally.

The monitored compound, or a precursor, should also be administered to the biological system under study, such as a perfused organ, a tissue homogenate, a cell culture or the entire organism. For compounds existing in the blood stream or excreted into urine, for example, registered levels should increase after administration of either the substance itself or a parent compound. A linear dose−response correlation may however not necessarily be expected, due to the complexity of the metabolizing systems involved.

The opposite study is perhaps even more important: the induction of decreases in the levels of the monitored compound by administration of an inhibitor of its biosynthesis. This must be done in *in vitro* as well as *in vivo* systems. Lack of a recorded decreasing effect of a well-known inhibitory drug, such as aspirin or indomethacin, should draw the attention to the possibility of serious sources of error in the RIA method. It is sometimes seen in the literature that such lack of an expected decrease − without any further investigation — is interpreted as due to an 'aspirin-resistant cyclo-oxygenase'.

It may however be difficult to perform appropriate inhibition experiments starting from basal levels of a compound, if it normally exists in amounts close to the detection limit of the assay. The inhibition experiment must then be designed in some other way. For example, if a previously registered increase in the monitored compound, seen after administration of a precursor, disappears when the system is pre-treated with a suitable inhibitor, then this is a good indicator of the validity of the assay.

However, even if the results from all the above mentioned studies are satisfactory, RIA data should always be interpreted with caution and preferably be backed up by other methods — if possible, by g.c./m.s. techniques. If such reference methods are not available, it is often possible to obtain qualitative and semi-quantitative information using isotope-labelled substances in the biological system under study. *In vitro* systems, such as cell cultures, should be studied, for instance with a radiolabelled precursor, to establish that the measured compound is really formed. It is often reported in the literature that a certain cell line produces specified prostaglandins or thromboxanes, based only on RIA measurements. In view of the inherent non-specificity of immunological methods, such statements may be somewhat unreliable.

4. COMMON PROBLEMS IN EICOSANOID RADIOIMMUNOASSAY

4.1 Instability of the target substance

One of the most common and important problems in eicosanoid assay concerns the possible degradation of the monitored compound. Naturally, this aspect is not specific for RIA but concerns all analytical methods. Breakdown of a product may be a metabolic phenomenon, and a stable metabolite may thus be preferable as target for measurements. This aspect was discussed in some detail in Chapter 2, and will not be further dealt with here.

Instead, a related problem will be addressed: the possible *chemical* instability of the monitored eicosanoid. Several of the eicosanoids are chemically unstable, some of them extremely so (TXA_2, PGI_2). For such compounds, assay methods requiring stability are naturally always aimed instead at stable decomposition products or derivatives. With compounds that are somewhat more stable, however, such as PGE_2 and PGD_2, attempts are often made to assay them as such. Several RIAs have been published for prostaglandins of the E type (see 2,4), and a few also for PGD_2 (31,32). Technical problems however limit their use (see ref. 4 and references therein). Both for PGEs and Ds, two types of degradative reactions take place, which are particularly pronounced in biological material such as plasma. One reaction is isomerization of the side chain alpha to the keto group (the carboxyl and methyl side chains in PGE and PGD, respectively) during enolization of this substituent. The second and more serious reaction is dehydration of the sensitive β-ketol group of the ring, leading to PGA or PGB compounds from PGEs, and to the analogous dehydration products of PGDs (33–35) (*Figure 3*). The chemical instability of particularly PGD compounds is rather pronounced, and a number of different degradation products rapidly appear (*Figure 3*). These reactions are catalysed by albumins (34,35), and thus, in all work with biological material, a partial decomposition of the unstable parent PGD should always be kept in mind.

Several of the decomposition products formed may be even more unstable than the

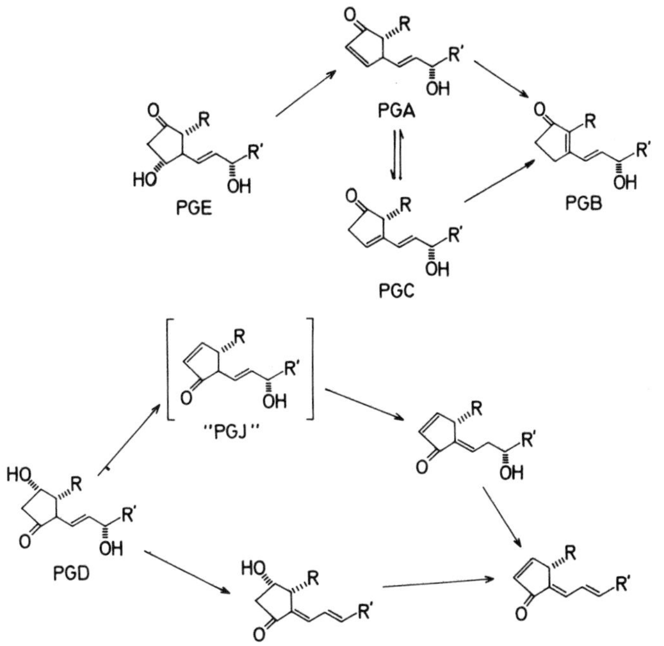

Figure 3. Degradation of prostaglandins of the E and D type in aqueous media. No convincing proof has as yet been provided for the initial formation of the compound designed PGJ; hence, it is shown within brackets (cf. ref. 67).

parent compound. This is the case for example with PGAs: the Δ^{10}-double bond formed is susceptible to nucleophilic attack at the activated C-11 (Michael addition; see 36). Various water-soluble conjugates with proteins, peptides and other compounds may thus be formed and escape detection by an eicosanoid assay.

Naturally, such chemical instability implies the same problems, regardless of the analytical method employed. It is discussed in this context for two reasons. First, degradation is often more pronounced in RIA. All RIAs are based on an incubation of the compound with the antibody in aqueous environment, and this incubation is often carried out in the presence of relatively large amounts of proteins (unextracted plasma or other biological material; carrier γ-globulins, etc.) during relatively long times, and sometimes even at elevated temperatures.

Second, when working with compounds susceptible to dehydration, it must be borne in mind that the immunogen — the eicosanoid coupled to a large carrier molecule — is usually prepared employing dehydrating conditions to facilitate peptide bond formation. This may explain the common finding that an antibody intended to recognize only PGEs often cross-reacts extensively also with the corresponding PGAs and PGBs (4).

There are several possible approaches to avoid problems caused by chemical instability of the target substance. Attempts are often made to minimize degradation by using short incubation times, low temperatures and a pH where the compound is more stable. If protein has to be present (such as carrier proteins for the precipitation step), it may be added immediately before, or together with, the precipitating agent. Such methods are often used successfully in RIAs for PGE compounds.

An entirely different, but also widely used solution to the problem is to quantitatively convert the unstable prostanoid into a stable derivative or degradation product, and then assay the compound in this form instead. PGEs have earlier been converted into PGBs by alkali treatment prior to RIA (37), or into PGFs by reduction with sodium borohydride (38). However, as mentioned, PGE is nowadays considered sufficiently stable for RIA as such, if proper precautions are taken.

The situation is somewhat different for certain PGE metabolites. If they retain the PGE ring structure, they, too, are susceptible to dehydration and may be more unstable than the parent compound (39,40). A major PGE_2 metabolite in the human circulation is 15-keto-13,14-dihydro-PGE_2 (41). This compound may form a bicyclic product after dehydration, 11-deoxy-13,14-dihydro-15-keto-11,16-cyclo-PGE_2 (see Figures 2 and 3 of Chapter 2), which has been found to be highly stable and suitable for monitoring. The compound is formed quantitatively in alkaline environment, and several RIAs have been developed for this product and are currently in use for monitoring PGE_2 production *in vivo* (42,43).

Corresponding β-oxidized metabolites of PGE compounds are found in the urine of many species (Chapter 2). A similar approach has been employed in immunological methods for 11α-hydroxy-9,15-diketo-2,3,4,5-tetranorprostane-1,20-dioic acid, a major urinary PGE metabolite in the human (41). This compound is converted into the corresponding bicyclic product by alkali treatment and can then be assayed by RIA or EIA (44).

So far, relatively few assays exist for PGD compounds, which may perhaps be explained by its instability. Recently, an RIA was developed against the stable O-methyl oxime (methoxime) derivative of the compound (45), an approach that has also been used for 6-keto-$PGF_{1\alpha}$ (46).

A different kind of chemical instability is the presence of several forms of a compound in equilibrium with each other. This phenomenon is known for many substances in this area, such as PGEs, PGDs (isomerization of the side chains, as mentioned above), tetranor PGF metabolites, 11-dehydro-TXBs, and many products of the 5-lipoxygenase pathway (δ-lactonization), 6-keto-$PGF_{1\alpha}$ (lactol formation). *Figure 4* shows some of these different forms of eicosanoids. Usually, the formation of these different forms occurs in aqueous media, and should thus be borne in mind particularly when RIA is employed. The phenomenon may be without significance for quantitation, either if the analytical method measures all forms of the compound in question with equal accuracy, or if the conditions of the assay procedure lead to the formation of mainly one of the forms. Under other circumstances, however, the phenomenon may give rise to serious errors, particularly if the procedure requires a purification step where the different forms separate and one or more may be lost.

4.2 Problems related to the preparation of the immunogen

As mentioned in Section 4.1, coupling of the hapten to a carrier normally takes place under dehydrating conditions, which may lead to degradation of a susceptible molecule. In addition to this problem, other difficulties may arise at this step.

Certain compounds with a hydroxyl group delta to a carboxyl are prone to δ-lacton-

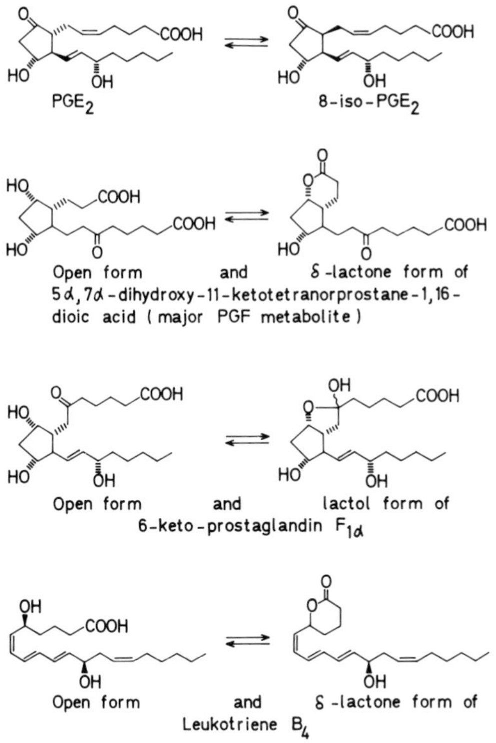

Figure 4. Occurrence of different chemical forms of some eicosanoids in equilibrium in aqueous media.

ization, which is also favoured by dehydrating conditions. If the carboxyl group is the only one in the molecule, as is the case in 5-HETE, LTB$_4$ and other related substances (*Figure 4*), coupling to the carrier protein may thus be inhibited extensively and the yield of the conjugate insufficient. This is likely to be the reason for the paucity of published RIAs for such compounds, for example LTB$_4$ (47−50).

To solve this problem, several approaches have been tried. Blocking the 5-hydroxyl group by derivatization (for example by acetylation) is one possibility, but is difficult to achieve without simultaneous induction of the lactonization one wishes to avoid. Derivatization of the carboxyl into some other form which is still possible to conjugate to a protein is another possibility, for example conversion into a hydrazide (51). The best solution is probably the introduction of a spacer arm, which increases the distance between the 5-hydroxyl and the carboxyl and prevents lactonization. Such approaches were recently described, and two different conjugates of LTB$_4$ with BSA or KLH were prepared, employing 1,3-diaminopropane and 6-N-maleimidohexanoic acid as spacers, respectively (51). Another immunogen was prepared by conjugating lysine amino groups of BSA to the 12-oxy function of LTB$_4$ (49).

With certain other compounds, however, this side effect of δ-lactonization during coupling may be an advantage (see below).

A different problem arises when the hapten contains several carboxyl groups. Ex-

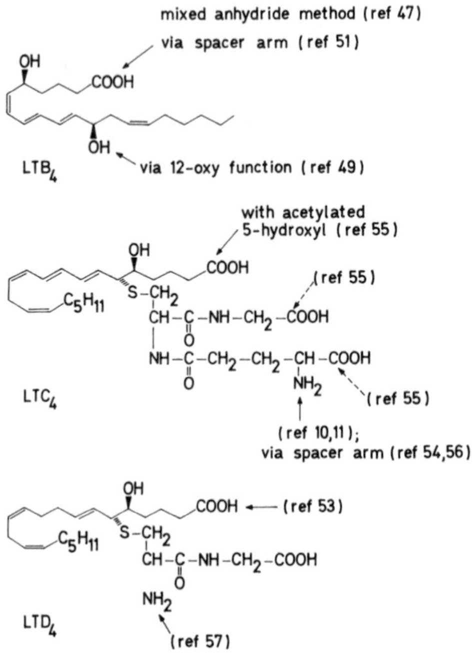

Figure 5. Structures of leukotrienes B$_4$, C$_4$ and D$_4$ and some immunogenic conjugates of these compounds prepared by different methods (refs. 10, 11, 47−51, 53−58).

amples of such compounds are the ω-oxidized, dicarboxylic degradation products of prostanoids, which often dominate the urinary profile of metabolites. Other such compounds are the cysteinyl-containing leukotrienes (*Figure 5*). Although it is possible that one carboxyl may be more reactive than the other(s) in such compounds, it is by no means certain that the desired, homogeneous conjugate would result. Coupling at random at either carboxyl should be avoided, since it would yield a mixture of antibodies with different specificities.

Various solutions to this problem have been tried for different compounds. Antibodies against the tetranor-PGF metabolites were raised against a conjugate prepared by coupling exclusively at the ω-carboxyl (52). To achieve this, advantage was taken of the facile δ-lactonization at the alpha end of the molecule, which could be induced by prior acid treatment, but which also occurred spontaneously during coupling: the problem, thus, in fact solved itself.

However, this approach could not be applied to the analogous PGE metabolite, which has a keto group as the corresponding ring substituent and thus cannot form a δ-lactone. A similar conjugate, coupled at the ω-end, was instead prepared using a synthetic monomethyl ester of the metabolite as starting material (44).

A major circulating as well as urinary metabolite of TXB$_2$ was recently shown to be 11-dehydro-TXB$_2$ (Chapter 2). Dehydrogenation at C-11 converts the thromboxane ring into a carboxylic side chain, and the compound is actually a dioic acid. Conjugation to a protein carrier might thus theoretically take place at either the C-1 or the

C-11 carboxyl; however, the compound is not likely to exist in the acyclic form during coupling, for the same reason as above.

The cysteinyl-containing leukotrienes, LTC_4, D_4 and E_4, contain three, two and two carboxyls, respectively (*Figure 5*). Antibodies against immunogenic conjugates of these compounds have been raised in different laboratories (10,11,48,53–58). None of these have taken advantage of the δ-lactonization to block the eicosanoid carboxyl but instead used other approaches. In some cases, the free *amino* group of the leukotriene was coupled to amino groups on the protein, using either glutaraldehyde (10), dimethyl-pimelindiimidate (11), or 1,5-difluoro-2,4-dinitrobenzene (54,57) as coupling reagent. A different approach employed 6-N-maleimidohexanoic acid (54,56): in those cases, the amino group of the leukotriene was coupled to thiol groups on the protein. The latter two techniques also lead to the introduction of a spacer arm. A conjugate between BSA and LTD_4 (or presumably 11-*trans*-LTD_4) was prepared synthetically with the eicosanoid carboxyl coupled to the protein: the glycine carboxyl was esterified during the procedure (53). Another immunogenic conjugate (55) was prepared using the common procedure (with the eicosanoid carboxyl coupled to protein amino groups). No particular precautions were however taken to induce coupling preferentially at one of the three carboxyls; instead the leukotriene was first subjected to acetylation, which may have prevented lactonization.

The resulting antibodies against these different leukotriene conjugates displayed somewhat differing specificities for the various cysteinyl-containing compounds. In general, specificities were rather low, at least in comparison with prostaglandin and thromboxane antibodies. The most specific antiserum against LTC_4 was obtained by Wynalda *et al.* (58), who used a slightly different method: instead of using the natural hapten, they employed synthetic hexahydro-7-*cis*-LTC_4, which was presumably resistant to metabolic degradation in the antibody-producing animal.

4.3 Problems related to the preparation of tracer

As was mentioned above, many multiply tritium-labelled eicosanoids are commercially available. Their specific activities are often over 100–150 Ci/mmol, which renders them suitable for RIA purposes.

When the monitored compound is not available, it may have to be prepared in the scientist's own laboratory. Total chemical syntheses of these complex molecules is normally beyond the capacity of most laboratories, and the average scientist has to resort to biosynthetic methods, employing a biological system and a tritium-labelled precursor.

Two different problems may then arise. First, the compound may be formed in large amounts by the biological system employed, resulting in a considerable dilution with endogenous material and, consequently, an unacceptably low specific activity. Sometimes it may be possible to prevent this dilution by including an inhibitor of an early enzymatic step in the pathway in question, and employing a labelled precursor distal to that step. For example, $[^3H_8]TXB_2$ may be prepared by incubating platelets with $[^3H_8]$-arachidonic acid, but the specific activity may not be sufficiently high for use in RIA. A better preparation of $[^3H_8]TXB_2$ may instead be obtained in high yield from $[^3H_8]$-PGH_2 incubated with aspirin-treated platelets. Another example is the preparation *in vivo* of urinary prostaglandin F metabolites, which can be successfully achieved in indomethacin-pre-treated volunteers receiving injections of $[^3H_7]PGF_{2\alpha}$ (52). In both these cases, the endogenous dilution was kept at a minimum by inhibition of the cyclo-oxygenase step.

The second difficulty is encountered in the leukotriene field. Very few biological systems are known that can produce leukotrienes in acceptable amounts, such as chopped guinea-pig lungs or leukocytes of different types and species. It has however been found that some of these systems do not readily accept exogenous substrate but instead convert mainly the endogenous precursor fatty acid. Addition of $[^3H_8]$arachidonic acid to such a system thus results in the formation of the desired compounds only in very low yield and with unacceptably low specific activities − even though conversion of the endogenous precursor acid is high.

The endogenous contribution may be minimized by employing a purified enzyme system. For example, the undesired release of endogenous arachidonate metabolites from platelets during $[^3H_8]TXB_2$ preparation may be avoided by the use of a purified thromboxane synthetase (59). Similarly, the yield of tritium-labelled products of the 5-lipoxygenase pathway might be improved by using the purified 5-lipoxygenase instead of intact cells or tissues (60). Another possibility is to by-pass the critical step(s) and to start the preparation of more 'distal' products using, for example, commercially available $[^3H]LTA_4$ as starting material. It should be pointed out, however, that most available leukotrienes are only labelled with tritium in the 14 and 15 positions, and thus their specific activity is rather low (20−60 Ci/mmol). The only exception to this so far is LTB_4, which can be obtained octa-tritiated.

If it is impossible for some reason to prepare the proper tracer with sufficiently high specific activity, other alternatives may be tried. A possible solution to the problem is to use a heterologous tracer. The first example of the use of such tracers was when prostaglandins of the 1-series were employed as tracers in RIAs for compounds of the 2-series. The Δ^5-double bond had then been reduced with tritium gas (i.e. the compounds were $5,6-^3H_2$-labelled) (6). A different approach is often used successfully today: the monitored eicosanoid is coupled at the carboxyl to an amino acid, an amine, or some similar compound that can be iodinated using ^{125}I (61). Such tracers can be prepared with extremely high specific activities, around 2000 Ci/mmol, which may render the assay extremely sensitive. The antibody usually accepts such a compound readily as a ligand, since it has distinct similarities with the immunogen used to produce the antibody. Success in the assay may however also depend on whether the 'proper' ligand can displace this heterologous ligand from the antibody binding sites. This is not always readily done (61).

There are however certain draw-backs with the use of ^{125}I-labelled tracers in RIA. Due to the short half-life of this isotope, preparation of the tracer may have to be done with short intervals. Furthermore, because of the high energy of γ-radiation, it is not advisable to use radioiodine in a laboratory where work with small amounts of β-emitters is simultaneously going on. The toxicity of γ-emitters should also be borne in mind.

An alternative approach is possible: instead of introducing a substituent that can be labelled with radioiodine, the unlabelled prostanoid can be coupled to a compound that is already labelled with tritium. Suitable compounds for this purpose are tritium-labelled

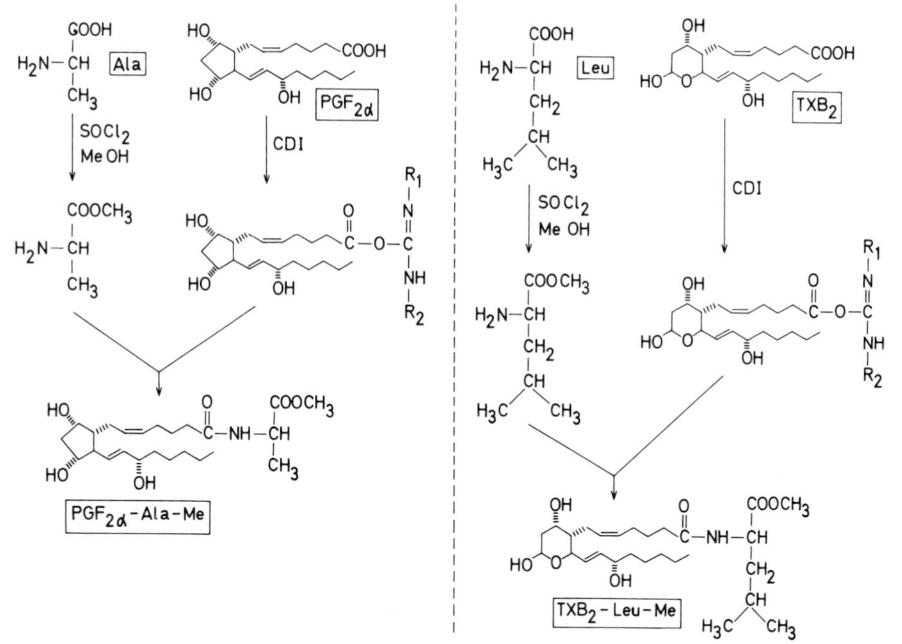

Figure 6. Preparation and structures of tritium-labelled amino acid−prostanoid conjugates for use as heterologous tracers in RIA.

amino acids, which can be obtained with high specific activities. Conjugation is done in the usual way between the eicosanoid carboxyl and the amino group of the amino acid (62). *Figure 6* shows two examples of such tracers. Leucine was found to be a particularly good substitutent: this amino acid can be obtained labelled with tritium in the 3, 4 and 5 position, and the specific activity is then over 140 Ci/mmol (62).

4.4 Deterioration of assay performance with time

A distinct disadvantage with an extensive automatization of the RIA is that the scientist may not detect an insiduously developing deterioration of the assay. This is particularly the case when data are obtained directly on-line during the final counting of radioactivity. Several factors must be kept in firm control, which pertain to the RIA itself, and not to the quality or processing of the samples (see below, Section 5).

As was mentioned above (Section 2.6), most researchers working with RIA prefer to employ conditions giving B_0/T values of about 0.5, since this usually gives the best balance between precision and sensitivity. This is represented by curve A in *Figure 7*. One of these factors can be increased, but only at the expense of the other (see also *Figure 1*). However, even when the optimal conditions have been satisfactorily established, the assay usually begins to deteriorate after some time. Usually, the antibody binding of the tracer decreases, giving gradually higher radioactivity values in the free fraction: in our example above thus increasing the B_0 values (panel B in *Figure 7*). Since T remains constant, the effect is a more shallow slope of the standard curve,

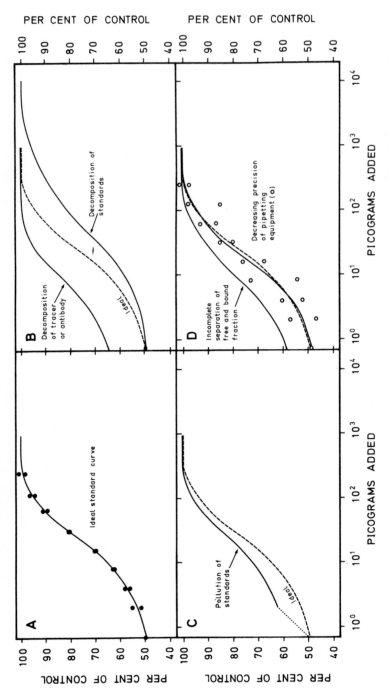

Figure 7. Some examples of malfunction in radioimmunoassays (standard curves), caused by aging of reagents or equipment. **Panel A** shows the standard curve obtained under optimal conditions, and the same curve is inserted also in the other panels (broken line). **Panel B** shows the effect of decomposition of tracer and standards, respectively. **Panel C** shows the effect of contamination of a set of standards, exposed to frequent pipetting with plastic tips (the standards were used ~ 50 times). **Panel D** shows the effects of wear and tear of pipetting equipment. The scattered data of the lower curve indicate that the former 'high precision' pipette no longer deserves this designation. The upper of the two curves shows the effect of incomplete separation of antibody-bound and free fraction, in this case caused by an undetected leakage of the precipitating reagent (PEG) from a Cornwall syringe with an old refill unit.

similar to the shape obtained with a higher antibody dilution (see *Figure 1*).

One of the most common causes of such decreased ligand binding is decomposition of the compound. Chemical decomposition (Section 4.1) is often enhanced in dilute solutions, such as are commonly used in standard and tracer preparations. In the latter case, internal radiation damage further adds to the problem.

Many scientists prefer to prepare fresh solutions every day to minimize this problem. This may however substantially increase the cost of the assay, and may thus not be possible for everybody. Furthermore, if fresh solutions of all reagents are prepared for every assay, the inter-assay variation inevitably increases. In addition, decomposition of the assayed compound may often occur even in stock solutions, which is sometimes overlooked, and for tracers the radiation damage is, in fact, more pronounced in concentrated solutions than in dilute ones.

It is, however, obviously of utmost importance to establish whether the monitored compound is chemically stable under the storage and assay conditions employed. In our experience, PGFs and most PGF metabolites, TXB_2 and 11-dehydro-TXB_2, and the bicyclic degradation product of 15-keto-13,14-dihydro-PGE_2 are all sufficiently stable to be kept and used even in dilute solutions for at least several weeks. Radiation damage of tracers should be checked regularly, for example by a simple extraction and/or a chromatographic step. Most such degradation products are highly polar and will then remain in the aqueous phase.

A rather deceptive situation occurs if the tracer preparation is of recent date — and thus the B_0/T value is satisfactory — whereas a certain decomposition of the standards may have occurred. This is seen as a shift to the right of the standard curve (panel B in *Figure 7*), that is, larger nominal amounts of the standard have to be added before displacement of the tracer takes place. Assayed biological samples will then give values somewhat higher than the actual ones.

If the same set of standard dilutions is used in several RIAs, the possible contamination of these solutions must also be kept in mind. Impurities may, for example, be introduced from the plastic tips of the pipettes, and if the whole series of standards is similarly affected, this source of error may be difficult to detect. The slope and shape of the standard curve remain essentially 'normal', although it is slightly shifted to the left (panel C in *Figure 7*). The effect of such a pollution is that biological samples then tend to give lower values — which is generally welcomed by the scientist, who may believe he has managed to improve his assay (most sources of error tend to give too high values in RIA). The simplest way to detect such contamination is to include 'zero standards' in the standard curves: that is, a buffer solution of the same age and exposed to the same number of pipettings as the standards. There should not be any difference between the radioactivity values from those 'zeros' and from the maximal binding tubes (B_0). Any contamination of the standards will immediately be seen as a difference beteen those two sets of B_0 tubes, and as a 'jump' at the low end of the curve (panel C, *Figure 7*).

Antibodies are usually quite stable and may be stored frozen for many years. Working dilutions are usually kept in the refrigerator and are, in our experience, also sufficiently stable for normal use (at least several months). However, decomposition of such preparations is occasionally seen. A possible explanation is the presence of proteases in the immunized animal's blood. If degradation of the antibody occurs, the situation will naturally be exactly the same as if a more diluted antibody solution was used (see *Figure 1*: with this condition, an increased B_0 value and a more shallow slope of the standard curve are seen.

It should be mentioned in this context that scientists using only commercial RIA kits normally do not encounter any of these difficulties, since the material supplied in the kits is usually only sufficient for a small number of assays. This may seem to be an advantage; however, it must be pointed out that the material is also insufficient for optimization of the method. We strongly recommend each scientist in this area to set up his/her own assay, and to maintain the method at optimal conditions by keeping a sharp look-out for the above mentioned phenomena.

A different problem concerns the equipment employed. Naturally, high precision pipettes should be used at all steps; however, such utensils are not immune to aging. The inevitable consequence is loss of precision, which can be detected as increased scattering of data, most easily seen from the duplicates or triplicates of the standard curve (panel D, *Figure 7*).

A convenient method to evaluate the precision of the equipment, once the method is established, is to calculate the so-called 'goodness of fit' for the set of standards. Each point is then calculated back against the standard curve. One or two deviating B/T values may be regarded as technical mistakes and deleted from the standard curve. However, if the whole set of standards has a high coefficient of variation (scattered data, panel D, *Figure 7*), something must be wrong and the error sought.

Another possibility is to calculate the intra-assay coefficient of variation for sample pools (with low and high concentrations) as well as from replicate measurements. If the intra-assay coefficient of variation is high, a careful control of the equipment should be done.

The last curve shown in panel D, *Figure 7*, is similar to the curve obtained with a high dilution of the antibody (*Figure 1* (or a degraded antibody), or the one seen with a partially degraded tracer preparation (panel B, *Figure 7*). In the experiment shown in panel D, however, the reason was a different one: the precipitation of the antibody-bound fraction was incomplete, due to leakage from an old automatic pipette used for the addition of PEG. The same artifact may be seen if the temperature is somewhat too high at this step, or if the amount of added carrier γ-globulin is insufficient. This type of shift of the standard curve is thus a rather common one and can obviously have many causes. The inexperienced assayist may be tempted to compensate for the decreased binding of the tracer (B_0) by using a more concentrated antibody solution. We do not recommend such arbitrary modifications of the method: instead, the source of error should be identified and the appropriate measures taken.

5. MAJOR SOURCES OF ERROR IN EICOSANOID RADIOIMMUNOASSAY

Ever since this methodology was introduced in the eicosanoid field some 15 years ago, there has been considerable controversy concerning the reliability of RIA results (reviews, 6,63). In general, so called 'basal' eicosanoid biosynthesis in many biological systems tends to be overestimated, when based on RIA data, and sometimes even far too high to be compatible with the healthy organism. This has often been found in blood, urine or tissue analyses, as well as in assays of other biological materials. The development and increasing use of highly specific g.c./m.s. methods, which give levels only fractions of those of RIA, however focused the attention on these discrepancies and gradually convinced many scientists in this field. Thus, RIA data are nowadays often carefully reported as 'immunoreactive PG' ('iPG') or 'PG-like immunoreactivity', instead of specifically stating absolute levels of a certain compound.

Cross-reactions with structurally related eicosanoids may no doubt contribute to an unrealistically high measured level of a compound. In particular, this may pertain to attempts to measure very small amounts of a compound that occurs together with other eicosanoids of far higher concentrations (for example, primary prostaglandins in human urine are found in amounts of a few hundred nanograms in 24 h, whereas several tens of micrograms, or even more, of their β-oxidized metabolites are excreted in the same time).

However, true cross-reactions of this kind probably cannot explain more than a minor part of the falsely high RIA values obtained in, for example, blood plasma, where no eicosanoid seems to exist in any higher amounts. Other explanations must be sought. In this context it must be emphasized, that all that RIA does is to give information about *the extent of inhibition of the binding between the antibody and the labelled ligand*. This inhibition can be brought about by true displacement of the tracer: by the 'proper' unlabelled substance or a structurally related compound. This is a genuine immunological inhibition of the tracer binding. However, also *non-immunological* inhibition of this binding can occur. Such inhibition may be caused by totally unrelated factors, such as variations in protein concentration, ionic strength, pH, the presence of impurities, and so on. A well-known inhibitor of antigen – antibody binding in general is, for example, heparin, although the nature of this interaction remains obscure.

It should perhaps also be mentioned here that all scientists working with eicosanoid RIA do not accept these two concepts of immunological versus non-immunological inhibition of the antigen – antibody binding. In our opinion, however, it is useful to separate the two phenomena: we find them somewhat similar to the competitive and non-competitive types of enzyme inhibition.

The non-immunological inhibition − whether this is the correct designation or not − is a particularly serious source of error for several reasons: it is very common, it may be very pronounced and many scientists are not even aware of it.

Since the assayist hopefully has complete control over the quality of the RIA reagents, some of these interfering factors must originate in the biological samples. Obviously, a complex biological material may contain a multitude of interfering compounds. Prior purification of the sample could thus be expected to eliminate this problem. Unfortunately, however, processing of the samples may introduce more problems than it solves. The matter of whether − and how − biological samples should be processed prior to RIA is in fact an often debated issue, and there is still considerable controversy over this point.

There are many advantages with a direct RIA, applied to unextracted samples (for example, blood plasma).

(i)   The simplicity of the method gives a high sample capacity.

(ii)   The reproducibility is high: when analysing a series of blood samples taken from the same subject, essentially identical assay conditions are thus obtained in all samples, and registered differences in the levels of the monitored compound are likely to reflect true fluctuations.

(iii)   Without extraction and purification, there are no problems with estimation of and variations in recovery (see below).

(iv)   One advantage which is more seldom recognized is that the presence of albumin may exert a beneficial effect on the assay, and thus, lipophilic extraction of blood samples, which removes albumin, may give highly erroneous results (63,64). A likely explanation is the release of large amounts of albumin-bound lipophilic substances, which may occur in concentrations several orders of magnitude higher than those of the eicosanoids, such as free fatty acids. Addition of an albumin solution to albumin-free samples may in fact greatly improve the assay accuracy (63,64). The deleterious effect of albumin on certain unstable eicosanoids should however also be kept in mind (see above, Section 4.1).

Unfortunately, there are however also a number of draw-backs with direct RIA of unextracted samples, in addition to the possible cross-reactions with related compounds discussed above. Direct RIA of urinary samples, in contrast to blood, may imply large differences in assay conditions, since diuresis may vary over a wide range with large variations in ionic strength, excretion of eicosanoids and numerous other factors as a consequence. Even a series of urinary samples taken from the same subject usually displays these fluctuations. Since antibodies may be very sensitive to such variations, the final results from a series of samples may show large differences, which are then only illusory.

Furthermore, if the monitored compound occurs in very low amounts, below the detection limit of the assay, direct RIA is not possible. The samples must then at least be concentrated.

A peculiar phenomenon encountered with some antibodies is an *enhancement* of the antigen−antibody binding in the presence of unextracted plasma and also some other complex biological materials. The explanation is unknown: it is not caused by non-specific binding of the ligand by the plasma but occurs only as a synergism between the antibody and some component(s) in the assayed sample (6,23). The phenomenon is seen even with very small amounts of plasma, as little as a few nanolitres. This synergism is usually maximal in the presence of as little as $1-2$ μl of unextracted plasma, and the binding of the tracer may then be increased by as much as 10%. If the assay is not tested with such small amounts (most scientists work with direct RIA assay plasma volumes of around $50-100$ μl or more), this very serious source of error may go un-noticed. The result is that all U/T values decrease, and may even fall below the standard curve. The presence of such interfering factor(s) thus completely precludes the assay of unextracted samples. There are two possible solutions to this problem: either the biological samples must be extracted and purified (see below), or a small amount of a plasma pool ($1-2$ μl) is added to all tubes, including the standards.

Many scientists are thus in favour of purification of RIA samples. The earliest pro-cedures usually consisted of solvent extraction, followed by some relatively crude chromatographic step, which gave at least group separation of the eicosanoids. Such measures should have eliminated some of the cross-reacting substances; however, unexpectedly, measured levels were often considerably above those of direct assay (6). Part of the explanation may be the above-mentioned stripping of interfering material from albumin. Further contributions were no doubt provided by the procedure itself (6,63,65): from solvents, column material, plastic tubing, gas tanks, etc. Extraction, chromatography, pooling of chromatographic fractions and evaporation of the solvent under a gas stream is a very common procedure in eicosanoid RIA, but the contribution of interfering material from the procedure employed is unfortunately rarely checked.

The identities of such introduced impurities are generally unknown. A few substances are however known to interfere. For example, a resin often used for extraction of eicosanoids, Amberlite XAD-2, has long been recognized as a highly interfering substance (6,65), and this method thus cannot be employed in RIA. Another substance with similar effects is the ubiquitous bis(2-ethyl-hexyl)phthalate ('dioctylphthalate'), which unfortunately is a component of many materials commonly used in a laboratory.

The use of modern h.p.l.c. techniques for purification of RIA samples has improved the situation considerably, first, because of the higher quality of stationary phases and solvents, and second, because the monitored compound is often eluted in a very small volume. However, RIA results even from such procedures cannot automatically be trusted, and what is often called 'immunoreactive material' may be detected in many fractions other than the expected one(s).

The sensitivity of different antibody preparations to such influence of impurities may vary greatly (66). It could thus be worthwhile to devote some effort to finding an antibody less susceptible to such non-immunological interference. Unfortunately this is seldom done. Commercial preparations are manufactured with detailed information about cross-reactions with structurally related compounds. That the antibody may also be inhibited by totally unrelated factors to an extent that virtually precludes the use of the assay is however seldom mentioned.

Another difficulty with purified RIA samples concerns the recovery of the monitored compound. First, it may be quite variable, particularly if the compound exists in different chemical forms with different physico-chemical properties (Section 4.1; *Figure 4*). Second, a small amount of the labelled compound must be added to the sample for estimation of recovery, and this will naturally influence the final RIA results. It is sometimes argued that addition of a different compound with similar properties but which is not bound by the antibody would be a safer method; however, there would still be the extra added radioactivity to consider, and even closely related compounds may have entirely different chromatographic properties [for example, TXB_2 is not a suitable tracer during purification of its metabolite, 11-dehydro-TXB_2 (23)].

Thus, there is no universal answer to the problem of the best treatment of RIA samples. We would like to draw attention to the fact that biological samples − processed or not − can never be assayed under exactly the same conditions as the standards. Addition of biological material to the standards in order to mimic the samples may improve the situation but does not guarantee identical conditions. The best thing we can recommend is that the scientist using RIA is aware of the possibility that a certain or even a major part of the inhibition of the antibody−tracer binding may be caused by factors other than the assayed substance. RIA is always an uncertain method for measuring *absolute* amounts of a compound. The great value of the method is that it provides a simple tool for detecting *changes* in the levels of the monitored compound during physiological or pathological events.

6. ACKNOWLEDGEMENTS

Supported in part by a grant from the Swedish Medical Research Council (project no. 03X-05915).

7. REFERENCES

1. Lieberman,S., Erlanger,B.F., Beiser,S.M. and Agate,F.J.,Jr. (1959) *Recent Prog. Hormone Res.*, **15**, 165.
2. Dray,F., Charbonnel,B. and Maclouf,J. (1975) *Eur. J. Clin. Invest.*; **5**, 311.
3. Caldwell,B., Burstein,S., Brock,W. and Speroff,L. (1971) *J. Clin. Endocrinol. Metab.*, **33**, 171.
4. Dray,F., Mamas,S. and Bizzini,B. (1982) In *Methods in Enzymology*. Lands,W.E.M. and Smith,W.L. (eds), Academic Press, New York, Vol. 86, p. 258.
5. Axen,U. (1974) *Prostaglandins*, **5**, 45.
6. Granström,E. and Kindahl,H. (1978) *Adv. Prostaglandin Thromboxane Res.*, **5**, 119.
7. Kirton,K.T., Cornette,J.C. and Barr,K.L. (1972) *Biochem. Biophys. Res. Commun.*, **47**, 903.
8. Anderson,G.W., Zimmerman,J.E. and Callahan,F.M. (1964) *J. Am. Chem. Soc.*, **86**, 1839.
9. Pradelles,P., Grassi,J. and Maclouf,J. (1985) *Anal. Chem.*, **57**, 1170.
10. Aehringhaus,U., Wölbling,R.H., König,W., Patrono,C., Peskar,B.M. and Peskar,B.A. (1982) *FEBS Lett.*, **146**, 111.
11. Peskar,B.A., Hoppe,U., Simmet,T. and Peskar,B.M. (1986) *Proceedings, INSERM-NATO Advanced Workshop: Biology of Icosanoids and Related Substances in Blood and Vascular Cells.* Lagarde,M. (ed.) INSERM Symposium, Lyon, France.
12. Köhler,G. and Milstein,C. (1975) *Nature*, **256**, 495.
13. David,F., Somme,G., Provost-Wisner,A., Theze,J. and Dray,F. (1985) *Adv. Prostaglandin Thromboxane Leukotriene Res.*, **15**, 23.
14. Tanaka,T., Ito,S., Hiroshima,O., Hayashi,H. and Hayaishi,O. (1985) *Biochim. Biophys. Acta*, **836**, 125.
15. Lee,J.Y., Chernov,T. and Goetzl,E.J. (1984) *Biochem. Biophys. Res. Commun.*, **123**, 944.
16. DeWitt,D.L., Day,J.S., Gauger,J.A. and Smith,W.L. (1982) In *Methods in Enzymology*. Lands,W.E.M. and Smith,W.L. (eds), Academic Press, New York, Vol. 86, p. 229.
17. Hamberg,M., Svensson,J. and Samuelsson,B. (1975) *Proc. Natl. Acad. Sci. USA*, **72**, 2994.
18. Moonen,P., Klok,G. and Keirse,M.J.N.C. (1983) *Prostaglandins*, **26**, 797.
19. Scatchard,G. (1949) *Ann. N.Y. Acad. Sci.*, **51**, 660.
20. Ciabattoni,G., Maclouf,J., Catella,F., FitzGerald,G.A. and Patrono,C. (1987) *Biochim. Biophys. Acta*, in press.
21. Roberts,L.J.,II, Sweetman,B.J. and Oates,J.A. (1981) *J. Biol. Chem.*, **256**, 8384.
22. Westlund,P., Kumlin,M., Nordenström,A. and Granström,E. (1986) *Prostaglandins*, **31**, 413.
23. Kumlin,M. and Granström,E. (1986) *Prostaglandins*, **32**, 741.
24. Granström,E., Diczfalusy,U. and Hamberg,M. (1983) In *Prostaglandins and Related Substances*. Pace-Asciak,C.R. and Granström,E. (eds), New Comprehensive Biochemistry, Elsevier Science Publishers, Amsterdam, Vol. 5, p. 45.
25. Desbuquois,B. and Aurbach,G. (1971) *J. Clin. Endocrinol.*, **33**, 732.
26. Kirkham,K. and Hunter,W., eds (1971) *Radioimmunoassay Methods*. Churchill Livingstone, Edinburgh.
27. Fitzpatrick,F.A. and Wynalda,M.A. (1976) *Anal. Biochem.*, **73**, 198.
28. Rodbard,D., Bridson,W. and Rayford,P. (1969) *J. Lab. Clin. Med.*, **74**, 770.
29. Davis,S.E., Munson,P.J., Jaffe,M.L. and Rodbard,D. (1980) *J. Immunoassay*, **1**, 15.
30. Murata,A., Ogawa,M., Matsuda,K., Kitahara,T., Nishibe,S., Kurokawa,E. and Kosaki,G. (1983) *J. Immunoassay*, **4**, 407.
31. Anhut,H., Peskar,B.A., Wachter,W., Gräbling,B. and Peskar,B.M. (1978) *Experientia*, **34**, 1494.
32. Narumiya,S., Ogorochi,T., Nakao,K. and Hayaishi,O. (1982) *Life Sci.*, **31**, 2093.
33. Stehle,R.G. (1982) In *Methods in Enzymology*. Lands,W.E.M. and Smith,W.L. (eds), Academic Press, New York, Vol. 86, p. 436.
34. Fitzpatrick,F.A. and Wynalda,M.A. (1983) *J. Biol. Chem.*, **258**, 11713.
35. Kikawa,Y., Narumiya,S., Fukushima,M., Wakatsuka,H. and Hayaishi,O. (1984) *Proc. Natl. Acad. Sci. USA*, **81**, 1317.
36. Cagen,L., Pisano,J., Ketley,J., Habig,W. and Jakoby,W. (1975) *Biochim. Biophys. Acta*, **398**, 205.

37. Levine,L., Gutierrez Cernosek,R.M. and Van Vunakis,H. (1971) *J. Biol. Chem.*, **246**, 6782.
38. Lindgren,J.Å., Kindahl,H. and Hammarström,S. (1974) *FEBS Lett.*, **48**, 22.
39. Fitzpatrick,F.A., Aguirre,R., Pike,J.E. and Lincoln,F.H. (1980) *Prostaglandins*, **19**, 917.
40. Granström,E., Hamberg,M., Hansson,G. and Kindahl,H. (1980) *Prostaglandins*, **19**, 933.
41. Hamberg,M. and Samuelsson,B. (1971) *J. Biol. Chem.*, **246**, 6713.
42. Granström,E., Fitzpatrick,F.A. and Kindahl,H. (1982) In *Methods in Enzymology*. Lands,W.E.M. and Smith,W.L. (eds), Academic Press, New York, Vol. 86, p. 306.
43. Starczewski,M., Voigtmann,R., Peskar,B.A. and Peskar,B.M. (1984) *Prostaglandins Leukotrienes Med.*, **13**, 249.
44. Inagawa,T., Imai,K., Masuda,K., Morikawa,Y., Hirata,F. and Tsuboshima,M. (1983) *Adv. Prostaglandin Thromboxane Leukotriene Res.*, **11**, 196.
45. Maclouf,J., Corvazier,E. and Wang,Z. (1986) *Prostaglandins*, **31**, 123.
46. Oliw,E. (1980) *Prostaglandins*, **19**, 271.
47. Salmon,J.A., Simmons,P.M. and Palmer,R.M.J. (1982) *Prostaglandins*, **24**, 225.
48. Rokach,J., Hayes,E.C., Girard,Y., Lombardo,D.L., Maycock,A.L., Rosenthal,A.S., Young,R.N., Zamboni,R. and Zweerink,H.J. (1984) *Prostaglandins Leukotrienes Med.*, **13**, 21.
49. Lewis,R.A., Mencia-Huerta,J.-M., Soberman,R.J., Hoover,D., Marfat,A., Corey,E.J. and Austen,K.F. (1982) *Proc. Natl. Acad. Sci. USA*, **79**, 7904.
50. Phillips,M.J., Gold,W.M. and Goetzl,E.J. (1983) *J. Immunol.*, **131**, 906.
51. Young,R.N., Zamboni,R. and Rokach,J. (1983) *Prostaglandins*, **26**, 605.
52. Granström,E. and Kindahl,H. (1976) *Prostaglandins*, **12**, 759.
53. Levine,L., Morgan,R.A., Lewis,R.A., Austen,K.F., Clark,D.A., Marfat,A. and Corey,E.J. (1981) *Proc. Natl. Acad. Sci. USA*, **78**, 7692.
54. Young,R.N., Kakushima,M. and Rokach,J. (1982) *Prostaglandins*, **23**, 603.
55. Lindgren,J.-Å., Hammarström,S. and Goetzl,E.J. (1983) *FEBS Lett.*, **152**, 83.
56. Hayes,E.C., Lombardo,D.L., Girard,Y., Maycock,A.L., Rokach,J., Rosenthal,A.S., Young,R.N., Egan,R.W. and Zweerink,H.J. (1983) *J. Immunol.*, **131**, 429.
57. Aharony,D., Dobson,P., Bernstein,P.R., Kusner,E.J., Krell,R.D. and Smith,J.B. (1983) *Biochem. Biophys. Res. Commun.*, **117**, 574.
58. Wynalda,M.A., Brashler,J.R., Bach,M.K., Morton,D.R. and Fitzpatrick,F.A. (1984) *Anal. Chem.*, **56**, 1862.
59. Hammarström,S. and Falardeau,P. (1977) *Proc. Natl. Acad. Sci. USA*, **74**, 3691.
60. Rouzer,C. and Samuelsson,B. (1986) *Proc. Natl. Acad. Sci. USA*, **82**, 6040.
61. Dray,F. (1982) In *Methods in Enzymology*. Lands,W.E.M. and Smith,W.L. (eds), Academic Press, New York, Vol. 86, p. 297.
62. Sautebin,L., Kindahl,H., Kumlin,M. and Granström,E. (1985) *Prostaglandins*, **30**, 435.
63. Granström,E. and Lindgren,J.-Å. (1986) In *Handbook of Biology and Chemistry of Prostaglandins and Related Metabolites of Polyunsaturated Fatty Acids*. Curtis-Prior,P.B. (ed.), Churchill Livingstone, Edinburgh, in press.
64. Granström,E. and Kindahl,H. (1982) In *Methods in Enzymology*. Lands,W.E.M. and Smith,W.L. (eds), Academic Press, New York, Vol. 86, p. 320.
65. Granström,E. (1980) In *Radioimmunoassay of Drugs and Hormones in Cardiovascular Medicine*. Albertini,E., DaPrada,M. and Peskar,B.A. (eds), Elsevier/North Holland Biomedical Press, p. 229.
66. Patrono,C., Pugliese,F., Ciabattoni,G., Patrignani,P., Maseri,A., Chierchia,S., Peskar,B.A., Cinotti,G.A., Simonetti,B.M. and Pierucci,A. (1982) *J. Clin. Invest.*, **69**, 231.
67. Fukushima,M., Kato,T., Ota,K., Arai,Y., Narumiya,S. and Hayaishi,O. (1982) *Biochem. Biophys. Res. Commun.*, **109**, 626.

CHAPTER 11

Enzyme immunoassay

SHOZO YAMAMOTO, KAZUSHIGE YOKOTA,
TAKEHARU TONAI, FUMIAKI SHONO and YOKO HAYASHI

1. INTRODUCTION

Radioimmunoassay (RIA) has been widely utilized in the routine assay of prostaglandins (PGs) as a sensitive and specific method (1). However, the use of radioactive labels is associated with problems of environmental pollution. Moreover, chemical or enzymatic synthesis of radioactive antigens, with a high enough specific radioactivity to enable sensitive assays, may not always be feasible. In view of these intrinsic disadvantages of RIAs we have attempted to apply techniques of enzyme immunoassay (EIA) to the determination of various arachidonate metabolites. The technique of EIA is a non-isotopic method which uses an enzyme protein as a label (2−4). As shown in *Figure 1*, the antigen molecule is linked to enzymes such as β-galactosidase or peroxidase. The enzyme-labelled antigen and the sample to be assayed are allowed to react with an antibody in a competitive manner. Then, the immunocomplex is separated from free antigen by the double-antibody method or the solid-phase method. The enzyme activity of the immunocomplex is determined and correlated with the amount of the antigen. Since our earlier attempts to develop an EIA for $PGF_{2\alpha}$ (5), a number of authors have described EIAs of various arachidonate metabolites as listed in *Table 1*. In some of these, the enzyme as a label is bound to antibody rather than antigen. Various methods are utilized to separate the immunocomplex. The enzyme activity is assayed by the measurement of fluorescence, absorption in the visible region or by chemiluminescence.

This chapter deals with EIAs by the solid-phase method in relation to two important arachidonate metabolites, 6-keto-$PGF_{1\alpha}$ and thromboxane (TX) B_2. The former compound is a stable degradation product of anti-aggregatory and vasodilating PGI_2 (prostacyclin), and the latter is a product of the pro-aggregatory and vasoconstricting TXA_2.

2. ENZYME IMMUNOASSAY OF 6-KETO-$PGF_{1\alpha}$

2.1 Outline of the assay

6-Keto-$PGF_{1\alpha}$ is labelled with β-galactosidase. As shown in *Figure 2*, antiserum is bound to a polystyrene tube, and the enzyme-labelled and unlabelled 6-keto-$PGF_{1\alpha}$ are allowed to react with the immobilized antibody in a competitive manner. The immunologically bound β-galactosidase is incubated with 4-methylumbelliferyl-β-D-galactoside as substrate, and the measured enzyme activity is correlated inversely with

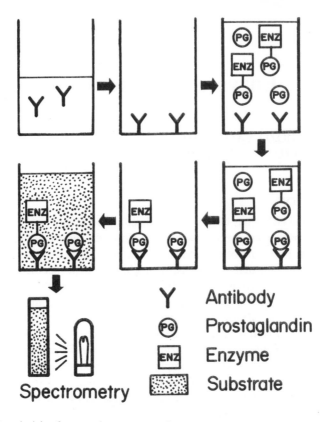

Figure 1. The principle of enzyme immunoassay of prostaglandins.

the amount of unlabelled 6-keto-PGF$_{1\alpha}$. The method has been published in refs 9 and 20.

2.2 Preparation of anti-6-keto-PGF$_{1\alpha}$ antiserum

The carboxyl group of 6-keto-PGF$_{1\alpha}$ is conjugated to amino groups of bovine serum albumin (BSA) by the N-succinimidyl ester method (21).

(i) Dissolve 6-keto-PGF$_{1\alpha}$ (2 mg) in 50 μl of 80% dioxane containing 3 mg of 1-ethyl-3-(3-dimethylaminopropyl)carbodiimide-HCl.

(ii) Keep the mixture at 25°C for 3 h, and then dilute it with 1 ml of water.

(iii) Extract with 2 ml of ethyl acetate twice, then wash the organic layer with water and dry it over anhydrous sodium sulphate.

(iv) Evaporate the solvent, and mix the dried residue (N-succinimidyl ester of 6-keto-PGF$_{1\alpha}$) with 10 mg of BSA dissolved in 0.2 ml of 50 mM sodium phosphate buffer at pH 7.3.

(v) Incubate the mixture overnight at 4°C, and then apply the resulting emulsion to a Sephadex G-25 column (1.1 × 33 cm).

(vi) Elute with 50 mM sodium phosphate buffer, pH 7.3, and collect fractions containing protein (conjugate of 6-keto-PGF$_{1\alpha}$ to BSA), as monitored by absorption at 280 nm.

Table 1. Enzyme immunoassays of prostaglandins and lipoxygenase products.

Compounds	Labels	Labelled compounds	Bound/Free separation	Detection methods	Minimum detection limit (fmol)	References
PGD_2	peroxidase	antigen	immobilized antibody	fluorescence	10	6
PGE_2	peroxidase	antigen	immobilized antibody	fluorescence	300	7
$PGF_{2\alpha}$	β-galactosidase	antigen	double antibodies	absorption	500	5
	β-galactosidase	antigen	double antibodies	fluorescence	30	8
6-Keto-$PGF_{1\alpha}$	β-galactosidase	antigen	immobilized antibody	fluorescence	30	9
	alkaline phosphatase	antibody	immobilized antigen	absorption	1000 (IC_{50})	10
TXB_2	β-galactosidase	antigen	double antibodies	fluorescence	100	11
	β-galactosidase	antigen	immobilized antibody	fluorescence	20	12
	β-galactosidase	antigen	double antibodies	fluorescence	2	13
			immobilized antibody			
13,14-Dihydro-15-keto-$PGF_{2\alpha}$	alkaline phosphatase	antibody	immobilized antigen	absorption	400 (IC_{50})	10
	β-galactosidase	antigen	immobilized antibody	fluorescence	10	14
5α,7α-Dihydroxy-11-keto-tetranorprostane-1,16-dioic acid	β-galactosidase	antigen	immobilized second antibody	fluorescence	30	15
11-Deoxy-15-keto-13,14-dihydro-11,16-cyclo-PGE_2	catalase	antigen	immobilized antibody	chemiluminescence	1	16
19-Carboxy-11-deoxy-13,14-dihydro-15-dehydro-2,3,4,5,20-pentanor-11β-16ξ-cyclo-PGE_1	β-galactosidase	antigen	double antibodies	fluorescence	1.6	17
	β-galactosidase	antigen	immobilized second antibody	fluorescence	1.6	15
LTB_4	alkaline phosphatase	antibody	immobilized antigen	absorption	10 000 (IC_{50})	10
	β-galactosidase	antigen	double antibodies	fluorescence	4	18
LTC_4	β-galactosidase	antigen	immobilized antibody	fluoresence	16	19
	alkaline phosphatase	antibody	immobilized antigen	absorption	200 (IC_{50})	10

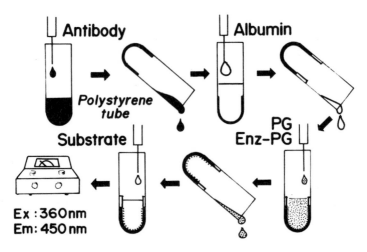

Figure 2. Illustration of the procedures of enzyme immunoassay for prostanoids by the solid-phase technique.

(vii)   Adjust the protein concentration of the conjugate to 0.5 mg/ml, and emulsify the conjugate (1 mg protein) in an equal volume of Freund's complete adjuvant (for the first injection) or incomplete adjuvant (for later injections).

(viii) Inject the emulsion subcutaneously into several sites on the back of a female New Zealand white rabbit (~2 kg body weight) every second week for a total of seven times for about 3 months. Titration of antibody is carried out by RIA (9).

(ix)   Collect whole blood from the carotid artery, and leave it at room temperature for 2 h.

(x)   Centrifuge it at 1200 g for 20 min at 4°C, and store the supernatant (antiserum) at −20°C.

2.3 Conjugation of 6-keto-PGF$_{1\alpha}$ and β-galactosidase

(i)   Dissolve 6-keto-PGF$_{1\alpha}$ (15 μg) and [5,8,9,11,12,14,15-^{3}H(N)]6-keto-PGF$_{1\alpha}$ (0.75 μCi) in 50 μl of 80% dioxane containing 2.25 mg of 1-ethyl-3-(3-dimethyl-aminopropyl)carbodiimide-HCl and 1.5 mg of N-hydroxysuccinimide (21).

(ii)   Keep the mixture at 25°C for 3 h, and dilute it with 1 ml of water, followed by extraction twice with 2 ml of ethyl acetate.

(iii)   Wash the organic layer with water, and dry it over anhydrous sodium sulphate.

(iv)   Evaporate the solvent, and mix the dried residue (N-succinimidyl ester of 6-keto-PGF$_{1\alpha}$) with 0.5 mg of β-galactosidase from *Escherichia coli* (Boehringer Mannheim, 300 U/mg) dissolved in 0.2 ml of 50 mM sodium phosphate buffer, pH 7.3.

(v)   After incubating the mixture overnight at 4°C, apply the resulting emulsion to a Sephadex G-25 column (1.1 × 33 cm), and elute with 50 mM sodium phosphate buffer, pH 7.3.

(vi)   Combine fractions showing β-galactosidase activity, and adjust the protein concentration to 50 μg/ml with buffer B (see below).

On the basis of the molecular weight of the enzyme (518 000) and the specific radioactivity of [^{3}H]6-keto-PGF$_{1\alpha}$ (22 600 c.p.m./nmol), about 5.4 mol of 6-keto-PGF$_{1\alpha}$ are bound per mol of β-galactosidase. The antigenicity of 6-keto-PGF$_{1\alpha}$ and the affinity of β-galactosidase for substrate are little affected by the conjugation described above (see reference 9 for details). The conjugate can be stored at 4°C as a solution for at least 2 years without appreciable loss of immunogenicity and enzyme activity.

2.4 Reagents

(i)   Incubation buffer A: 50 mM sodium phosphate buffer at pH 7.3 containing 0.1 M NaCl, 1 mM MgCl$_2$ and 0.1% NaN$_3$.
(ii)   Incubation buffer B: buffer A containing 0.1% ovalbumin.
(iii)   0.5% BSA dissolved in buffer A.
(iv)   Enzyme-labelled 6-keto-PGF$_{1\alpha}$ dissolved in buffer B (enzyme, 2.5 ng/ml; 6-keto-PGF$_{1\alpha}$, 26 fmol/ml) stored in a refrigerator at 4°C.
(v)   Standard solution of 6-keto-PGF$_{1\alpha}$: dissolve 1 mg of 6-keto-PGF$_{1\alpha}$ in 1 ml of acetone. Dilute the solution with buffer A to prepare working standards of various concentrations.
(vi)   0.1 mM 4-methylumbelliferyl-β-D-galactoside: 9.47 mg dissolved in 1 ml of dimethylformamide and then diluted to 280 ml with buffer B. The solution should be prepared every week, and stored in a dark bottle at 4°C.
(vii)   0.1 M glycine-NaOH buffer, pH 10.3.
(viii) 1 μM Quinine sulphate: 7.8 mg dissolved in 10 ml of 50 mM H$_2$SO$_4$ and then diluted 1000-fold with 50 mM H$_2$SO$_4$. Since 4-methylumbelliferone (product of the β-galactosidase reaction) is unstable, quinine sulphate (1 μM equivalent to 1.54 μM 4-methylumbelliferone) is used as a reference compound in fluorimetry.
(ix)   Anti-6-keto-PGF$_{1\alpha}$ antiserum: diluted 1000-fold with buffer A.

2.5 Standard assay conditions

To optimize the detectability and the sensitivity of the assay, the amount of antiserum and enzyme-labelled antigen and the incubation time of each component must be examined (see ref 9 for details).
(i)   Place antiserum diluted 1000-fold (200 μl) at the bottom of a polystyrene tube (Falcon 2052, Becton Dickinson, Cockeysville).
(ii)   Incubate it for 1 h to allow binding to antibody to the tube, then decant the contents and wash the tube with 1 ml of buffer B.
(iii)   Add 0.5 ml of 0.5% solution of BSA to the tube and incubate it for 30 min at 37°C.
(iv)   Decant the contents and wash the tube with 1 ml of buffer B.
(v)   Add 200 μl of authentic 6-keto-PGF$_{1\alpha}$ or a sample to be tested to the tube.
(vi)   After 5 min, add enzyme-labelled 6-keto-PGF$_{1\alpha}$ (50 μl; equivalent to 1.3 fmol of 6-keto-PGF$_{1\alpha}$ and 125 pg of β-galactosidase).
(vii)   Shake the tube at 26°C for 2 h, followed by two washings of the tube with 1 ml of buffer B.
(viii) React the bound β-galactosidase with 300 μl of 0.1 mM 4-methylumbelliferyl-β-D-galactoside at 30°C for 1 h and terminate the reaction by the addition of 2.5 ml of 0.1 M glycine-NaOH buffer at pH 10.3.

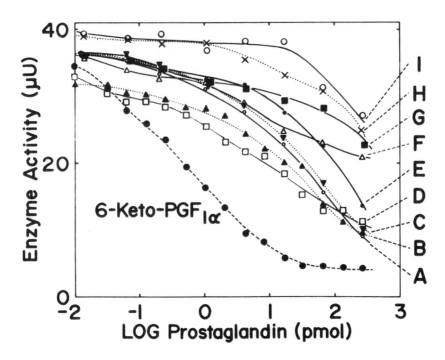

Figure 3. Calibration curve of 6-keto-PGF$_{1\alpha}$ and cross-reactivity of anti-6-keto-PGF$_{1\alpha}$ antibody. The standard amount of enzyme-labelled 6-keto-PGF$_{1\alpha}$ is mixed with various amounts of 6-keto-PGF$_{1\alpha}$ (closed circles and broken line) or one of the following arachidonate metabolites for the standard enzyme immunoassay: (**A**) PGE$_1$, (**B**) PGF$_{2\alpha}$, (**C**) PGE$_2$, (**D**) PGF$_{1\alpha}$, (**E**) PGD$_2$, (**F**) TXB$_2$, (**G**) PGB$_2$, (**H**) 13,14-dihydro-15-keto-PGF$_{2\alpha}$ and (**I**) 13,14-dihydro-15-keto-PGE$_2$.

(ix) Measure the fluorescence intensity of 4-methylumbelliferone released using a spectrofluorimeter such as a Hitachi model MPF 2A; set the excitation wavelength at 360 nm, and the emission wavelength at 450 nm and use cuvettes with 10-mm lightpath. Quinine sulphate (1 μM) is appropriate as the standard.

In our assay 1 unit of β-galactosidase is defined as that amount of enzyme which produces 1 μmol of 4-methylumbelliferone per min under the conditions described above.

2.6 Calibration curve and cross-reactivity

When the EIA is performed with various amounts of 6-keto-PGF$_{1\alpha}$ in competition with the standard amount of enzyme-labelled 6-keto-PGF$_{1\alpha}$, the plots of β-galactosidase activity versus log dose of 6-keto-PGF$_{1\alpha}$ give a calibration curve as shown in *Figure 3*. The minimum detectable amount of 6-keto-PGF$_{1\alpha}$ (90% of maximum binding of the enzyme-labelled antigen) is 30 fmol, and the maximum detectable amount (10% of maximum binding) is 10 pmol. Cross-reactivities of the antibody with other arachidonate metabolites are as follows: PGF$_{1\alpha}$ (3.7%), PGF$_{2\alpha}$ (2.0%), PGE$_1$ (0.9%), PGE$_2$ (1.0%), PGD$_2$ (0.68%), TXB$_2$ (0.17%), PGB$_2$ (<0.1%), 13,14-dihydro-15-keto-PGF$_{2\alpha}$ (<0.1%), and 13,14-dihydro-15-keto-PGE$_2$ (<0.1%).

2.7 **Validity of the assay**

The intra-assay coefficient of variation of the EIA is 8.0% ($n = 10$), and the inter-assay coefficient of variation is 2.0% ($n = 5$). When the purified material from human serum (see below) is mixed with various amounts of authentic 6-keto-PGF$_{1\alpha}$ and subjected to both EIA (x) and RIA (y), a satisfactory correlation is observed between the two assays ($y = 1.009x + 0.069$, $r = 0.994$) (see ref. 9 for details).

2.8 **Application to human serum**

Since the prostaglandin content in human blood is very low, the prostaglandins must be extracted from the serum and concentrated to comply with the sensitivity of the assay. The method of Powell (22) using a Sep-Pak C$_{18}$ cartridge (Waters) is a convenient technique for PG extraction.

(i)   Wash a Sep-Pak C$_{18}$ column with 20 ml of methanol and 20 ml of water, and apply human serum (10 ml) acidified to pH 3.2 with 2 M HCl to the column.

(ii)   Wash the column with 20 ml of water, and elute the polar lipids and fatty acids with 15% ethanol (20 ml) and petroleum ether (20 ml), respectively.

(iii)   Elute the prostaglandins and TXB$_2$ with ethyl acetate (10 ml) instead of methyl formate used in the original method.

(iv)   Apply the extract derived from 40 ml of serum to a silicic acid column (0.6 g) according to the method of Siess and Dray (23).

(v)   Purify the eluate derived from 20 ml of serum by h.p.l.c. using a μBondapak C$_{18}$ column (3.9 × 330 mm). The solvent system is acetonitrile/water/acetic acid (30:70:0.1, v/v) at a flow-rate of 1 ml/min. 6-Keto-PGF$_{1\alpha}$ elutes after $9-12$ min.

When the amount of 6-keto-PGF$_{1\alpha}$ in the Sep-Pak C$_{18}$ extract is determined by EIA, an unusually high value ($50-60$ pmol/ml of human serum) is obtained. A larger amount of the Sep-Pak extract gives a higher value of 6-keto-PGF$_{1\alpha}$ per unit volume of human serum. The findings suggest the presence of a certain compound(s) which interferes with the EIA and gives an apparently high value of 6-keto-PGF$_{1\alpha}$. When 6-keto-PGF$_{1\alpha}$ is eluted from the h.p.l.c. column described above, the interfering compound is retained and separated from 6-keto-PGF$_{1\alpha}$ (see ref. 9 for details). As tested with ^{3}H-labelled 6-keto-PGF$_{1\alpha}$ as an internal standard, the recovery of 6-keto-PGF$_{1\alpha}$ is 95% at the step of Sep-Pak C$_{18}$ extraction, 81% upon silicic acid chromatography and 53% after h.p.l.c.

An example of 6-keto-PGF$_{1\alpha}$ determination by EIA is as follows (see ref. 9 for details). Starting with 60 ml of human serum, 6-keto-PGF$_{1\alpha}$ was extracted and purified by the three-step chromatographic procedure mentioned above. The purified material equivalent to 2 ml of serum was mixed with $0-0.54$ pmol of 6-keto-PGF$_{1\alpha}$, and each mixture was subjected to the standard EIA. The measured values were plotted against the amount of added 6-keto-PGF$_{1\alpha}$, and the level of 6-keto-PGF$_{1\alpha}$ in human serum was estimated from the intercept to be 56 ± 12 fmol/ml.

3. ENZYME IMMUNOASSAY OF TXB$_2$

3.1 Outline of the assay

As described above for 6-keto-PGF$_{1\alpha}$, TXB$_2$ can also be labelled with β-galactosidase. A competitive reaction of the enzyme-labelled TXB$_2$ and the sample to be tested is carried out with the immobilized antibody (*Figure 2*). The method has been published in refs 12 and 24.

3.2 Preparation of anti-TXB$_2$ IgG

The carboxyl group of TXB$_2$ is conjugated to amino groups of BSA by the mixed anhydride method (25).

(i)   Dissolve TXB$_2$ (6 mg) in 0.5 ml of dioxane, and mix the solution with 10 μl of tri-n-butylamine and 2 μl of isobutyl chloroformate.

(ii)   Keep the mixture at $10-12°C$ for 30 min, and then add it dropwise (each time in a 10-μl aliquot) to BSA (20 mg) dissolved in 0.6 ml of 0.5% sodium hydrogen carbonate.

(iii)   Stir the mixture at 4°C for 4 h after addition of 0.5 ml of dioxane and dialyse it against 500 ml of 50% dioxane at 4°C for 2 h and then twice against 1 l of sodium phosphate buffer, pH 7.3, at 4°C for 12 h.

(iv)   Adjust the protein concentration to 2 mg/ml with the same buffer, and emulsify the conjugate (1 mg protein) in an equal volume of Freund's complete adjuvant.

(v)   Inject the emulsion subcutaneously at several sites in the back of a male New Zealand white rabbit (2 kg body weight). Injections are carried out every second week, for a total of seven times for about 3 months. Titration of antibody is performed by RIA (12).

(vi)   Collect whole blood from the carotid artery, and leave it at room temperature for 30 min.

(vii)   Store the supernatant (antiserum) at $-20°C$ after centrifuging at 1200 g for 20 min at 4°C.

(viii) Mix the antiserum (0.5 ml) with 156 mg of ammonium sulphate (50% saturation), and centrifuge the mixture at 17 000 g for 20 min.

(ix)   Dissolve the precipitate in 200 μl of 50 mM Tris-HCl buffer, pH 8.6, containing 0.15 M NaCl and 0.02% NaN$_3$, and dialyse against the same buffer.

(x)   Apply the dialysate to a column of protein A$-$Sepharose (Pharmacia), preconditioned with the same buffer.

(xi)   Wash the column with 50 ml of the equilibration buffer, and elute the IgG fraction with 20 ml of 0.1 M glycine-HCl buffer at pH 3.0.

(xii)   Collect the eluate in 0.5-ml fractions in tubes containing 1 ml of 1 M Tris-HCl buffer, pH 7.4, and dialyse against incubation buffer A (see below).

(xiii) Concentrate the dialysate to 5 ml (0.58 mg IgG/ml), and store at $-20°C$.

(xiv)   Determine the protein concentration of the IgG fraction by the use of $A_{280}^{1\%} = 13.8$ (26).

3.3 Conjugation of TXB$_2$ and β-galactosidase

(i)   Dissolve TXB$_2$ (200 μg) and [5,6,8,9,11,12,14,15(N)-^{3}H]TXB$_2$ (3.0 × 10^5 c.p.m.) in 50 μl of 80% dioxane containing 300 μg of 1-ethyl-3-(3-dimethyl-aminopropyl)-carbodiimide and 200 μg of N-hydroxysuccinimide (21).

(ii)   Keep the mixture at 30°C for 2 h, and dilute it with 2 ml of water, followed by extraction twice with 2 ml of ethyl acetate.

(iii) Evaporate the organic layer and mix the dried residue (N-succinimidyl ester of TXB$_2$) with 1 mg of β-galactosidase (see Section 2.3) dissolved in 0.2 ml of 10 mM sodium phosphate buffer at pH 7.3.

(iv)   After incubating overnight at 4°C, dialyse the mixture against 500 ml of 50% dioxane, twice against 500 ml of 10 mM sodium phosphate buffer at pH 7.3 and against 500 ml of incubation buffer A, each for 2 h at 4°C.

(v)   Adjust the protein concentration to 173 μg/ml with buffer B (see below).

On the basis of the molecular weight of the enzyme (518 000) and the specific radioactivity of [^{3}H]TXB$_2$ (5.5 × 10^5 c.p.m./μmol), about 33.8 mol of TXB$_2$ are bound per mol of β-galactosidase. The antigenicity of TXB$_2$ is reduced 60% by its conjugation to β-galactosidase (12). The K_m value of the enzyme for substrate is almost unaffected (12). The solution of the β-galactosidase-labelled TXB$_2$ (173 μg protein/ml of buffer B) retains its original enzyme activity after 1-year storage at 4°C.

3.4 Reagents

(i)   Incubation buffer A: 10 mM sodium phosphate buffer at pH 7.0 containing 0.1 M NaCl, 1 mM MgCl$_2$ and 0.1% NaN$_3$.

(ii)   Incubation buffer B: buffer A containing 0.1% ovalbumin.

(iii)   0.5% BSA dissolved in buffer A.

(iv)   Enzyme-labelled TXB$_2$ dissolved in buffer B (enzyme, 1.3 ng/100 μl; TXB$_2$, 86 fmol/100 μl) stored in a refrigerator at 4°C.

(v)   Standard solution of TXB$_2$: dissolve 1 mg of TXB$_2$ in 1 ml of ethanol. Dilute the solution with buffer A to prepare working standards of various concentrations.

(vi)   0.1 mM 4-methylumbelliferyl-β-D-galactoside: see Section 2.4.

(vii)   0.1 M glycine-NaOH buffer, pH 10.3.

(viii) 1 μM Quinine sulphate: see Section 2.4

(ix)   Anti-TXB$_2$ antibody: dilute the stock solution to a protein concentration of 290 ng/ml with buffer A.

3.5 Standard assay conditions

Experiments to establish the standard conditions are described in ref. 12.

(i)   Place anti-TXB$_2$ IgG solution (58 ng in 200 μl) at the bottom of a polystyrene tube (Falcon 2008, Becton Dickinson, Cockeysville).

(ii)   Incubate it for 1 h at 37°C to allow binding of the antibody to the tube, and then add a 0.5% solution of BSA, and incubate the mixture for 30 min at 37°C.

(iii)   Discard the liquid contents and wash the tube twice with 1 ml of buffer B.

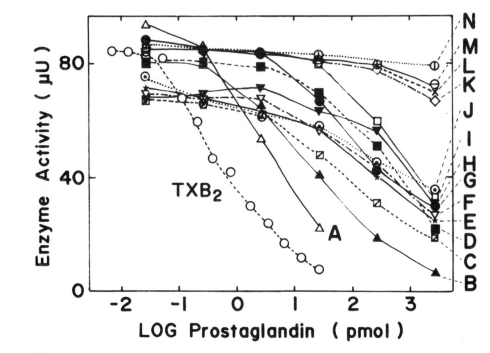

Figure 4. Calibration curve of TXB_2 and cross-reactivity of anti-TXB_2 antibody. The standard amount of enzyme-labelled TXB_2 is mixed with various amounts of TXB_2 (open circles and broken line) or one of the following arachidonate metabolites for the standard enzyme immunoassay: (**A**) 2,3-dinor-TXB_2, (**B**) 15-keto-$PGF_{2\alpha}$, (**C**) $PGF_{1\alpha}$, (**D**) PGD_2, (**E**) PGE_1, (**F**) PGB_2, (**G**) 2,3,4,5-tetranor-TXB_2, (**H**) PGA_2, (**I**) $PGF_{2\alpha}$, (**J**) PGE_2, (**K**) 13,14-dihydro-15-keto-$PGF_{2\alpha}$, (**L**) 5α, 7α-dihydroxy-11-keto-tetranorprostane-1, 16-dioic acid, (**M**) 6-keto-$PGF_{1\alpha}$ and (**N**) 13,14-dihydro-15-keto-PGE_2.

(iv)   Add a solution (100 μl) of authentic TXB_2, or the sample to be tested, to the tube.

(v)   After 5 min mix the solution with enzyme-labelled TXB_2 (100 μl, equivalent to 86 fmol of TXB_2 and 1.3 ng of β-galactosidase).

(vi)   Incubate the mixture at 26°C for 2 h and then at 4°C for more than 12 h.

(vii)   Wash the tube twice with 1 ml of buffer B.

(viii)   Allow the bound β-galactosidase to react with 300 μl of 0.1 mM 4-methylumbelliferyl-β-D-galactoside at 30°C for 1 h, and terminate the reaction by the addition of 2.5 ml of 0.1 M glycine-NaOH buffer at pH 10.3.

(ix)   Determine the fluorescence intensity as described for 6-keto-$PGF_{1\alpha}$.

3.6 Calibration curve and cross-reactivity

A calibration curve obtained by the standard EIA is shown in *Figure 4*. The minimum and maximum detectability levels of TXB_2 (defined as the amounts of unlabelled TXB_2 required to displace the maximum binding of the enzyme-labelled TXB_2 by 10% and 90%) are 20 fmol and 14 pmol, respectively. Cross-reactivities of the antibody with 2,3-dinor-TXB_2 and 15-keto-$PGF_{2\alpha}$ are 18.6% and 4.6%. The following arachidonate metabolites show cross-reactivities of less than 1%: 2,3,4,5-tetranor-TXB_2, PGA_2,

PGB$_2$, PGD$_2$, PGE$_1$, PGE$_2$, PGF$_{1\alpha}$, PGF$_{2\alpha}$, 6-keto-PGF$_{1\alpha}$, 13,14-dihydro-15-keto-PGE$_2$, 13,14-dihydro-15-keto-PGF$_{2\alpha}$ and 5α,7α-dihydroxy-11-keto-tetranorprostane-1,16-dioic acid.

3.7 Validity of the assay

The intra-assay coefficient of variation of the EIA (0.11 pmol of TXB$_2$) is 5.5% (n = 10), and the inter-assay coefficient of variation is 11.5% (n = 6). When the purified material from human serum (see below) is mixed with various amounts of authentic TXB$_2$ and subjected to both EIA (y) and RIA (x), a good correlation is observed between the two assays ($y = 0.75x + 0.11$, $r = 0.979$).

3.8 Application to human blood and urine

Since the content of TXB$_2$ in human blood and urine is very low, TXB$_2$ must be extracted and concentrated to meet the detectability of the assay. As described in detail for 6-keto-PGF$_{1\alpha}$, Sep-Pak C$_{18}$ extraction (88% yield) and h.p.l.c. are necessary to remove endogenous interfering substance(s) (see ref. 12 for details).

For the determination of the endogenous level of TXB$_2$ in peripheral blood, the use of an anti-coagulant procedure such as the addition of indomethacin and EDTA during the blood withdrawal is recommended.

When EIA is carried out for urinary TXB$_2$, it should be noted that anti-TXB$_2$ antibody may cross-react with 2,3-dinor-TXB$_2$, which is present in a considerable amount in urine (12).

As an example of EIA of TXB$_2$ in human plasma (prepared in the presence of indomethacin and EDTA), the material purified by h.p.l.c. was mixed with various amounts of TXB$_2$, and subjected to EIA. The endogenous level of TXB$_2$ estimated by the intercept of the plots (measured TXB$_2$ versus added TXB$_2$) was 0.21 pmol/ml of human plasma (12).

4. REFERENCES

1. Granström,E. and Kindahl,H. (1978) In *Advances in Prostaglandin and Thromboxane Research*. Frölich,J.C. (ed.), Raven Press, New York, Vol. 5, p. 119.
2. Schuurs,A.H.W.M. and van Weemen,B.K. (1977) *Clin. Chim. Acta*, **81**, 1.
3. Wisdom,G.B. (1976) *Clin. Chem.*, **22**, 1243.
4. Ishikawa,E., Imagawa,M., Hashida,S., Yoshitake,S., Hamaguchi,Y. and Ueno,T. (1983) *J. Immunoassay*, **4**, 209.
5. Hayashi,Y., Yano,T. and Yamamoto,S. (1981) *Biochim. Biophys. Acta*, **663**, 661.
6. Hiroshima,O., Hayashi,H., Ito,S. and Hayaishi,O. (1986) *Prostaglandins*, **32**, 63.
7. Tanaka,T., Ito,S., Hiroshima,O., Hayashi,H. and Hayaishi,O. (1985) *Biochim. Biophys. Acta*, **836**, 125.
8. Yano,T., Hayashi,Y. and Yamamoto,S. (1981) *J. Biochem.*, **90**, 773.
9. Tonai,T., Yokota,K., Yano,T., Hayashi,Y., Yamamoto,S., Yamashita,K. and Miyazaki,H. (1985) *Biochim. Biophys. Acta*, **836**, 335.
10. Miller,D.K., Sodowski,S., DeSousa,D., Maycock,A.L., Lombardo,D.L., Young,R.N. and Hayes,E.C. (1985) *J. Immunol. Methods*, **81**, 169.
11. Hayashi,Y., Ueda,N., Yokota,K., Kawamura,S., Ogushi,F., Yamamoto,Y., Yamamoto,S., Nakamura,K., Yamashita,K., Miyazaki,H., Kato,K. and Terao,S. (1983) *Biochim. Biophys. Acta*, **750**, 322.
12. Shono,F., Yokota,K. and Yamamoto,S. (1985) *J. Biochem.*, **98**, 1069.
13. Sawada,M., Inagawa,T. and Frölich,J.C. (1985) *Prostaglandins*, **29**, 1039.
14. Yokota,K., Horie,K., Hayashi,Y., Yamamoto,S., Yamashita,K. and Miyazaki,H. (1986) *Biochim. Biophys. Acta*, **879**, 322.

15. Shimizu,H., Taniguchi,K., Uchida,S., Kira,H., and Kawasaki,A. (1986) In *Challenging Frontiers for Prostaglandin Research*. Katori,M., Yamamoto,S. and Hayaishi,O. (eds), Gendai-Iryosha, Tokyo, p. 229.
16. Lange,K., Simmet,T. and Peskar,B.A. (1985) In *Advances in Prostaglandin, Thromboxane, and Leukotriene Research*. Hayaishi,O. and Yamamoto,S. (eds), Raven Press, New York, Vol. 15, p. 85.
17. Inagawa,T., Imaki,K., Masuda,H., Morikawa,Y., Hirata,F. and Tsuboshima,M. (1983) In *Advances in Prostaglandin, Thromboxane, and Leukotriene Research*. Samuelsson,B., Paoletti,R. and Ramwell,P. (eds), Raven Press, New York, Vol. 11, p. 191.
18. Sawada,M. and Frölich,J.C. (1986) In *Challenging Frontiers for Prostaglandin Research*. Katori,M., Yamamoto,S. and Hayaishi,O. (eds), Gendai-Iryosha, Tokyo, p. 224.
19. Taniguchi,K., Uchida,S., Shimizu,H., Kira,H. and Kawasaki,A. (1986) In *Challenging Frontiers for Prostaglandin Research*. Katori,M., Yamamoto,S. and Hayaishi,O. (eds), Gendai-Iryosha, Tokyo, p. 230.
20. Yamamoto,S., Tonai,T. and Yokota,K. (1985) In *Methods of Enzymatic Analysis*. Bergmeyer,H.U. (ed.), VCH Verlagsgesellschaft, Weinheim, Vol. 8, p. 40.
21. Hosoda,H., Kawamura,N. and Nambara,T. (1981) *Chem. Pharm. Bull.*, **29**, 1969.
22. Powell,W.S. (1982) In *Methods in Enzymology*. Lands,W.E.M. and Smith,W.L. (eds), Academic Press, New York, Vol. 86, p. 467.
23. Siess,W. and Dray,F. (1982) *J. Lab. Clin. Med.*, **99**, 388.
24. Yokota,K., Shono,F. and Yamamoto,S. (1985) In *Methods of Enzymatic Analysis*. Bergmeyer,H.U. (ed.), VCH Verlagsgesellschaft, Weinheim, Vol. 8, p. 50.
25. Erlanger,B.F., Borek,F., Beiser,S.M. and Lieberman,S. (1959) *J. Biol. Chem.*, **234**, 1090.
26. Sober,H.A., ed. (1968) *Handbook of Biochemistry*. The Chemical Rubber Co., Cleveland, C-1-C-193.

CHAPTER 12

Cyclo-oxygenase:
measurement, purification and properties

RICHARD J.KULMACZ and WILLIAM E.M.LANDS

1. INTRODUCTION

The cyclo-oxygenase activity of prostaglandin H (PGH) synthase catalyses the transformation of a polyunsaturated fatty acid, such as arachidonic acid (20:4), to prostaglandin G:

$$20:4 + 2O_2 \; - - \rightarrow PGG_2$$

The purified cyclo-oxygenase activity of PGH synthase is accompanied by a peroxidase activity that can convert PGG_2 to PGH_2. The retention of this combination of activities in the same holoenzyme molecule apparently confers some survival value for the many animal species conserving this arrangement. A synergistic interaction occurs between the peroxidase activity and the cyclo-oxygenase activity in the same molecule that does not occur when the two activities are on separate molecules (1). This interaction permits the cyclo-oxygenase to respond explosively to small triggering levels of hydroperoxide activator. The mechanism of the cyclo-oxygenase thus has some features that depend on the peroxidase activity, and investigators must be careful to separate primary and secondary aspects when studying the detailed kinetic behaviour of the cyclo-oxygenase.

2. MEASUREMENT OF CYCLO-OXYGENASE ACTIVITY

The cyclo-oxygenase reaction is commonly monitored either by quantitating the amount of prostaglandin produced from radiolabelled arachidonate at fixed reaction intervals, or by continuously monitoring the consumption of oxygen or the co-oxidation of a peroxidase co-substrate. The radiotracer method can be made very sensitive and it works in crude systems. However, measurement of oxygen or co-substrate consumption is much more convenient when sufficient activity is available, and it furnishes a more detailed and continuous record of the reaction kinetics. The choice between the two methods depends on the amount of cyclo-oxygenase and the instrumentation available, the degree to which the product prostaglandins need to be characterized and the amount of kinetic details that need to be controlled. Several general aspects that are common to all of the assay techniques will be discussed first.

2.1 General features of the assay

2.1.1 *Choice of buffer*

The cyclo-oxygenase from sheep seminal vesicles has an optimum pH near pH 7 (2), and its activity declines to about 50% of optimal at pH 8.5. Accordingly, we generally use 0.1 M potassium phosphate, pH 7.2 as the assay buffer.

2.1.2 *Stimulatory additives*

Many compounds have been found to stimulate the cyclo-oxygenase activity (3). Most of the stimulatory agents appear to serve as co-substrate for the peroxidase activity of the synthase. The extent of stimulation (several-fold) appears to be roughly the same for all, but the optimal concentration varies from compound to compound, with some compounds being inhibitory at higher levels. Phenol (1 mM) stimulates the cyclo-oxygenase about 5-fold at pH 7.2 and 3-fold at pH 8.5, and it provides a convenient way to maximize cyclo-oxygenase activity for kinetic assays.

2.1.3 *Preparation of substrate fatty acid*

The peroxides which accumulate spontaneously in stored samples of polyunsaturated fatty acids have distinct effects on the kinetics of the cyclo-oxygenase reaction, and they may prevent obtaining the evidence for the requirement of the enzyme for hydroperoxide activators. The peroxides can be chemically reduced by treating the stock solution of fatty acid in toluene with sodium borohydride. After washing with water to remove excess borohydride, formation of further peroxides can be inhibited by addition of a small amount of an anti-oxidant such as butylated hydroxytoluene (BHT). The anti-oxidant should be present at less than 1 mol per 50 mol fatty acid to avoid interfering with the oxygenase kinetics (4). The concentration of fatty acid in the stock solution can be determined by standard gas chromatographic techniques. We have found that the fatty acid solution can be stored for several months in sealed ampules at $-20°C$. Each day the cyclo-oxygenase assay is to be run, a suitable aliquot of the stock solution is dried under a stream of nitrogen, and the residue dissolved in either ethanol or 0.1 M Tris-HCl, pH 8.5, to provide a working stock of 20 mM fatty acid. Small volumes of this working fatty acid stock are added to each cyclo-oxygenase reaction with a microsyringe. Amounts of ethanol below 5% in the final assay mixture generally do not inhibit the cyclo-oxygenase reaction, but this must be checked directly in each system studied. A more rapid acceleration of the cyclo-oxygenase has been observed in some systems in which ethanol was added.

2.2 Assay of cyclo-oxygenase with the polarographic oxygen electrode

For an example of the use of the polarographic oxygen electrode in the assay of the cyclo-oxygenase activity, see ref. 5.

2.2.1 *Components of the oxygen electrode system*

The electrode, membrane, cuvette, stirrer magnet, water bath and monitor can be purchased from Yellow Springs Instruments (Model 53). The operating principles and basic design of the electrode are described by Beechey and Ribbons (6). Briefly, a potential of about 0.8 V is maintained between the two electrodes on the end of the sensor probe. Oxygen diffuses to, and is consumed at, the surface of the cathode, setting up a current between the electrodes. The current is limited by the rate of diffusion of oxygen to the cathode surface, and thus is proportional to the oxygen tension in the surrounding solution. It is the current between the electrodes that is detected by the electronics of the oxygen monitor, amplified, and converted into a $0-100$ mV d.c. signal for display on a chart recorder or other device.

The surface of the metal electrodes is easily fouled by protein, etc. and so it is moistened with a very small volume ($2-3$ μl) of electrolyte solution and covered with a thin sheet of Teflon film. The Teflon is permeable to oxygen, allowing the gas to diffuse from the reaction cuvette into the electrolyte solution to replace the oxygen consumed at the cathode. The finite permeability of the Teflon film dampens the oxygen monitor's response to changes in the oxygen tension in the reaction cuvette outside the membrane. This dampening effect can introduce considerable distortion into the record of oxygen levels reported by the monitor when the concentration changes are rapid, as with many cyclo-oxygenase reactions (7). We believe that the most consistent performance is obtained when the electrode surfaces are cleaned with an eraser and a fresh Teflon membrane put on each day.

We have modified the monitor to include an offset circuit for the output to the chart recorder. With this modification, a 5 or 10% decrease in oxygen from initial levels (~ 230 μM) can give a full-scale deflection of a chart recorder set at 5 mV or 10 mV full scale. This gives a very sensitive indication of changes in the oxygen concentration. Another helpful modification is to replace the bath assembly stirring motor with a faster one that is combined with a rheostat and an on/off switch. These changes permit closer control of the behaviour of the stirrer magnet in the reaction cuvette. This helps avoid the stirrer 'wobble' seen at low speeds that causes electromagnetic noise in the assay system, without rotating the driving magnet faster than the stirring magnet in the cuvette can follow.

(i)   Place a stirring magnet into a clean cuvette, and add the reaction buffer (usually 3.0 ml of 0.1 M potassium phosphate, pH 7.2/1 mM phenol).

(ii)   Secure the cuvette and its contents in the bath assembly and turn the stirrer motor on.

(iii)   After a few minutes of equilibration at the desired temperature, shut off the stirrer motor long enough to allow the oxygen sensor to be inserted over the liquid in the cuvette so as to exclude air bubbles that interfere with detecting the dissolved oxygen.

(iv)   Switch on the stirrer and the monitor, and examine the recorder output to make sure the system has stabilized.

(v)   Add any additional reaction components at this time through the capillary slot in the probe, using a microsyringe with a 4 inch long needle (or a normal needle fitted with an extension of narrow-bore Teflon tubing).

2.2.2 *Graphical analysis of oxygen versus time trace*

A typical chart recorder tracing of the monitor output as a function of time is shown

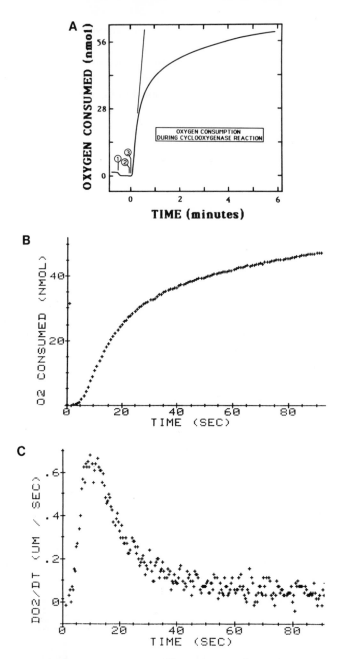

Figure 1. Oxygen electrode assay of cyclo-oxygenase activity. (**A**) Chart recorder tracing of oxygen consumption in a reaction cuvette containing 3 ml of 0.1 M potassium phosphate, pH 7.2 and 1 mM phenol. Indomethacin was added at point 1, pure synthase holoenzyme at point 2 and arachidonate at point 3. The straight line is tangent to the curve at its steepest point, and is used to calculate the optimal velocity of the cyclo-oxygenase. (**B**) Oxygen consumption data from the same cyclo-oxygenase reaction after conversion to digital form as described in the text. Every second data point is shown. The point of addition of arachidonate is taken as 0 time. (**C**) Cyclo-oxygenase velocities during the reaction, obtained by differentiation of the digitized record shown in panel **B**.

in *Figure 1A*. The reaction cuvette initially contained 3.0 ml of 0.1 M potassium phosphate, pH 7.2, with 1 mM phenol. The reaction is commonly initiated by the addition of the cyclo-oxygenase, but it can also be accomplished by addition of the fatty acid substrate. In the latter case, the investigator will benefit from careful rinsing of cuvettes to avoid carry-over of arachidonate from previous incubations (see below). The point of each addition can be indicated with the chart recorder's event marker (or by momentarily shorting the monitor output to perturb the recorder tracing).

In the example shown, an aliquot of indomethacin was added at point 1, the holoenzyme was added at point 2 and the reaction was initiated after a short period of preincubation by injection of arachidonate at point 3 (0 time). There was an initial lag period before oxygen consumption becomes apparent, as the enzyme bound its substrates and began to generate its activator hydroperoxide. The lag period was longer for the indomethacin-treated synthase than for untreated enzyme (8). The rate of oxygen consumption then increased to a maximum before falling off due to self-inactivation of the enzyme. Thus the cyclo-oxygenase reaction has no single characteristic velocity but varies continuously.

To estimate the optimal velocity reached in a given reaction, place a ruler tangential to the curve at its steepest point, and mark the chart paper with a pencil to record the ruler's position. The slope of the ruler's edge can then be converted to enzyme units (e.g. nmol oxygen/min) by taking into account the chart speed and full scale setting of the recorder, the full scale output of the monitor, and the initial oxygen concentration in the reaction cuvette at the temperature used. An example of this calculation (for the reaction shown in *Figure 1A*) is as follows:
the slope indicates a pen deflection of 57% of full scale in 1cm, which converts to

$$0.57 \text{ full scale/cm} \times 3 \text{ cm/min} \times 10 \text{ mV/full scale} \times 232 \ \mu M \ O_2/100 \text{ mV}$$
$$= 40 \ \mu M \ O_2/min \qquad\qquad \text{Equation 1}$$

This can also be expressed as 0.67 $\mu M \ O_2$/sec or 120 nmol O_2/min (reaction volume is 3 ml).

2.2.3 *Conversion of data to digital form and computer analysis*

Digitizing the analogue output from the oxygen electrode monitor allows a more detailed analysis of the cyclo-oxygenase reaction kinetics than does graphical examination of the chart recorder trace. Such a detailed analysis can include calculation of the first derivative to obtain displays of the cyclo-oxygenase velocity as a function of time. An added sophistication is to make a correction for the finite diffusion coefficient of the Teflon membrane covering the electrode surface so as to convert the recorded changes in electrode response to changes in oxygen concentration in the reaction cuvette.

Several suitable A/D converters and microcomputers are commercially available. They vary considerably in cost and in the level of programming expertise required in their operation. We use the Smartface programmable A/D converter (Analytical Parameters, Chicago, IL) in conjunction with an Apple II + microcomputer (Apple Computer Co., Cupertino, CA). The analogue signal (typically −10 to 0 mV) from the oxygen electrode monitor is converted to a digital data stream of up to 20 points/sec during the cyclo-oxygenase reaction and held temporarily in the computer. After the reaction is over, the data can be averaged (or otherwise smoothed), differentiated, etc. and the results displayed on the video monitor and/or printer, and written to a magnetic diskette for a permanent record. A printout of the digitized record of the reaction in *Figure 1A* is shown in *Figure 1B* and that of the differentiated file in *Figure 1C*.

2.2.4 *Sources of interference*

The tendency of some proteins to bind fatty acid should be borne in mind when interpreting cyclo-oxygenase assay results. Cytosol from several sources has been found to inhibit the velocity, but not the extent, of the cyclo-oxygenase reaction with pure ovine PGH synthase. The inhibition was apparent with as little as 1 mg of cytosolic protein/ml present in the reaction. Increasing the arachidonic acid concentration overcame this inhibition in a manner that suggested a competition between the synthase and cytosolic proteins for binding arachidonate.

It is important to clean the probe and the Teflon membrane covering the electrode before it is transferred to a fresh reaction cuvette. This can conveniently be accomplished using plastic wash bottles to rinse with a 70% ethanol solution and then with distilled water. Cuvettes (with stir bars removed) are washed with a brush and soapy water, rinsed several times with tap water and de-ionized water, and finally rinsed twice with acetone. The stir bars are washed separately in similar fashion, *except ethanol is substituted for acetone* to avoid damaging the plastic coating. Cuvettes and stir bars are allowed to air dry before use.

2.3 **Assay of cyclo-oxygenase with radioisotope**

For an example of the use of radioisotope for the assay of the cyclo-oxygenase, see Miyamoto *et al.* (3).

2.3.1 *Substrate*

[1-^{14}C]arachidonic acid, which is available at a specific activity of more than 50 Ci/mol, has been found to be a convenient substrate for the radiochemical assay of the cyclo-oxygenase. Although ^{3}H-labelled materials are available at higher specific activity, the ^{14}C is more easily detected by the thin layer radiochromatogram scanner (Berthold Instruments, Pittsburgh, PA) we use. The radioactive fatty acid is diluted with the desired amount of unlabelled fatty acid (in 0.1 M Tris, pH 8.5), and added in a small volume to a reaction mixture containing 0.1 M potassium phosphate, pH 7.2, 1 μM haem, and the enzyme. The final volume of the reaction is typically about 0.20 ml.

2.3.2 *Quenching reaction and extraction of lipids*

(i)   Add three volumes of a pre-chilled ($-20°C$) mixture of ethyl ether/methanol/0.2 M citric acid (30/4/1) to the reaction mixture, vigorously agitate the contents, and allow the phases to separate in an ice bath for a few minutes.

(ii) Remove the upper phase to a clean tube, and add about 100 mg of anhydrous sodium sulphate to absorb water from the solvent.

2.3.3 *Separation and quantitation of products*

An aliquot of the extract is applied at 4°C to the pre-absorbent layer of a silica gel G thin-layer chromatography plate (Uniplates, Analtech, Inc., Newark, DE), and the plate developed at 4°C with ethyl acetate/isooctane/acetic acid (10/10/0.1). The relative amounts of arachidonate, PGG_2, PGH_2 and more polar products (identified by reference to standard materials as described by Graff; ref. 9) are determined by scanning the thin layer plate with a Berthold TLC Scanner, and integrating the areas under the appropriate peaks. Smaller amounts of radioactivity can be more precisely quantitated by scraping the silica from the appropriate bands into glass vials for liquid scintillation counting.

2.4 **Assay of cyclo-oxygenase with spectrophotometry**

For an example, see Takeguchi and Sih (10).

This method has many features that parallel the continuous assay with the oxygen electrode. The spectrophotometric (or colorimetric) monitoring is based on sequential reactions of the cyclo-oxygenase (generating PGG_2) and the peroxidase (converting PGG_2 to PGH_2) activities contained in the PGH synthase, with the peroxidase activity being the one actually measured. Its success depends upon the peroxidase co-substrate being converted to a relatively stable chromophore in a predictable stoichiometric relationship to the reduction of PGG, on the absence of competing non-chromogenic co-substrates, and on the absence of other peroxide-generating or peroxide-removing activities. We have found N,N,N′,N′-tetramethylphenylenediamine (TMPD) to be a convenient co-substrate for use in the assay.

(i) Place 2 ml of 0.1 M Tris-HCl, pH 8.5 in a spectrophotometer cuvette, followed by 20 μl of 4 mg/ml TMPD and the aliquot of enzyme to be assayed. Continuous stirring of the cuvette contents with a magnetic stir bar is desirable if the enzyme is particulate.

(ii) Record the absorbance at 611 nm as a function of time for about 1 min to establish the background rate of TMPD oxidation then add 5 μl of 20 mM arachidonate, and record the absorbance changes for another 3 min or so.

The changes in absorbance at 611 nm with time observed in this reaction system with the pure synthase roughly resemble the changes in oxygen consumption seen when the oxygen electrode is used to monitor the cyclo-oxygenase reaction (*Figure 1A*). As was done for the oxygen electrode data, the optimal velocity of absorbance change can be obtained by graphical analysis of the chart recorder tracing. The rate of absorbance change before addition of arachidonate should be subtracted from the optimal velocity value. Conversion from units of absorbance per time to those of concentration of peroxide reduced per time can be accomplished using an extinction coefficient of 13.5 (mM TMPD oxidized)$^{-1}$cm^{-1} (R.Kulmacz, unpublished observations) and a stoichiometry of 2 mol TMPD oxidized/mol PGG_2 reduced (11).

3. PURIFICATION OF CYCLO-OXYGENASE

Homogeneous PGH synthase can be purified from sheep seminal vesicles in considerable amounts; 20 mg per 250 g batch of tissue is typical (12). The procedure we use was adapted from that described by van der Ouderaa *et al.* (13), and involves detergent solubilization of the microsomal enzyme followed by gel-filtration chromatography and isoelectric focusing. The result of this 3.5 day procedure is an electrophoretically homogeneous preparation of the synthase, essentially free of its haem prosthetic group (exhibiting a 20-fold stimulation of cyclo-oxygenase activity by added haem), with a specific activity of up to 150 nmol O_2/min/mg protein. Other purification schemes have been reported that are less time consuming (e.g. ref. 14), but the reported cyclo-oxygenase specific activities are considerably lower than we observe. Inactive synthase protein is likely to be a contaminant of most synthase preparations and the probable cause of the wide range of cyclo-oxygenase specific activities that have been reported for electrophoretically homogeneous preparations of the synthase. Details of the purification procedure that we use are given below. All steps are done at $0-4°C$.

(i)   Chisel frozen ($-70°C$) ram seminal vesicles (250 g) into 3 cm cubes and homogenize in a Waring blender with 350 ml of 50 mM Tris-HCl (pH 8.0)/5 mM EDTA/5 mM diethyldithiocarbamate/1 mM phenol for about 2 min.

(ii)   Pour the homogenate into large plastic bottles and centrifuge in a Sorvall GSA rotor at 8000 r.p.m. for 10 min.

(iii)   Pour off the supernatant liquid from beneath the fatty, fibrous mat at the top of centrifuge bottle, filter through several layers of cheesecloth, and centrifuge for 45 min at 50 000 r.p.m. in a Beckman Ti 60 rotor.

(iv)   Aspirate the supernatant liquid using a Pasteur pipette connected to a water aspirator, and resuspend the microsomal pellet in 200 ml of 50 mM Tris-HCl (pH 8.0)/0.1 M $NaClO_4$/1 mM EDTA/0.1 mM diethyldithiocarbamate/0.5 mM phenol, and centrifuge again at 50 000 r.p.m. for 45 min.

(v)   Resuspend the washed microsomes in 180 ml of 50 mM Tris-HCl (pH 8.0)/0.1 mM EDTA/1 mM phenol and add 20 ml of 10% Tween 20 dropwise, with continuous stirring.

(vi)   Continue stirring for 20 min before the undissolved microsomal material is removed by centrifugation at 50 000 r.p.m. for 1 h. The supernatant liquid at this point contains the solubilized PGH synthase, and it can be collected by gentle aspiration into a clean vacuum flask.

(vii)   Concentrate the detergent-solubilized synthase solution to about 30 ml by ultrafiltration on an Amicon XM-50 membrane, and then load on a 5 × 60 cm column of AcA34 (an agarose—acrylamide gel filtration matrix). The equilibration and elution buffer is 50 mM Tris—HCl (pH 8.0)/0.1 mM EDTA/0.2 mM phenol/0.1% Tween 20/0.01% NaN_3 and the flow-rate about 75 ml/h. A considerable amount of milky material emerges at the void volume, well separated from the fractions with cyclo-oxygenase activity.

(viii) Combine the active fractions, concentrate to about 20 ml by ultrafiltration on an XM-50 membrane, and wash with two 50 ml portions of water on the same membrane to lower the ionic strength of the solution. The volume should be reduced to about 3 ml prior to isoelectric focusing.

Preparative isoelectric focusing is done in a horizontal bed of purified dextran (Ultrodex, from LKB Instruments).

(i)   Prepare the gel by pouring a slurry containing 5 g of Ultrodex, 4.2 ml of pH 5−8 ampholytes, 0.7 ml of pH 3.5−10 ampholytes, 10 ml of glycerol, 500 mg of octyl glucoside and 95 ml of water into a casting tray, and then allow the water to evaporate until the weight of the slurry has decreased by 20%.

(ii)   Transfer the gel tray to a cooling plate maintained at 0°C.

(iii)   The gel can be pre-focused at 6 W power level for 3 h before loading the sample.

(iv)   Gently pipette the sample onto the surface of the gel about one third of the way from the cathode end, and mix into the gel with a spatula, before focusing is started. A power level of 6 W is maintained throughout the 16 h of focusing. The pH gradient of the focused gel can be sampled with a surface pH electrode if desired. The cyclo-oxygenase activity is found in a broad peak centered at a pH of 6.5.

(v)   Fractionate the gel by pushing a 30-row grid into the gel, thus dividing it along its length into 30 separate fractions.

(vi)   Transfer each of the fractions to a small column with a spatula, and elute any protein with 6 ml of 10% glycerol/0.1% octyl glucoside.

(vii)   Concentrate the active fractions from isoelectric focusing to about 5 ml by ultrafiltration on an XM-50 membrane and load on a 1.6 × 75 cm column of either AcA 34 or Sephacryl S-300.

(viii) Elute with 50 mM Tris-HCl (pH 8.0)/0.1 M NaCl/0.1% octyl glucoside/0.1 mM EDTA/0.01% NaN_3.

(ix)   Pool the fractions containing cyclo-oxygenase activity and concentrate to about 10 ml by ultrafiltration on an XM-50 membrane.

(x)   Add glycerol (0.5 vol) as a cryoprotectant and divide up the solution into small aliquots for freezing on dry ice and subsequent storage at −70°C. The frozen synthase retains full cyclo-oxygenase activity for several years under these conditions.

The cyclo-oxygenase activity at each stage of the purification is monitored with the oxygen electrode assay. The assays are run in the presence and absence of haem to estimate the ratio of apoenzyme to total enzyme. Protein concentrations are assayed with the modification of the Lowry method described by Peterson (15). The homogeneity of the synthase preparation is assessed by standard electrophoretic techniques in polyacrylamide gels (16).

4. PROPERTIES OF CYCLO-OXYGENASE

4.1 Size of the synthase and its subunit composition

The pure PGH synthase exhibits a single band with a molecular weight of around 72 000 daltons when denatured with sodium dodecyl sulphate and analysed by polyacrylamide gel electrophoresis (17,18). Gel-filtration chromatography of the synthase in the presence of 6 M guanidinium-HCl also indicated a single polypeptide component, with molecular weight of 68 000 daltons (19).

The size of the native synthase has been assessed by both gel-filtration chromatography and by analytical ultracentrifugation (19). These methods indicate the protein molecular weight to be about 126 000−132 000 daltons, making it very likely that the native protein is a, made up of two subunits of about 70 000 daltons each. Cross-linking studies have supported the dimeric arrangement of the detergent-solubilized synthase (20), but the arrangement of the synthase in cellular membranes *in vivo* is not known. The synthase purified in Tween 20 was found to have 0.69 g detergent/g protein, whereas that purified in octyl glucoside had only 0.11 g detergent/g protein (19).

4.2 Haem requirement

Both catalytic activities of the synthase have been found to require a haem, iron protoporphyrin IX (3,17,18). Several haem analogs have also been tested. Haem a and iron mesoporphyrin IX promote both cyclo-oxygenase activity and peroxidase activity, whereas mangano protoporphyrin IX appears to promote the cyclo-oxygenase activity rather selectively (21). Myoglobin and haemoglobin are able to stimulate both activities of the synthase, but this has been found to be due to the haem released from these proteins (22).

The haem requirement of the two catalytic activities of the synthase can be assessed by monitoring the changes in the catalytic activities as a known portion of the apoenzyme is titrated with a concentrated solution of haem (22). The binding of haem to the synthase can also be monitored by the absorbance changes in the 410 nm region. One problem encountered with using absorbance measurements to quantitate binding is the large amount of non-specific binding of haem to the hydrophobic synthase − detergent complex that occurs, making any endpoint difficult to discern. In this respect, the use of dimethyl sulphoxide as the solvent for the haem has been found to help reduce non-specific binding in these titrations. The haem can be conveniently dissolved in dimethyl sulphoxide at a concentration of 5 mM.

From the results of many individual titrations of the synthase with haem, we concluded that only one haem is required per synthase dimer for full catalytic activity, although there appears to be one haem binding site on each subunit. One consequence of this unexpected stoichiometry of one haem per functional dimer is that the two polypeptide chains of the synthase are not functionally identical, although the two subunits appear very similar on the basis of electrophoretic analyses and N-terminal sequencing. Another consequence of the haem stoichiometry, with implications for the peroxidase and cyclo-oxygenase reaction mechanisms, is that the two catalytic activities of the synthase use the same molecule of haem as prosthetic group.

To reconstitute the holoenzyme, a concentrated solution of haem is added to the apoenzyme to give a haem/subunit ratio of 1 (a 2-fold excess), and the mixture incubated for about 30 min at room temperature. We have found recently that the addition of a peroxidase co-substrate (e.g. phenol or tryptophan) is not necessary to protect the pure cyclo-oxygenase activity from haem-dependent destruction as reported earlier (21, 24), but apoenzyme prepared by other methods may be different in this regard. Once reconstituted, the holoenzyme can be refrozen for storage.

4.3 Absorbance spectrum of the synthase

The synthase holoenzyme has been found to have an absorbance spectrum typical of a haemoprotein in the ferric state (25,26). A sample of synthase with very high cyclo-

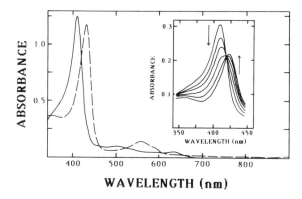

WAVELENGTH (nm)

Figure 2. Absorbance spectrum of the pure PGH synthase holoenzyme. The synthase was reconstituted with haem as described in the text. The solid line is the absorbance spectrum obtained from the resting (ferric) synthase; the broken line is that obtained after reduction of the synthase with dithionite. **Insert:** changes in the absorbance spectrum of the synthase at several points during a titration with NaCN. The arrows indicate the direction of the changes as the cyanide concentration was increased.

oxygenase specific activity (150 μmol O_2/min/mg; 5.4 μM haem; 11.4 μM subunit) was used to obtain the spectra shown in *Figure 2*. The main features of the spectrum of the resting synthase are the peak at 411 nm (extinction coefficient = 230 mM haem^{-1}cm^{-1}), the broad band at 500 nm and the charge-transfer band centered around 634 nm. The extinction coefficient at 411 nm has been found to vary considerably in different batches of the synthase, and may reflect a variable amount of haem binding sites with lower extinction coefficients in the various preparations. Treatment of the synthase with a small amount of the reductant sodium dithionite under an argon atmosphere (to avoid destruction of the haem, see ref. 27) converts the synthase to the ferrous form, with absorbance bands at 432 nm and 557 nm, and a shoulder at 591 nm (*Figure 2*).

Haem ligands, such as cyanide, have distinct effects on the cyclo-oxygenase and peroxidase activities (11,13,28) and on the absorbance spectrum of the synthase. An example of these absorbance changes is shown in the insert to *Figure 2*. The resting synthase was titrated with a solution of sodium cyanide, and the absorbance spectrum in the Soret region recorded after each addition of ligand. A progressive shift is seen from the initial peak at 410 nm to one with a lower extinction coefficient at 424 nm, with an isosbestic point at 420 nm. The fraction of the enzyme with bound ligand can be calculated from the absorbance at 410 nm, using the following equation:

$$[E \cdot CN]/[E_{total}] = 1 - (A_{410} - A_{410} \, final)/(A_{410} \, initial - A_{410} \, final). \qquad \text{Equation 2}$$

From the definition of the dissociation constant of the synthase·CN complex given in Equation 3

$$K_d = [E][CN]/[E \cdot CN] \qquad \text{Equation 3}$$

we can obtain the relationship shown in Equation 4

$$[E_{total}]/[E \cdot CN] = (K_d/[CN]) + 1 \qquad \text{Equation 4}$$

A plot of the ratio of total synthase to synthase haem complex (calculated using Equation 1) versus the reciprocal of the corresponding cyanide concentrations then allows estimation of the dissociation constant of the synthase·cyanide complex, which we have found to be about 0.2 mM (12).

4.4 **Protease sensitivity**

Proteases can be quite useful probes of an enzyme's structure. Protease digests of the native enzyme often give information about the topological arrangement of the component polypeptides, and digests of the denatured protein afford peptides useful for determining the primary sequence of the polypeptide. The synthase subunits are reasonably large polypeptides (over 500 amino acid residues), and only very limited regions ($\sim 5\%$ of the residues) have been sequenced to date. The response of the native synthase to trypsin does however give some clues to its topological arrangement. Although over 50 basic amino acids are present in each subunit (18,20), we found that at a synthase/trypsin ratio of 10 the apoenzyme appears to be cut only once by trypsin, and the holoenzyme is left untouched (29). Both catalytic activities are lost in concert from the apoenzyme upon hydrolysis by protease, and the addition of haem during the course of a digestion spares any remaining activity. In addition, the fragments appear to remain bound to each other after the apoenzyme is hydrolysed by trypsin, even though no disulphide bridges are present. Thus, the lysine and arginine residues are likely to be sequestered within the three-dimensional structure of the native synthase, and strong intra- and interpeptide bonding is likely to be present.

Some batches of the apoenzyme have been found to be more resistant to trypsin digestion than others. The source of this variability is not known, but it does not appear to be due to the residual haem in the preparations.

4.5 **Requirement for hydroperoxide initiator**

It has been known for 15 years that glutathione peroxidase, an enzyme that reduces hydroperoxides to the corresponding alcohols at the expense of oxidizing glutathione, is an effective inhibitor of the cyclo-oxygenase (30). The product of the cyclo-oxygenase reaction is the hydroperoxide, PGG_2, that can further stimulate the reaction (31), and glutathione peroxidase converts it to the non-stimulatory PGH_2. In the past few years it has become possible to quantitate the level of hydroperoxide needed to sustain the cyclo-oxygenase reaction *in vitro*, and to describe in biochemical terms parts of the sequence that leads to initiation of the cyclo-oxygenase reaction by hydroperoxide.

4.5.1 *Quantitation of the hydroperoxide requirement using glutathione peroxidase*

A method has been used that utilizes a competition between the cyclo-oxygenase and glutathione peroxidase for hydroperoxides to quantitate how much hydroperoxide is required to sustain the cyclo-oxygenase reaction. Fixed amounts of the synthase are reacted with arachidonic acid in the presence of increasing amounts of glutathione peroxidase, and the velocities of the cyclo-oxygenase reaction are determined. The result, when the percentage of remaining cyclo-oxygenase activity is plotted against the amount of glutathione peroxidase added, is generally a downwardly sloping straight line, as indicated by the solid symbols in *Figure 3*. It would be anticipated that the higher the requirement (K_p) of the cyclo-oxygenase for hydroperoxide, the less would be the

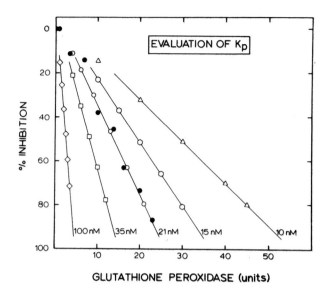

Figure 3. Evaluation of the requirement for activator hydroperoxide (K_p). The solid symbols represent the inhibition of the cyclo-oxygenase activity observed with the indicated levels of glutathione peroxidase. The various open symbols represent the computer-simulated results obtained when the indicated values of K_p were used in the calculations, as described in the text.

glutathione peroxidase needed for its inhibition, and thus the slope of the line shown in *Figure 3* should have the information necessary to determine the value of K_p. To convert the slope of this line to a K_p value, it is first necessary to set up a simple mathematical model for the reaction system containing the cyclo-oxygenase, the synthase peroxidase and the glutathione peroxidase (32). The model assumes all three enzyme activities follow Michaelis–Menten kinetic patterns, with velocities calculated from the following equations:

$$\text{Cyclo-oxygenase } V = [\text{synthase}] \times \text{cyclo-oxygenase } V_{max}/(1 + K_p/P)$$

Equation 5

$$\text{Synthase peroxidase } V = [\text{synthase}] \times \text{peroxidase } V_{max}/(1 + \text{peroxidase } K_m/P)$$

Equation 6

$$\text{Glutathione peroxidase } V = [\text{GSP}] \times \text{GSP } V_{max}/(1 + \text{GSP } K_m/P)$$

Equation 7

The values used in the model for the K_m of the synthase peroxidase for peroxide (2.5 μM), the cyclo-oxygenase V_{max} (45 nM PGG/sec/nM synthase) and the V_{max} of the synthase peroxidase (163 nM PGG/sec/nM synthase) are those determined experimentally. The value of the GSP K_m used is 1.5 μM and the level of synthase is 8.4 nM.

The three equations are then written into a computer program (Applesoft BASIC language for an Apple II + microcomputer) so that the three enzyme velocities can be evaluated rapidly and repeatedly, using small time intervals for each iteration, and a simulated reaction profile is generated. A value of K_p is chosen for each simulated

221

titration of the cyclo-oxygenase with glutathione peroxidase, and the simulated reaction is run with each of a series of increasing amounts of glutathione peroxidase. At the start of each simulated reaction, the hydroperoxide concentration (P) is assumed to be 1 nM, and the velocities of the three reactions are calculated for a 0.1 sec interval. The amounts of peroxide generated or consumed in the interval are tallied up, the peroxide concentration updated, and the calculations repeated for the next 0.1 sec interval. To mimic the self-catalysed inactivation observed with the actual enzyme, the amount of synthase was decreased by 1/1200 of the amount of cyclo-oxygenase and peroxidase turnover by the synthase during each interval.

The model predicts a linear decrease in cyclo-oxygenase velocity as the glutathione peroxidase level is increased (*Figure 3*), just as is observed for the real enzyme. By running the simulator program with several different values of K_p, it is possible to arrive at a value that fits the actual glutathione peroxidase titration data quite well. In the illustration in *Figure 3*, a good agreement is seen between the simulations (open symbols) and the experimental data (solid symbols) when the K_p value is 21 nM. A hyperbolic relationship exists between the value of K_p and the amount of glutathione peroxidase predicted to be needed for complete inhibition of the cyclo-oxygenase (12), allowing the value of K_p to be evaluated from the inhibition of the cyclo-oxygenase by glutathione peroxidase under different reaction conditions.

4.5.2 *Response of systems with an impaired cyclo-oxygenase to additions of hydroperoxide*

A value for K_p can also be evaluated from the response of the reaction kinetics of an impaired cyclo-oxygenase to additions of exogenous hydroperoxide (33). This method has the virtue of being usable for hydroperoxides other than PGG, including HOOH. The basic principle of this method for evaluating K_p is the faster acceleration of cyclo-oxygenase activity in the very early stages of the cyclo-oxygenase reaction if the initial level of hydroperoxide is increased (34). To make quantitation of these changes in the accelerative phase of the reaction more precise, it is necessary to impair the cyclo-oxygenase, so as to lengthen the duration of this phase from the control value of 5 sec to some 30−60 sec. A combination of 1 mM phenol and 5 mM cyanide has been found to give a suitable impairment of the cyclo-oxygenase.

The changes in the appearance of the cyclo-oxygenase reaction profile that result from impairment of the cyclo-oxygenase by phenol/cyanide, and from addition of hydroperoxide to the impaired system, are shown schematically in *Figure 4*. One indicator of the relative acceleration of the cyclo-oxygenase reaction, the lag (time at which the optimal cyclo-oxygenase velocity is reached), is indicated for each of the reactions with a dotted line. To quantitate the changes in the acceleration of the cyclo-oxygenase brought about by the addition of hydroperoxide, they are expressed as a fractional activation (FA) based on the following relationship:

$$FA = [\text{lag}_{(CN/phenol)} - \text{lag}_{(CN/phenol + sample)}]/[\text{lag}_{(CN/phenol)} - \text{lag}_{(phenol)}]$$

Equation 8

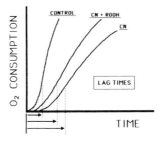

Figure 4. Changes in cyclo-oxygenase reaction kinetics upon addition of cyanide and hydroperoxide. Shown are schematic representations of the oxygen consumption versus time traces in cyclo-oxygenase reactions containing phenol alone (control), phenol and cyanide (+CN), and phenol, cyanide, and added lipid hydroperoxide (CN + ROOH). The dotted line indicates the lag time before the optimal cyclo-oxygenase velocity is reached in each of the three reactions.

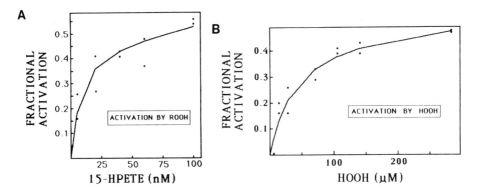

Figure 5. Activation of an impaired cyclo-oxygenase reaction system by added hydroperoxide. The responses of a cyanide/phenol-impaired cyclo-oxygenase reaction system to the indicated levels of added 15-HPETE (**A**) and HOOH (**B**) were quantitated as Fractional Activation values as described in the text.

For those fatty acid hydroperoxides and HOOH that have been examined in detail, the value of FA appears to be a saturable function of the concentration of hydroperoxide added (P) with the form:

$$FA = FA_{max}/(1 + K/P) \qquad \text{Equation 9}$$

where FA_{max} is the FA value at saturating levels of hydroperoxide.

In the case of 15-hydroperoxyeicosatetraenoic acid (HPETE), the value of K arrived at in this fashion (*Figure 5A*) is quite close to the 21 nM estimated for the K_p value of PGG_2 (another fatty acid hydroperoxide) by the competition with glutathione peroxidase described earlier, lending support to the idea that both K_p and K are measures of the hydroperoxide level required for sustained cyclo-oxygenase initiation. In contrast, the value of K for HOOH is of the order of 50 μM (*Figure 5B*), making it a much less effective initiator of the cyclo-oxygenase.

4.6 **Substrate requirements**

4.6.1 *Fatty acid*

The apparent accessibility of a fatty acid substrate to its enzyme reaction site is significantly influenced by binding to other proteins and other hydrophobic molecules and surfaces. Thus lower concentrations of substrate fatty acids can give maximal cyclo-oxygenase velocity when highly purified enzyme is used. Results obtained with the pure enzyme do not, however, give a clear indication of the accessibility to enzyme in cellular cytosol or in intracellular membranes. Nevertheless, K_s and K_i values permit some comparisons of the relative accessibility of different fatty acids to the substrate binding site. Crude preparations of PGH synthase have a K_s value for arachidonate (20:4 *n*-6) of $5-10$ μM, and some reported (35) K_i values are:

Fatty acid	K_i (μM)
18:1 *n*-9	22
18:3 *n*-3	15
20:3 *n*-3	6
20:5 *n*-3	2.5
22:6 *n*-3	1.7

The homologue of arachidonic acid, 20:3 *n*-6 reacts more rapidly than arachidonate in some systems, but the *n*-3 series of fatty acids are poor cyclo-oxygenase substrates, especially when hydroperoxide levels are kept low in the reaction system.

4.6.2 *Oxygen*

To examine the oxygen dependence of the cyclo-oxygenase reaction, the oxygen content in the reaction cuvette can be decreased by slightly raising the electrode and flushing the headspace with a stream of nitrogen gas, with the stirrer running. When the desired level of oxygen is reached, the flow of nitrogen and the stirrer are shut off and the electrode lowered back to the surface of the liquid, displacing the gas in the head space. As an alternative that avoids long equilibration times in the cuvette, a large volume of the reaction buffer in a flask can be saturated with the nitrogen by bubbling the gas through the buffer for 10 min or so, and an aliquot of the treated buffer quickly transferred to the reaction cuvette. When a wide range of oxygen concentrations were studied in this manner, it was found that the cyclo-oxygenase activity of a crude synthase preparation was relatively unaffected at values about 30 μM, and had half-maximal activity at about 5 μM (36). More recently, we have found the cyclo-oxygenase activity of the pure synthase to have a somewhat higher requirement for oxygen, with half-maximal activity at about 20 μM. The lower apparent oxygen requirement of the crude synthase may reflect the presence of oxygen-binding components that form a pool of oxygen that is not free to interact with the electrode, but is still available as substrate for the cyclo-oxygenase.

4.7 **Interaction with cyclo-oxygenase inhibitors**

4.7.1 *Time-dependent inhibitors*

The ability of non-steroidal anti-inflammatory drugs (NSAID) to inhibit the cyclo-oxygenase activity (36) has opened many new experimental approaches to studying the role of prostaglandins in physiological events. Aspirin and indomethacin cause a time-dependent loss of cyclo-oxygenase activity (38) that does not occur with the methyl esters of these agents (39). The time-dependent inactivation follows simple, first-order kinetics that has a decay rate characteristic for each agent and is linearly dependent on the concentration of the agent. As a result, the oxygenation rate observed after the enzyme has a 5 or 10 min pre-incubation with these agents is much less than when the enzyme is added to a mixture of agent and substrate. A comparison of these two types of response in drug screening programs permits a facile recognition of any agents with a time-dependent effect.

The selective action of NSAIDs on the cyclo-oxygenase leaves the peroxidase activity of the synthase uninhibited. In fact, these drugs have been found to stabilize the peroxidase activity to extremes of pH and heat (40). Titration of the synthase with small additions of time-dependent inhibitor gave linear decreases in the cyclo-oxygenase activity (measured after 5 min exposure), with maximal inhibition observed when about 1.2 mol of inhibitor had been added per mol of synthase dimer (8). Some $4-10\%$ of the original cyclo-oxygenase velocity remained even when excess drug had been added. Calibration of the routine protein assay with the synthase protein itself rather than using bovine serum albumin as the reference material made the calculations of stoichiometry more reliable. The sharp end-point in these titrations indicated a very high affinity of the synthase for the three drugs tested. The interaction of the synthase with the drugs was interpreted with the following paradigm:

$$E + I \underset{\longrightarrow}{\overset{K_i}{\longleftarrow}} EI \overset{k}{\longrightarrow} \text{inactive E}$$

Inactivation rate constants (k) ranged from 3 to 17 min^{-1} for the compounds studied (8), and K_i values ranged from 0.1 to 1.7 μM. The observed stoichiometry of 1 mol drug/mol of synthase dimer indicates that the two subunits of the synthase are distinct, and it echoes the observation that only one haem is required per dimer for full cyclo-oxygenase activity (23). Because the synthase apoenzyme and holoenzyme were found to require similar amounts of indomethacin for maximal inhibition of the cyclo-oxygenase, the difference between the two subunits in inhibitor binding is unlikely to result from binding of haem.

A lack of absorbance change around 410 nm in the spectrum when the synthase holoenzyme was treated with flurbiprofen indicated that any conformational change induced in the synthase by the binding of flurbiprofen did not alter the interaction between the synthase and its haem prosthetic group. The actions of the time-dependent agents on the cyclo-oxygenase are therefore likely to result from their actions at a site other than the haem.

Quantitative recovery of intact indomethacin from a stoichiometric mixture with the synthase that had an inhibited cyclo-oxygenase activity demonstrated convincingly that the inhibitory effect of the drug does not involve its covalent reaction with the enzyme. Rather, incubation of the synthase with the time-dependent inhibitors seemed to form a relatively stable variant of cyclo-oxygenase that had a considerably restrained catalytic velocity, but whose temporal catalytic lifespan was proportionately extended. The sigmoidal shape of the early portion of the cyclo-oxygenase time course was accentuated for the synthase treated with the time-dependent agents. The sigmoidal shape is evidence of the autoaccelerative nature of the cyclo-oxygenase reaction that has been shown to be a consequence of the requirement for hydroperoxide initiator. The treated synthase can be shown to retain a requirement for initiator by adding glutathione peroxidase and observing the inhibition of the cyclo-oxygenase activity. The well-established pharmacological effectiveness of the agents like indomethacin, may result from an inability of the catalytically slowed cyclo-oxygenase to generate a sustaining level of initiator hydroperoxide in the face of the full, unimpaired, activity of tissue peroxidases, including the peroxidase activity of the synthase itself.

4.7.2 *Rapidly reversible inhibitors*

Two other forms of inhibition observed with the cyclo-oxygenase involve interference with substrate binding (competitive inhibition) and antagonism of hydroperoxide activation (non-competitive inhibition). The former type is exhibited by all fatty acids, and also by many carboxylic NSAIDs. The latter type is exhibited by many phenolic and anti-oxidant molecules. Under assay conditions where the hydroperoxide levels are unrestrained, non-competitive agents of this type tend to be poor inhibitors (and sometimes they are even activators). They are increasingly effective inhibitors in the presence of hydroperoxide scavenging agents (41). The fact that inhibition by acetamidophenol can be observed only under assay conditions in which the concentration of hydroperoxides is suppressed has led to a hypothesis (42) that the successful use of acetamidophenol as an analgesic agent indicates that tissue hydroperoxide levels in human hyperalgesic states are not as high as those found in acute inflammatory states. We might thus expect hydroperoxide-antagonizing agents such as acetamidophenol to be more effective in relieving a general hyperalgesic state than a severe inflammatory condition.

5. ACKNOWLEDGEMENTS

Some of this work was supported by a grant from the United States Public Health Service, GM 30509.

6. REFERENCES

1. Kulmacz,R.J., Miller,J.F.,Jr. and Lands,W.E.M. (1985) *Biochem. Biophys. Res. Commun.*, **130**, 918.
2. Kulmacz,R.J. and Lands,W.E.M. (1983) *Adv. Prostaglandins Thromboxane Leukotriene Res.*, **11**, 93.
3. Miyamoto,T., Ogino,N., Yamamoto,S. and Hayaishi,O. (1976) *J. Biol. Chem.*, **251**, 2629.
4. Vanderhoek,J.Y. and Lands,W.E.M. (1973) *Biochim. Biophys. Acta*, **296**, 382.
5. Vanderhoek,J.Y. and Lands,W.E.M. (1973) *Biochim. Biophys. Acta*, **296**, 374.
6. Beechey,R.B. and Ribbons,D.W. (1972) *Methods Microbiol.*, **6B**, 25.
7. Cook,H.W., Ford,G. and Lands,W.E.M. (1979) *Anal. Biochem.*, **96**, 341.
8. Kulmacz,R.J. and Lands,W.E.M. (1985) *J. Biol. Chem.*, **260**, 12572.
9. Graff,G. (1982) In *Methods in Enzymology*. Lands,W.E.M. and Smith,W.L. (eds), Academic Press, New York, Vol. 86, p. 376.
10. Takeguchi,C. and Sih,C.J. (1972) *Prostaglandins*, **2**, 169.
11. Reed,G.A., Lasker,J.M., Eling,T.E. and Sivarajah,K. (1985) *Prostaglandins*, **30**, 153.
12. Kulmacz,R.J. and Lands,W.E.M. (1985) *Prostaglandins*, **29**, 175.
13. van der Ouderaa,F.J., Buytenhek,M., Slikkerveer,F.J. and van Dorp,D.A. (1979) *Biochim. Biophys. Acta*, **572**, 29.
14. Mevkh,A.T., Sudina,G.F., Golub,N.B. and Varfolomeev,S.D. (1985) *Anal. Biochem.*, **150**, 91.
15. Peterson,G.L. (1979) *Anal. Biochem.*, **100**, 201.

16. Laemmli,U.K. (1970) *Nature*, **227**, 680.
17. Hemler,M., Lands,W.E.M. and Smith,W.L. (1976) *J. Biol. Chem.*, **251**, 5575.
18. van der Ouderaa,F.J., Buytenhek,M., Nugteren,D.H. and van Dorp,D.A. (1977) *Biochim. Biophys. Acta*, **487**, 315.
19. van der Ouderaa,F.J.G. and Buytenhek,M. (1982) In *Methods in Enzymology*. Lands,W.E.M. and Smith, W.L. (eds), Academic Press, New York, Vol. 86, p. 60.
20. Roth,G.J., Siok,C.J. and Ozols,J. (1980) *J. Biol. Chem.*, **255**, 1301.
21. Ogino,N., Ohki,S., Yamamoto,S. and Hayaishi,O. (1978) *J. Biol. Chem.*, **253**, 5061.
22. Ueno,R., Shimizu,T., Kondo,K. and Hayaishi,O. (1982) *J. Biol. Chem.*, **257**, 5584.
23. Kulmacz,R.J. and Lands,W.E.M. (1984) *J. Biol. Chem.*, **259**, 6358.
24. Hemler,M.E. and Lands,W.E.M. (1980) *Arch. Biochem. Biophys.*, **201**, 586.
25. van der Ouderaa,F.J., Buytenhek,M. and van Dorp,D.A. (1980) *Adv. Prostaglandin Thromboxane Res.*, **6**, 139.
26. Roth,G.J., Machuga,E.T. and Strittmatter,P. (1981) *J. Biol. Chem.*, **256**, 10018.
27. Titus,B.G., Kulmacz,R.J. and Lands,W.E.M. (1982) *Arch. Biochem. Biophys.*, **214**, 824.
28. Hemler,M.E. and Lands,W.E.M. (1980) *J. Biol. Chem.*, **255**, 6253.
29. Kulmacz,R.J. and Lands,W.E.M. (1982) *Biochem. Biophys. Res. Commun.*, **104**, 758.
30. Lands,W., Lee,R. and Smith,W. (1971) *Ann. N.Y. Acad. Sci.*, **180**, 107.
31. Hemler,M.E., Graff,G. and Lands,W.E.M. (1978) *Biochem. Biophys. Res. Commun.*, **85**, 1325.
32. Kulmacz,R.J. and Lands,W.E.M. (1983) *Prostaglandins*, **25**, 531.
33. Marshall,P.J., Warso,M.A. and Lands,W.E.M. (1985) *Anal. Biochem.*, **145**, 192.
34. Hemler,M.E., Cook,H.W. and Lands,W.E.M. (1979) *Arch. Biochem. Biophys.*, **193**, 340.
35. Lands,W.E.M., LeTellier,P.R., Rome,L.H. and Vanderhoek,J.Y. (1973) *Adv. Biosci.*, **9**, 15.
36. Lands,W.E.M., Sauter,J. and Stone,G.W. (1978) *Prostaglandin Med.*, **1**, 117.
36. Vane,J.R. (1971) *Nature*, **231**, 232.
38. Smith,W.L. and Lands,W.E.M. (1971) *J. Biol. Chem.*, **246**, 6700.
39. Rome,L.H. and Lands,W.E.M. (1975) *Proc. Natl. Acad. Sci. USA*, **72**, 4863.
40. Mizuno,K., Yamamoto,S. and Lands,W.E.M. (1982) *Prostaglandins*, **23**, 743.
41. Hanel,A.M. and Lands,W.E.M. (1982) *Biochem. Pharmacol.*, **31**, 3307.
42. Lands,W.E.M. and Hanel,A.M. (1982) *Prostaglandins*, **24**, 271.

CHAPTER 13

Lipoxygenases: measurement, characterization and properties

TANKRED SCHEWE, HARTMUT KÜHN and SAMUEL M.RAPOPORT

1. INTRODUCTION

Lipoxygenases constitute a family of non-haem iron-containing dioxygenases that are widely distributed in animals and in plants. They catalyse the reaction of a polyenoic fatty acid, containing at least one 1,4-*cis,cis*-pentadiene system, with dioxygen forming a 1-hydroperoxy-2,4-*trans,cis* derivative (*Scheme 1*). The most important substrate of animal lipoxygenases is arachidonic acid (5,8,11,14-all *cis*-eicosatetraenoic acid). According to the position of the hydroperoxy group introduced at least three types of lipoxygenases have been distinguished (arachidonate 5-, 12- and 15-lipoxygenases). For a more precise classification see (1). In mammalian cells they are key enzymes in the biosynthesis of a variety of bioregulatory compounds such as hydroxyeicosate-traenoic acids (HETEs), leukotrienes, lipoxins and hepoxylines (2−4). In reticulocytes a cell-specific lipoxygenase is involved in the maturational breakdown of mitochondria (5).

The interest in lipoxygenases has grown since it was found that lipoxygenase products play a role in a variety of disorders such as bronchial asthma and inflammation. The study of the lipoxygenase pathway may contribute to the understanding of the pathogenesis of these disorders. Also the search for new lipoxygenase inhibitors appears to be a promising approach to develop new drugs.

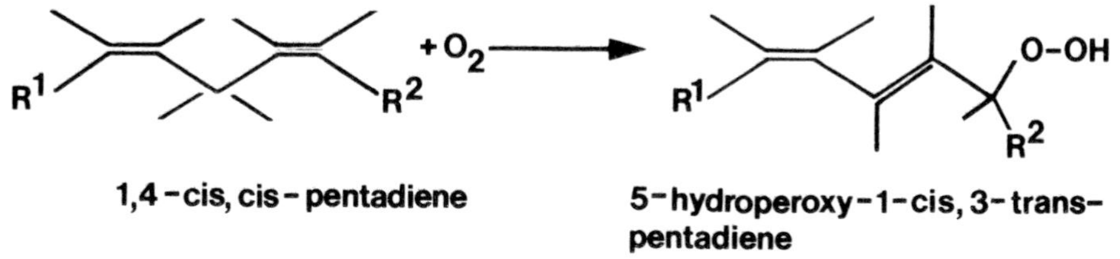

1,4-cis, cis-pentadiene   5-hydroperoxy-1-cis, 3-trans-
                                            pentadiene

Scheme 1. Scheme of dioxygenation reaction.

2. DETECTION AND ASSAY

The main methodological approach for the detection of lipoxygenases in animal systems has been the analysis of their products, mainly from labelled arachidonic acid. In cells generally the primarily formed hydroperoxides are reduced to the corresponding hydroxy compounds predominantly by the ubiquitous glutathione (GSH) peroxidase/GSSG reductase system. From the product pattern the type of lipoxygenase is deduced (for possible uncertainties and complications see Section 2.2). The quantification of lipoxygenase activities requires a purified system, since all methods are subject to interferences (see *Table 3*). Unfortunately, only a few animal lipoxygenases have been purified sufficiently to enable such quantitative analysis to be done.

2.1 Methods to measure lipoxygenase activity in purified systems

Generally three types of methods may be employed to follow lipoxygenase reactions:

(i)   measurement of the disappearance of one of the substrates (fatty acid or oxygen);
(ii)   measurement of the formation of primary products;
(iii) measurement of secondary products.

For kinetic studies, either oxygen consumption measured with a Clark electrode oxy-

Table 1. Selected substrates for the measurement of lipoxygenases.

Substrate	Use	Comments
Linoleic acid	Simplest natural substrate; few side-reactions.	(i) Stoichiometry between O_2 uptake and conjugated diene formation under suitable conditions. (ii) Poor substrate for some mammalian lipoxygenases. (iii) Haemoglobin exhibits 'quasi-lipoxygenase activity' exclusively with dienoic fatty acids.
Arachidonic acid	(i) Universal substrate. (ii) Physiological substrate for many mammalian lipoxygenases. (iii) Positional specificity can be determined by analysis of the reaction products(s).	Multiple dioxygenations and alternative reactions are possible; no stoichiometry between O_2 uptake and conjugated diene formation.
Other polyenoic fatty acids	Precise analysis of the positional specificity	–
Hydroperoxypolyenoic fatty acids (5-HPETE, 12-HPETE, 15-HPETE, 13-HPODE)	(i) Formation of epoxyleukotrienes (LTA_4 synthase activity) and lipoxins. (ii) Hydroperoxidase activities, formation of hepoxylines.	To avoid confusing an interference with multiple dioxygenations use anaerobic conditions (except for lipoxin formation)
Mono- and dihydroxy-eicosatetraenoic acids (5-HETE, 15-HETE, 5,15-DHETE)	Separate measurement of multiple dioxygenations; lipoxin formation.	Catalytic concentrations (1 μM) of a monohydroperoxypolyenoic fatty acid required.
Phospholipids (e.g. from soybeans, hen's eggs or mitochondria)	Selective for some arachidonate 15-lipoxygenases in the absence of phospholipase	Undefined reaction products, secondary oxygen-consuming processes.
Submitochondrial particles	Excellent substrate for reticulocyte lipoxygenase.	Inhibition of the respiratory chain provides a sensitive assay.

graphic method), or the formation of conjugated dienes absorbing at 234 nm (spectrophotometric method) are mostly used. The most important contaminants are haem compounds which should not exceed a concentration of 10^{-8} M in the assay mixture. A simple method to estimate the haem content is the recording of the spectrum in the range between 370 and 450 nm. A maximum at about 406 nm (Soret peak) is characteristic of haem compounds.

2.1.1 *Substrates and assay conditions*

A variety of substrates may be employed to measure lipoxygenase activity. The most commonly used substrates and their applications are compiled in *Table 1*. The choice depends on both the type of lipoxygenase and the aim of an investigation. Owing to certain peculiarities of lipoxygenase reactions some general rules that relate to lipoxygenase assay are recommended in *Table 2*. A particular problem is the poor water solubility of the fatty acids. It is improved by increasing the pH to about 9.0. However, the majority of mammalian lipoxygenases exhibit an optimum near the physiological pH range. At pH 7.2 most lipoxygenases show sufficient activity which can be further

Table 2. General rules to develop a lipoxygenase assay.

1.	If a polyenoic fatty acid is used as substrate, transform it first to its soap (potassium, sodium or ammonium salt).
2.	If a detergent is necessary (at pH <9; photometric assay), use 0.2% sodium cholate (analytical grade) as final concentration; avoid Triton (favours non-enzymatic lipid peroxidation).
3.	Take care that the assay mixture contains about 1 μM of a hydroperoxypolyenoic fatty acid before the addition of the enzyme (otherwise lag phase of unpredictable length).
4.	Measure at 2°C, but not above 25°C (strong self-inactivation).
5.	Take care that the oxygen concentration does not drop below 30 μM during the assay.
6.	Use buffers low in heavy metals (at least analytical grade).
7.	Avoid the presence of haem compounds.
8.	Test presumed lipoxygenase activity by the use of specific inhibitors (see Section 2.2).

Table 3. Comparison of the oxygraphic and the spectrophotometric methods.

Criterion	Oxygraphy	Spectrophotometry
Sensitivity	Low, unless special construction is used.	High, owing to molar absorption co-efficient of hydroperoxypolyenoic fatty acids ($\epsilon_{234} = 28\ 000\ \mathrm{M^{-1}cm^{-1}}$).
Susceptibility to interferences	(i) Competing or subsequent oxygen-consuming processes lead to overestimates.	(i) Secondary decomposition of hydro-peroxy fatty acids leads to underestimates.
	(ii) Sensitive to temperature fluctuations owing to high temperature coefficient of reduction potential of oxygen.	(ii) Additions absorbing near 234 nm; turbid substrates (requirement for dual-wavelength instruments).
Quantification	Calibration of the measuring scale required (see *Table 4*).	Directly from molar absorption coefficients.
Additional information	–	Measurement at other wavelengths (repeated scans) indicates secondary product formation (multiple dioxygenations, hydroperoxidase activity).

Table 4. NADH calibration of oxygraphic scale.

1.	Dissolve 20 mg of NADH (disodium salt) in 1 ml of 0.1 M phosphate buffer, pH 7.4 (not in water!).
2.	Determine the exact concentration of solution by measuring its absorbance at 340 nm (record the spectrum!); $\epsilon_{340} = 6.22 \times 10^6 \ \text{M}^{-1} \ \text{cm}^{-1}$.
3.	Add 5 μl of the NADH solution per ml of air-saturated buffer (without fatty acid!) in the oxygraphic vessel.
4.	Close the vessel, wait for 1 min until the baseline does not change further, and inject $20-50 \ \mu$l of a suspension of submitochondrial particles (50 mg protein per ml, prepared according to ref. 7 with the exception that disintegration of the mitochondria is performed preferably by sonication).
5.	Wait until the end of the reaction (usually 1 min).
6.	Add a further portion of submitochondrial particles; if necessary correct the change in scale value produced by the NADH/NADH oxidase system for the blank value of the submitochondrial particles.
7.	Evaluate oxygen consumption according to the equation: $$2 \ \text{NADH} + 2\text{H}^+ + \text{O}_2 \rightarrow 2 \ \text{NAD}^+ + 2\text{H}_2\text{O}$$

Table 5. Assay of reticulocyte lipoxygenase.

A. Recipe for substrate mixture

1.	Mix 0.2 ml of pure linoleic acid (or arachidonic acid) with 1 ml of freshly distilled methanol. Store this stock solution under nitrogen atmosphere at $-20°$C.
2.	Mix 20 μl of the stock solution with 20 μl of 0.54 M KOH or 0.54 M NH$_4$OH.
3.	Add this freshly prepared mixture to 2 ml of cold 0.1 M phosphate buffer, pH 7.4 containing 4% sodium cholate (analytical grade). Keep strict order of additions. Do not store the substrate mixture overnight.

B. Measuring procedure (preferably at $2-4°$C)

Spectrophotometry

1.	Put 0.95 ml of 0.1 M phosphate buffer, ph 7.4 in a pre-cooled quartz cuvette; add 50 μl of substrate mixture; mix gently.
2.	Start by addition of enzyme (usually $5-50 \ \mu$l).
3.	Record the absorbance at 234 nm for $2-3$ min.
4.	Evaluate the linear part of the trace.

Oxygraphy

1.	Mix 0.95 volumes of pre-cooled buffer and 0.05 volumes of substrate mixture.
2.	Fill the oxygraphic vessel and close with a stopper provided with a capillary outlet.
3.	Wait for $2-3$ min until the baseline remains constant.
4.	Start the reaction by adding enzyme (~ 2.5-fold amount as compared with spectrophotometry) through the outlet with a microsyringe.

Testing of inhibitors

1.	Dissolve the lipoxygenase inhibitor in methanol, ethanol or 2-methoxyethanol (methylglycol) as a 0.1 M solution. Add the inhibitor solution in the proper dilution in the same solvent in such a volume that the final concentration of the solvent does not exceed 2% of final volume. Add the same amount of solvent to identically handled control samples.
2.	Modify procedure; pre-incubate the enzyme with buffer and inhibitor for $5-10$ min at $20°$C. Start the reaction by adding substrate mixture.

enhanced by addition of a detergent. If sodium cholate is used, note that this detergent cannot be employed below pH 6.7. Clear substrate solutions at pH values between 7 and 8 can be obtained if they are made from the potassium or ammonium salts rather than from the free fatty acid. The substrates should not be exhausted during the assay;

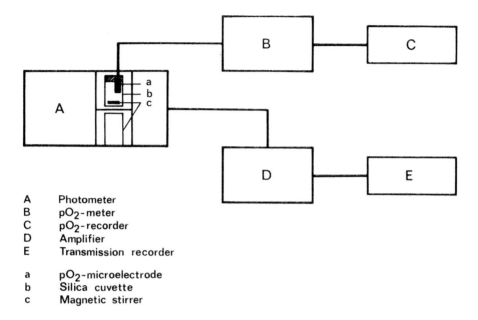

A	Photometer
B	pO₂-meter
C	pO₂-recorder
D	Amplifier
E	Transmission recorder

A Photometer
B pO_2-meter
C pO_2-recorder
D Amplifier
E Transmission recorder

a pO_2-microelectrode
b Silica cuvette
c Magnetic stirrer

Figure 1. Set-up for simultaneous oxygraphy and spectrophotometry.

otherwise alternative reactions take place such as aerobic hydroperoxidase reactions. At very high concentrations of substrate some lipoxygenases are subject to substrate inhibition. Sometimes the concentration of fatty acid in the assay is lowered by absorption on the vessel walls and phase separation. The actual concentration of lipoxygenase-accessible fatty acid can be easily determined, if the lipoxygenase is allowed to react up to substrate exhaustion and the concentration of the hydroperoxy fatty acid is measured photometrically at 234 nm.

2.1.2 *Oxygraphic and spectrophotometric measurement*

For most purposes either method is suitable to follow a lipoxygenase reaction. In *Table 3* their advantages and disadvantages are compared. There are however situations in which neither method alone gives reliable values of the lipoxygenase activity.

(i)   If crude enzyme preparations are used, where both secondary decomposition of hydroperoxy fatty acids (particularly in the presence of haem compounds) and alternative oxygen-consuming processes may occur.

(ii)   If the occurrence of aerobic hydroperoxidase activity of the lipoxygenase may be expected, for example at low oxygen concentrations (6).

A necessary but not sufficient criterion for the absence of interferences is the stoichiometry between the oxygen uptake and the formation of conjugated dienes. It may be checked by simultaneous measurement of both parameters (see Section 2.1.3).

From *Table 3* it may be concluded that the oxygraphic method is more suitable for the detection of lipoxygenase in crude systems, whereas the spectrophotometric procedure is more suitable with purified enzymes. For the study of lipoxygenase attack

233

on phospholipids and biological membranes the oxygraphic method is preferable. It is also indicated for the testing of lipoxygenase inhibitors which are often poorly soluble in water and absorb in the u.v.

The quantification of the oxygen uptake monitored by oxygraphy requires calibration. The measuring scale is obtained by two fix points, the upper one represented by the oxygen content of air-saturated water at the temperature of measurement (see physical-chemistry handbooks), the lower one by anaerobic conditions produced by the addition of a few grains of sodium dithionite. This calibration is only approximate, since the oxygen content of the assay mixture does not correspond to the value for pure water. Moreover, this method cannot be applied if the initial oxygen concentration desired deviates from that of air-saturated water. For precise studies calibration by NADH in the assay mixture is recommended (*Table 4*).

The same assay mixture may be applied for both the oxygraphic and the photometric method. As an example, the preparation of the assay mixture for reticulocyte lipoxygenase is given in *Table 5*.

2.1.3 Simultaneous measurement of oxygen uptake and conjugated diene formation

A special apparatus is recommended that permits the simultaneous monitoring of both parameters of the lipoxygenase reaction (*Figure 1*). The prerequisite of such a device is a highly sensitive micro Clark electrode coupled with an amplifier which permits the recording of an oxygen consumption of 2 nmol/min/ml. This value corresponds to an absorbance change at 234 nm of 0.05 min^{-1}.

2.2 Strategy to detect lipoxygenase activities in cells and tissues

The detection of lipoxygenase activities in complex systems faces the following difficulties:

(i)   the discrimination of a presumed lipoxygenase activity from other activities such as cyclo-oxygenase, cytochrome P-450-catalysed reactions (8), non-enzymatic lipid peroxidation, pseudo-lipoxygenase and quasi-lipoxygenase activities of haem compounds (9);

(ii)   the lability of lipoxygenases, in particular their tendency to self-inactivation;

(iii)   the masked state of some lipoxygenases, particularly arachidonate 15-lipoxygenases in many mammalian cells;

(iv)   alternative and consecutive reactions of both substrate fatty acids and the primary lipoxygenase products such as incorporation in esterified lipids, β-oxidation, ω-oxidation, etc;

(v)   the requirement for Ca^{2+} of the arachidonate 5-lipoxygenases (Ca^{2+} exerts a variety of other effects on the arachidonic acid metabolism).

2.2.1 Discrimination from alternative reactions

True lipoxygenase-catalysed reactions or lipoxygenase-derived products can be distinguished from related activities by means of criteria listed in *Table 6*. Important tools are inhibitors which are more or less specific (*Table 7*).

Table 6. Criteria for true lipoxygenase reactions.

1. Inhibition by 5,8,11,14-eicosatetraenoic acid (10^{-4} M)[a], nordihydroguaiaretic acid (10^{-5} M), 3-*t*-butyl-4-hydroxyanisole (10^{-3} M).

2. No inhibition by indomethacin (10^{-4} M), acetylsalicyclic acid (10^{-3} M)[a], 2,6-di-*t*-butyl-4-hydroxy-toluene (10^{-3} M)[b], metyrapone (10^{-4} M).

3. Stereospecificity of hydrogen abstraction (stereospecifically ^{3}H- or ^{2}H-labelled substrates required; ref. 10).

4. Positional specificity and stereospecificity of the primary products (application of chiral-phase h.p.l.c.)[c] (11).

[a]Pre-incubation required.
[b]Soybean lipoxygenase-1 is an exception.
[c]Pea lipoxygenase-1 is an exception.

Table 7. Effects of inhibitors on lipoxygenases and alternative reactions.

Inhibitor	Concentration (mM)	LOX	COX	Quasi-LOX activity	LPO	Cyt.P-450
ETYA	0.1	+	+	−	−	−
NDGA	0.01	+	+	+	+	n.t.
BHA	1	+	+	+	+	n.t.
BHT	1	−[a]	−	+	+	n.t.
BW 755C	0.1	+	+	n.t.	n.t.	n.t.
SHAM	1	+	+	+	n.t.	−
U-60275	0.05	+[b]	−	n.t.	n.t.	n.t.
AA 861	0.001	+[b]	−	n.t.	n.t.	n.t.
Acetylsalicylate	1	−	+	+	n.t.	−
Indomethacin	0.1	−	+	+	n.t.	−
Metyrapone	0.05	−	n.t.	n.t.	n.t.	+

[a]Some lipoxygenases are inhibited.
[b]Presumably specific for arachidonate 5-lipoxygenase.
n.t., not tested; LOX, lipoxygenase; COX, cyclo-oxygenase; LPO, lipid peroxidation; ETYA, 5,8,11,14-eicosatetraenoic acid; NDGA, nordihydroguaiaretic acid; BHA, 3-*t*-butyl-4-hydroxyanisole; BHT, 2,6-di-*t*-butyl-4-hydroxytoluene; BW 755C, 3-amino-1-/m-(trifluoromethyl)phenyl/-2-pyrazoline; SHAM, salicyl-hydroxamic acid; U-60275, 6,9-diepoxy-6,9-phenylimino-△6,8-prostaglandin I $_1$ (piriprost); AA 861, 2-(12-hydroxydodeca-5,10)-diynyl-3,5,6-trimethyl-1,4-benzoquinone.

2.2.2 *Methodological difficulties and their circumvention*

The self-inactivation of lipoxygenases (and also of cyclo-oxygenase) is favoured under conditions of strong liberation of free fatty acids such as damage to cells or activation of leukocytes and platelets. It may prevent the detection of lipoxygenase activity. Therefore care should be taken to avoid such situations during isolation of the cells. On the other hand, the unmasking of some lipoxygenases requires damage to cells (e.g. by freeze−thawing), which leads to the risk of activation of phospholipases.

The detection of the existence of a lipoxygenase pathway depends on the sensitivity of the procedures employed and the extent of reactions removing the lipoxygenase products as well as of those competing for the substrate. Interferences by reactions related to cell respiration are simply prevented by addition of antimycin A (10^{-5} M) which also inhibits β-oxidation and esterification of fatty acids.

Table 8. Procedure for isolation and analysis of hydroxypolyenoic fatty acids from cells.

1.	Resuspend at least 10^7 cells (leukocytes, lymphocytes, macrophages, mast cells, thrombocytes, reticulocytes, endothelial or smooth muscle cells or cells from various cell cultures, etc.) in 1 ml of Krebs−Ringer phosphate buffer or another suitable medium in a 5 ml glass-stoppered tube.
2.	Add 5 μl of a 0.2 M methanolic solution of linoleic or arachidonic acid to 5 ml of Krebs−Ringer phosphate buffer. Add 2.5 μCi of 1-^{14}C-labelled linoleic or arachidonic acid, respectively. Shake the substrate mixture frequently in a thermostat at 37°C. The substrate mixture is sufficient for five samples.
3.	Mix 1 ml of substrate mixture with 1 ml of the cell suspension. Add Ca^{2+} ionophore A23187 to a final concentration of 15 μM.
4.	Shake this mixture cautiously for 10 min at 37°C.
5.	Stop the reaction by rapid addition of the proper volume of 1 M sulphuric acid or citric acid to reach a pH of 3−4 (exactly to pH 4.5 in the case of red blood cells).
6.	Extract twice with 2 ml of ethylacetate, by means of a Vortex shaker (vibrator) for 1−2 min. If necessary, separate the solvent phases by centrifugation.
7.	Wash the combined ethylacetate extracts with saturated NaCl solution and dry by addition of anhydrous sodium sulphate.
8.	Evaporate the solvent under vacuum (rotary evaporator). Dissolve the residue in oxygen-free methanol. Add 1 p.p.m. of butylated hydroxytoluene (BHT) to protect the products from free radical-induced decomposition. Store under argon at −30°C.
9.	Apply aliquots to pre-coated silica gel t.l.c. plates in parallel with authentic standards. Develop in the solvent hexane-diethylether-glacial acetic acid (50:50:1 by vol). Scan radioactivity and evaluate the percentages of the fractions. Scrape off the silica gel from the regions of active fractions and extract with methanol or diethyl ether (for details see Chapter 5).
10.	Perform h.p.l.c. analysis (see Chapter 6 and ref. 11).

Since all lipoxygenases react preferentially with free fatty acids and the arachidonate 5-lipoxygenase only with them, activation of phospholipases is sometimes an essential pre-condition of detection of lipoxygenase activity. A high intracellular level of Ca^{2+}, which may be produced by the ionophore A23187, activates phospholipase A_2 and is essential for the arachidonate 5-lipoxygenase activity.

Interference by reactions removing lipoxygenase products is reduced by short incubation times. Low amounts of substrate are supplied so that they are exhausted within a few minutes. Such experiments may be classified as pulse-labelling.

2.2.3 *Detection of lipoxygenase activities in cells*

Usually the conversion of external radioactivity labelled polyenoic fatty acids to mono- and dihydroxypolyenoic fatty acids including leukotriene B_4 (a major lipoxygenase-derived eicosanoid in inflammatory cells) and to cysteinyl leukotrienes is studied. The hydroxypolyenoic acids (reduced species of the primary hydroperoxides) are simply isolated from the incubation mixture by one-step organic solvent extraction after acidification (for the isolation of the cysteinyl leukotrienes see Chapter 4). The organic solvent extract is analysed by quantitative radio t.l.c. or h.p.l.c. The procedure is described in *Table 8*. It is applicable to homogenates as well as to crude and purified enzyme preparations. The method is more sensitive than those described in Section 2.1, but not applicable for kinetic measurements. For homogenates it is recommended that the radioactive substrate is added immediately prior to or during the disintegration step,

Table 9. Recommendations for separation of lipoxygenases for activity staining.

1.	Pre-purify the lipoxygenase(s) as far as possible (e.g. by ammonium sulphate fractionation and anion-exchange chromatography). The higher the initial purity the sharper are the activity-stained bands. Crude extracts or cytosol fractions usually give diffuse bands, if any, after electrophoresis.
2.	Use a 5–10% gradient gel of polyacrylamide gel for disc electrophoresis. Omit a stacking gel.
3.	Isoelectric focusing in the pH range 5–7 is most versatile and discriminates different lipoxygenases.

Table 10. Procedure for the reaction step.

1.	If polyacrylamide gel electrophoresis at alkaline pH is used, be sure to rinse the gel with de-ionized water in a vessel of appropriate dimensions.
2.	Cover the gel with 0.1 M phosphate buffer, pH 6.8 and incubate for 15 min at 4°C.
3.	Freshly prepare the substrate mixture in an identical way as given in *Table 5* except that 0.1 M phosphate buffer, pH 6.8 containing 0.1% sodium cholate is used as basal medium.
4.	Pour off buffer and cover the gel with substrate mixture and allow reaction for 15 min at 4°C.

since otherwise a putative lipoxygenase activity may escape detection owing to self-inactivation.

With cells the following problems may arise.

(i)   The dilution of the exogenous labelled fatty acid by the pool of free fatty acids within the cells raises the threshold of detectability; in addition, the share of the lipoxygenase pathway may be underestimated.

(ii) The pattern of products found after pulse-labelling is strongly dependent on the time of incubation. The distribution of products can be determined from their specific radioactivities which can be calculated after h.p.l.c. separation from the absorbances at 234 nm (hydroxypolyenoic fatty acids) or 268 nm (leukotrienes). For this purpose a calibration of the h.p.l.c. elution scale by standard compounds is recommended.

(iii) The polyenoic fatty acid pools appear to be compartmentalized. Therefore external and endogenous polyenoic fatty acids may behave differently.

(iv) To test endogenous phospholipids as a source of lipoxygenase products, pre-labelling of the cells may be carried out; thereby the phospholipids are esterified with the radioactive fatty acid.

(v)   Some lipoxygenases are able to attack esterified fatty acids including phospholipids (5). The direct analysis of oxygenated phospholipid species requires special h.p.l.c. methods. Another approach is the use of $H_2^{18}O$ or $H_2^{17}O$. If the oxygenated phospholipids are subsequently hydrolysed in oxygen isotope-containing water, the isotope is introduced in the carboxylic group in contrast to the lipoxygenase products formed from free polyenoic fatty acids. .

2.3. Detection of lipoxygenases by activity staining

Lipoxygenases can be detected by specific staining of the protein bands for enzymic activity after separation by polyacrylamide gel electrophoresis, isoelectric focusing in polyacrylamide layers or related techniques. Some general experiences in the authors' hands are listed in *Table 9*.

Table 11. Procedure for the staining step.

A. Staining solution

1. Dissolve 0.1 g of *o*-dianisidine-HCl(3,3'-dimethoxybenzidine hydrochloride) in 10 ml of 96% ethanol with heating.
2. Add this solution to 90 ml of hot 0.1 M phosphate buffer, pH 6.8.
3. If necessary, decant after cooling from partially re-crystallized reagent.

B. Procedure

1. Rinse the gel thoroughly with de-ionized water.
2. Cover the gel with the staining solution.
3. Allow to stand for at least 2 h until reddish spots indicate the location of lipoxygenase activity.

The staining for activity includes two steps:

(i) incubation of the gel with a reaction mixture containing linoleic acid or arachidonic acid (reaction step);

(ii) localization of the lipoxygenase bands by a reagent to detect hydroperoxy compounds (staining step).

For the reaction step the guidelines given in Section 2.1.1 should be followed. The choice of the reaction mixture depends on the special properties of the lipoxygenase to be detected. The recipe given in *Table 10* has proved to be fairly universally applicable in our hands.

For the staining step *o*-dianisidine (3,3'-dimethoxybenzidine hydrochloride) is recommended (12). The procedure described in *Table 11* gives the best results. The main advantages are high sensitivity (comparable with the spectrophotometric lipoxygenase assay), negligible background colouring and stability of the colour. Ferrous thiocyanate (13) is also applicable, but with this reagent rapid background colouring can occur owing to its autoxidation. Potassium iodide-starch is not recommended, since the reaction is too slow and unspecific.

2.4 Immunological and molecular-biological detection of lipoxygenases

It is possible in some cases to analyse the amount and identity of lipoxygenase protein, its new synthesis and the mRNA coding for it. A pre-condition is the availability of antibodies, but only few of the mammalian lipoxygenases have been purified to the extent necessary for antibody production. Antibodies against a certain lipoxygenase may not be widely applicable; reticulocyte lipoxygenase, for example, is erythroid cell specific; its antibody does not cross-react with non-erythroid lipoxygenases.

For the immunological detection of reticulocyte lipoxygenase protein all standard techniques such as immuno-double-diffusion according to Ouchterlony or radial immuno-diffusion according to Mancini may be applied. A particularly useful technique is the 'Western' immunoblot procedure, which is applicable after sodium dodecylsulphate polyacrylamide gel electrophoresis (SDS−PAGE). After electrophoresis the unstained proteins are electrophoretically transferred to nitrocellulose paper, and the lipoxygenase is identified with an anti-lipoxygenase plus [^{125}I]protein A according to the procedure of Schmidt *et al.* (14).

Table 12. Guidelines to purify lipoxygenases.

A. Suitable methods

1. Ammonium sulphate fractionation (18).
2. Anion-exchange chromatography on DEAE Sephadex A-50 (18,21).
3. Isoelectric focusing (pH 5−7) (18).
4. F.p.l.c. techniques (19).
5. Affinity chromatography on the linoleic acid derivative of aminoethyl-Sepharose 4B under strictly anaerobic conditions (22).

B. General rules

1. Use heavy metal-free buffers; pass them through a Dowex A1 column; check for the absence of copper by extraction with dithizone reagent (0.001% in carbon tetrachloride) and for the absence of inorganic iron by bathophenanthroline reagent (0.1% in amyl alcohol).
2. Exclude O_2 during purification; use anaerobic buffers.
3. Avoid long standing between the preparation steps.
4. Store in liquid nitrogen.
5. Avoid Amicon filters for concentration of protein solutions.

In reticulocytes a new synthesis of lipoxygenase occurs which can be used for its detection in intact cells. They are incubated with [^{14}C]leucine or [^{35}S]methionine; thereafter the proteins of the cytosol are separated by SDS−PAGE, and the labelled polypeptide is visualized by autoradiography. The position of the lipoxygenase protein is localized by reference to purified enzyme or more specifically by double antibody precipitation (15). Lipoxygenases generally consist of a single polypeptide chain of more than 60 kd, so that they can be easily recognized among the synthesized polypeptides.

For the lipoxygenase mRNA of rabbit reticulocytes (16) and of pea seeds (17) clones of cDNA have been prepared. They can be used as probe for the presence of lipoxygenase mRNA.

3. PRINCIPLES OF ISOLATION AND PURIFICATION OF LIPOXYGENASES

All lipoxygenases except for soybean lipoxygenase-1 are extraordinarily labile. Therefore their purification is difficult: from animal sources the enzyme from rabbit reticulocytes can be obtained in comparatively large amounts (18). Recently, the arachidonate 5-lipoxygenase from human leukocytes and rat basophil leukaemia cells have also been purified to homogeneity although in very small amounts (19,20). Partial purification has been reported for the lipoxygenases of platelets, lungs, skin and testicles as well as for the arachidonate 12- and 15-lipoxygenases of white cells [for references see (5)]. Some general guidelines for purification of animal lipoxygenases are listed in *Table 12*.

4. CHARACTERIZATION OF LIPOXYGENASES

The characteristics of lipoxygenases with special reference to reticulocyte lipoxygenase are reviewed elsewhere (5). In this chapter only some methodological aspects are dealt with.

Table 13. Structural properties of DHETEs and on the mechanism of their formation.

Property	LTA₄ hydrolysis	Double dioxygenation
Positional isomerism	Obligatory occurrence of pairs of positional isomers (14,15- and 8,15-DHETE from 14,15-LTA$_4$, 5,6- and 5,12-DHETE from 5,6-LTA$_4$).	Usually preponderance of one positional isomer.
Configuration of chiral centres	Obligatory occurrence of diastereomers epimers at C_{14} and C_8 (14,15-LTA$_4$) or C_6 and C_{12} (5,6-LTA$_4$), respectively.	Stereospecific products.
Geometry of double bonds	All-*trans* conjugated triene in 8,15- and 5,12-DHETEs.	One double bond of the triene retains *cis* structure.
Isotopic composition	Incorporation of ^{18}O (^{17}O) from $H_2{}^{18}O$ ($H_2{}^{17}O$) in one of the OH groups.	Incorporation of $^{18}O_2$ ($^{17}O_2$) gas in both OH groups.

4.1 Positional and steric specificity

The lipoxygenase catalysis comprises two main steps:

(i)   abstraction of hydrogen from a double-allylic methylene group;

(ii)   introduction of dioxygen at an enzyme-bound, *cis,trans*-butadienyl radical.

Generally both steps proceed with a certain positional and steric specificity (1) with preponderance of the formation of a defined product. The stereospecificity of hydrogen abstraction can be directly determined by the use of stereospecifically ^2H- or ^3H-labelled polyenoic fatty acids (10). It may also be indirectly deduced from the stereospecificity of the dioxygen insertion which is established by analysis of the reaction product, since both steps of the catalytic cycle proceed anterofacially to each other. The positional isomers may be easily analysed by h.p.l.c. techniques (see Chapter 6). Either the free acids or their methyl esters are used. The latter are simply obtained by reaction with ethereal diazomethane (**Caution:** this reagent is strongly mutagenic; use gloves!). Although the hydroperoxypolyenoic fatty acids formed by purified lipoxygenases may be directly applied to h.p.l.c., it is recommended to reduce them immediately after the enzymatic reaction by either sodium borohydride (in water) or triphenyl phosphine (in organic solvents), since the hydroxypolyenoic fatty acids are more stable.

The analysis of the optical isomers requires micromolar amounts of substance as well as cumbersome chemical derivatizations (23−25). We have developed a chiral-phase h.p.l.c. method for the separation of both positional and optical isomers of lipoxygenase-derived hydroxy fatty acids (11). In addition to its simplicity this procedure is more sensitive by several orders of magnitude than the methods employed earlier; 10 pmol are sufficient for analysis.

4.2 Special lipoxygenase-catalysed reactions

In addition to the single dioxygenation of polyenoic fatty acids, lipoxygenases catalyse some further reactions such as double and triple dioxygenation, hydroperoxidase reactions and formation of epoxyleukotrienes from hydroperoxyeicosatetraenoic acids (HPETEs).

4.2.1 *Multiple dioxygenations*

Important lipoxygenase-derived dioxygenation products found in several animal cells are 5,15-, 8,15-, 5,12- and 14,15-dihydroxyeicosatetraenoic acids (DHETEs) (1,2). Except for 5,15-DHETE, these dihydroxyeicosanoids may also be formed by hydrolysis of epoxyleukotrienes (5,6-LTA$_4$ or 14,15-LTA$_4$, respectively). *Table 13* gives a comparison of the products formed by the two possible pathways. Unfortunately, the use of oxygen isotopes does not permit unequivocal discrimination, since dioxygen may be reduced in cells to superoxide (in particular in leukocytes) that attacks the epoxyleukotrienes as a nucleophile.

If 5-, 12- or 15-HETE are used as substrates, the product must in any case originate from double dioxygenation since both epoxyleukotriene formation and hydroperoxidase activities that require the presence of a hydroperoxy group are not possible. The reaction sample must contain about 2 μmol of a hydroperoxypolyenoic fatty acid, preferably 13-HPODE, as activator of the lipoxygenase (26).

5,15-DHETE is converted by reticulocyte lipoxygenase mainly to lipoxin-B which contains a conjugated tetraene system (27).

4.2.2 *Hydroperoxidase activities*

At low oxygen concentration lipoxygenases catalyse reactions of hydroperoxy fatty acids (e.g. HPODE) with the corresponding fatty acids. A complex mixture of products including oxooctadecadienoic acids, epoxyhydroxyoctadecenoic acids, linoleic acid dimers and pentane are formed [see (5)]. 12-HPETE is converted to hepoxylines (4), which have been suggested to mediate glucose-stimulated insulin secretion. Owing to the heterogeneity of products it is not possible to follow kinetically the whole hydroperoxidase reaction. Parts of it can be measured by following:

(i)   decrease in absorbance at 234 nm indicating formation of products other than dienes;

(ii)   increase in absorbance at 285 nm indicating formation of oxodienes. Here again repeated scans of the spectra are useful.

In combination with the chemical determination of the hydroperoxide content it is possible to evaluate the rough composition of the hydroperoxidase products.

4.2.3 *Leukotriene A$_4$ synthase activity*

Purified lipoxygenases are able to convert 5D$_S$- or 15L$_S$-HPETE to the unstable compounds 5,6-LTA$_4$- and 14,15-LTA$_4$, respectively. Partial steps of both dioxygenase and hydroperoxidase reactions may be involved in this reaction (1,5). The LTA$_4$ synthase activity can be measured kinetically under anaerobic conditions on account of the increase in absorbance at 270 nm owing to the formation of the conjugated triene system characteristic of leukotrienes. Anaerobiosis is necessary to avoid confounding with multiple dioxygenations (see also *Table 13*). A strong proof for the formation of an epoxytriene or epoxytetraene eicosanoid is the detection of methanolysis products of the highly unstable epoxide by h.p.l.c. and g.c./m.s. If methanolysis is performed with radioactive methanol one may dispense with mass spectroscopic identification (3,28).

5. ACKNOWLEDGEMENTS

We should like to thank Dr K.Pönicke (Institute of Pharmacology and Toxicology of the Martin-Luther-University Halle/Saale, GDR) for constructing the device for simultaneous measurement of oxygen consumption and conjugated diene formation as well as Gertrud Ryssowski for typing the manuscript.

6. REFERENCES

1. Kühn,H., Schewe,T. and Rapoport,S.M. (1986) In *Advances in Enzymology*. Meister,A. (ed.), John Wiley and Sons, New York, Vol. 58, p. 273.
2. Hansson,G., Malmsten,C. and Rådmark,O. (1983) In *Prostaglandins and Related Substances*. Pace-Asciak,C.R. and Granström,E. (eds), Elsevier Scientific Publishers, Amsterdam, p. 127.
3. Adams,J., Fitzsimmons,B.J., Girard,Y., Leblanc,Y., Evans,J.F. and Rokach,J. (1985) *J. Am. Chem. Soc.*, **107**, 464.
4. Pace-Asciak,C.R., Martin,J.M., Corey,E.J. and Su,W.-G. (1985) *Biochem. Biophys. Res. Commun.*, **128**, 942.
5. Schewe,T., Rapoport,S.M. and Kühn,H. (1986) In *Advances in Enzymology*. Meister,A. (ed.), John Wiley and Sons, New York, Vol. 58, p. 191.
6. Kühn,H., Salzmann-Reinhardt,U., Ludwig,P., Pönicke,K., Schewe,T. and Rapoport,S. (1986) *Biochim. Biophys. Acta*, **876**, 187.
7. Crane,F.L., Glenn,J.L. and Green,D.E. (1956) *Biochim. Biophys. Acta*, **22**, 475.
8. Capdevila,J., Marnett,L.J., Chacos,N., Prough,R.A. and Estabrook,R.W. (1982) *Proc. Natl. Acad. Sci. USA*, **79**, 767.
9. Kühn,H., Götze,R., Schewe,T. and Rapoport,S.M. (1981) *Eur. J. Biochem.*, **120**, 161.
10. Brash,A.R., Maas,R.L. and Oates,J.A. (1985) *J. Allerg. Clin. Immunol.*, **74**, 316.
11. Kühn,H., Wiesner,R., Lankin,V.Z., Nekrasov,A.A., Alder,L. and Schewe,T. (1987) *Anal. Biochem.*, **160**, 24.
12. DeLumen,B.D. and Kazeniak,S.J. (1976) *Anal. Biochem.*, **72**, 428.
13. Koch,R.B., Stern,B. and Ferrari,C.G. (1958) *Arch. Biochem. Biophys.*, **78**, 165.
14. Schmidt,J.R., Myers,A.M., Gillham,N.W. and Boynton,J.E. (1984) *Mol. Biol. Evol.*, **1**, 317.
15. Thiele,B.J., Belkner,J., Andree,H., Rapoport,T.A. and Rapoport,S.M. (1979) *Eur. J. Biochem.*, **96**, 563.
16. Affara,N., Fleming,J., Goldfarb,P.S., Black,E., Thiele,B. and Harrison,P.R. (1985) *Nucleic Acids Res.*, **13**, 5639.
17. Casey,R., Domoney,C. and Nielsen,N.C. (1985) *Biochem. J.*, **232**, 79.
18. Schewe,T., Wiesner,R. and Rapoport,S.M. (1981) In *Methods in Enzymology*. Lowenstein,J.M. (ed.), Academic Press, New York, Vol. 71, p. 430.
19. Goetze,A.M., Fayer,L., Bouska,J., Bornemeier,D. and Carter,G.W. (1985) *Prostaglandins*, **29**, 689.
20. Rouzer,C.A. and Samuelsson,B. (1985) *Proc. Natl. Acad. Sci. USA*, **82**, 6040.
21. Siegel,M.I., McConnel,R.T., Porter,N.A. and Cuatrecasas,P. (1980) *Proc. Natl. Acad. Sci. USA*, **77**, 308.
22. Grossman,S., Trop,M., Yawni,S. and Wilchek,M. (1972) *Biochim. Biophys. Acta*, **289**, 77.
23. Hamberg,M. (1981) *Anal. Biochem.*, **43**, 515.
24. Van Os,C.P.A., Rijke-Schilder,G.P.M., Kamerling,J.P., Gerwig,G.J. and Vliegenthart,J.F.G. (1980) *Biochim. Biophys. Acta*, **620**, 326.
25. Van Os,C.P.A., Rijke-Schilder,G.P.M., Van Halbeek,H., Verhagen,J. and Vliegenthart,J.F.G. (1981) *Biochim. Biophys. Acta*, **663**, 177.
26. Kühn,H., Wiesner,R., Lankin,V.Z., Nekrasov,A., Schewe,T. and Rapoport,S. (1986) *FEBS Lett.*, **203**, 247.
27. Kühn,H., Wiesner,R., Alder,L., Schewe,T. and Stender,H. (1986) *FEBS Lett.*, **208**, 248.
28. Bryant,R.W., Schewe,T., Bailey,J.M. and Rapoport,S.M. (1985) *J. Biol. Chem.*, **260**, 3548.

CHAPTER 14

Lipid peroxidation

TREVOR F.SLATER and KEVIN H.CHEESEMAN

1. INTRODUCTION

Lipid peroxidation is a free radical-mediated process that involves the peroxidative degradation of lipid material. In its broadest sense, the term 'lipid peroxidation' includes:

(i)   the peroxidative reactions of all types of lipid materials such as free fatty acids, phospholipids, triglycerides, cholesterol., etc.; and

(ii)   peroxidative mechanisms that may be non-enzymic in character, such as autoxidations, or enzyme-catalysed as with those reactions dependent on lipoxygenases (see Chapter 13) or cyclo-oxygenases (see Chapter 12).

In this chapter on practical aspects of lipid peroxidation, attention will be directed to only a few specific aspects of this broad set of reactions: indeed, some important topics will not be discussed at all, such as lipoxygenase (and cyclo-oxygenase) catalysed reactions, since these are dealt with elsewhere in this book. The peroxidation of cholesterol also will not be mentioned further here; a specialized review on this is by Smith (1). In fact, the main emphasis will be on the peroxidative degradations that can occur in membrane phospholipids, including any free fatty acids present, and where the initiation of peroxidation is by non-enzymic (radiation; metal-catalysed) and enzyme-catalysed mechanisms. Moreover, many of the examples will be given for rat liver endoplasmic reticulum (or 'microsomal' membranes) in order to make some detailed comparisons between the two different experimental approaches; references will be given, however, for peroxidative studies on other cellular membrane fractions.

The types of lipid peroxidation to be considered here are relatively unspecific in the sense that it is not too important whether the fatty acid is free or bound in phospholipids; moreover, the reactions can involve any unsaturated fatty acid although, in general, with the enzyme-catalysed reactions, the main changes are to arachidonate ($C_{20:4}$) and docosahexaenoic acid ($C_{22:6}$). The term 'lipid peroxidation' will be used in the remainder of this chapter with the understanding that the restrictions and comments made above are applied.

Lipid peroxidation is *initiated* by the attack of a reactive free radical ($R^{\cdot}$) on an unsaturated fatty acid (UFAH) such that a hydrogen-atom is abstracted and a carbon-centred fatty acid radical is formed:

$$R^{\cdot} + UFAH \rightarrow RH + UFA^{\cdot} \qquad \text{Equation 1}$$

243

The fatty acid radical can interact (usually very rapidly) with molecular oxygen to form the fatty acid peroxy-species:

$$UFA^{\cdot} + O_2 \rightarrow UFA\text{-}O\text{-}O^{\cdot} \qquad \text{Equation 2}$$

This peroxy-radical can oxidize its neighbouring molecules by hydrogen abstraction either from another molecule of fatty acid or from some other hydrogen donor (XH):

$$UFA\text{-}O\text{-}O^{\cdot} + UFAH \rightarrow UFA\text{-}OOH + UFA^{\cdot} \qquad \text{Equation 3}$$
$$+ \qquad XH \rightarrow UFA\text{-}OOH + X^{\cdot}$$

so that a chain reaction involving UFA$^{\cdot}$ is *propagated*. In biological materials there are always transition metal ions present, either endogenously or as contaminants that can catalyse the breakdown of the hydroperoxides to a complex variety of products including reactive free radicals such as the alkoxy-derivatives, UFA-O$^{\cdot}$:

$$\begin{cases} UFA\text{-}OOH \\ UFA\text{-}OO^{\cdot} \\ UFA\text{-}O^{\cdot} \end{cases} \xrightarrow{\text{metal ions}} \begin{array}{l} UFA\text{-}O^{\cdot} \\ UFA\text{-}OH \text{ (lipid alcohol)} \\ \text{Aldehydes, unsaturated aldehydes,} \\ \text{alkanes} \\ \text{shorter chain UFA-OOH,} \\ \text{epoxy-fatty acids, etc.} \end{array} \qquad \text{Equation 4}$$

Although Equation 4 gives some idea of the complexity of the reaction products of lipid peroxidation, it should also be noted that the complexity is compounded by:

(i)   the variety of unsaturated fatty acids present in biological samples that are susceptible to attack by free radical initiators;
(ii) the different stereo-isomeric products that can be produced from an initial hydrogen-atom abstraction of a polyunsaturated fatty acid (PUFAH):

$$R^{\cdot} + PUFA(H) \rightarrow RH + PUFA^{\cdot} \qquad \text{Equation 5}$$
$$PUFA^{\cdot} + XH \rightarrow \text{different diene isomers} \qquad \text{Equation 6}$$
$$PUFA^{\cdot} \xrightarrow{+O^{\cdot}_2 +XH} \text{different PUFA-OOH isomers} \qquad \text{Equation 7}$$

These reactions have been intensively studied, in particular by Porter and colleagues (2,3).

2. METHODS FOR MEASURING LIPID PEROXIDATION

The outline of lipid peroxidation that has been given above can be summarized for the case of a polyunsaturated fatty acid in a biomembrane as follows:

$$PUFA(H) + R^{\cdot} \rightarrow PUFA^{\cdot} + RH \qquad \text{Equation 8}$$
$$PUFA^{\cdot} \rightarrow \text{bond re-arrangements, appearance of} \qquad \text{Equation 9}$$
$$\text{diene conjugation bands}$$
$$PUFA^{\cdot} + O_2 \rightarrow PUFAO_2^{\cdot} \qquad \text{Equation 10}$$

$$\text{PUFAO}_2{}^{\cdot} + \text{PUFA(H) or XH} \rightarrow \text{PUFAOOH} \qquad \text{Equation 11}$$

PUFA-OOH, PUFAOO $\cdot$ $\xrightarrow{\text{metal ions}}$ products including	Equation 12
malonaldehyde,	
alkanals, alkenals,	Equation 13
4-hydroxy-alkenals	Equation 14
alkanes	Equation 15
epoxy-fatty acids	Equation 16
chemiluminescence	Equation 17
fluorescent	Equation 18
materials	

Each of the reactions shown in Equations 8−18 has been used to provide data on the extent of lipid peroxidation in biological systems. In Equation 8 the decrease in the content of the PUFAs during the reaction is a convenient procedure; in many cases, such as with liver microsomal suspensions, the major decrease is in $C_{20:4}$ and $C_{22:6}$ fatty acids. Equation 9 has often been used to detect the occurrence of lipid peroxidation by the demonstration of the appearance of diene-conjugation absorptions. Equation 10 is followed when oxygen uptake is monitored as an indicator of lipid peroxidation. Equation 11 can be used to provide data on the production of lipid hydroperoxides. Equations 12−18 reflect the complexity of breakdown products of which malonaldehyde is the one most frequently measured; exhalation of the alkanes ethane and pentane is a possible non-invasive whole body procedure for measuring lipid peroxidation. It is apparent that there are many different procedures available for detecting the occurrence of lipid peroxidation, and for measuring its extent. It is probably fair to say, however, that with biological samples none of the methods mentioned is without disadvantages: in consequence, wherever possible, more than one method should be used to provide confirmatory information. In this brief discussion it is not possible to provide detailed bibliography of all the methods quoted: an overview, with references, is by Slater (4) and many detailed descriptions of individual methods can be found in Packer (5). Some specific practical aspects are provided later in relation to the model systems described.

3. MODELS FOR STUDYING LIPID PEROXIDATION

Lipid peroxidation has been studied at many different levels of biological organization as well as in purely chemical systems: this section will describe a variety of models that have each provided valuable information on lipid peroxidation.

3.1 Homogeneous reactions

Studies on the interaction of initiating free radicals with pure PUFAs have provided data on the rates of such reactions (6,7) and on the variety of lipid hydroperoxide products (8). The kinetics of such reactions are best studied by pulse radiolysis (see 9) as the second-order rate constants are in the range $10^6 - 10^7$ M^{-1} sec^{-1} for free radicals such as $CCl_3OO^{\cdot}$, and considerably higher for $OH^{\cdot}$. An important study on the effects of vitamins E and C on the oxidation of unsaturated fatty acid in solution is by Niki *et al.* (10); see also Packer *et al.* (11).

3.2 **Purified enzymes and lipid micelles**

The autoxidation of unsaturated lipid in micelles and liposomes has been studied on numerous occasions: for background details on the autoxidation of phosphatidyl choline in liposomes, and for a study on the role of iron in ferritin- and haemosiderin-mediated lipid peroxidation in liposomes see (12,13).

The effects of radiation on PUFAs in lipid micelles have been studied, especially in relation to the evaluation of the cytotoxic effects of ionizing radiation. A recent elegant study with lipid micelles (14) provided data on the synergistic effets of α-tocopherol in combination with ascorbic acid on lipid peroxidation catalysed by an added peroxy radical-generating system. Purified enzymes, such as NADPH-cytochrome P_{450} reductase, have been investigated in relation to the effects of $O_2^{\cdot-}$ production and lipid peroxidation (see 15).

3.3 **Isolated organelles**

Details of the preparation of organelles mentioned below can be found in Chapter 3.

3.3.1 *Mitochondria*

It has been known for a long time that liver mitochondria peroxidize rather easily (see 16); a detailed review on mitochondrial peroxidation is by Vladimirov *et al.* (17). Of practical importance is the fact that liver mitochondria metabolize malonaldehyde (see 18); in consequence, the thiobarbituric acid reaction is not a suitable method for evaluating the rate of lipid peroxidation in mitochondrial suspensions, in homogenates or in whole cells.

3.3.2 *Nuclei*

A major practical problem here is the difficulty of obtaining really pure preparations of nuclei and nuclear membranes; since endoplasmic reticulum is very active in responding to the initiation of lipid peroxidation (see below) then relatively minor contamination of the nuclear membrane preparation with endoplasmic reticulum can give artefactual results. Pure samples of nuclear membranes, prepared from rat liver cells, are reported to undergo redox-cycling with the production of $O_2^{\cdot--}$ and lipid peroxidation (19,20); choline deficiency is also known to stimulate lipid peroxidation in rat liver nuclei (21,22).

3.3.3 *Endoplasmic reticulum*

Many more studies have been done on lipid peroxidation in the membranes of the endoplasmic reticulum (mostly *in vitro*, using microsomal suspensions) than with other organelles. Several important models are frequently studied in relation to microsomal lipid peroxidation, and these are summarized below.

(i) *Endogenous peroxidation of microsomal suspensions in buffer.* This is normally very slow and is principally a reflection of the 'contamination' of iron salts, the nutritional status of the animal (which affects the anti-oxidant content of the membranes), and the method of preparation that influences the endogenous level of lipid hydroperoxide. In general, this model of 'endogenous lipid peroxidation' is not very useful.

(ii) *NADPH-stimulated peroxidation.* This is appreciably faster than (i) and involves the enzymic reduction of Fe^{3+} by NADPH-cytochrome P_{450} reductase. If care and attention is paid during the preparation and handling of the microsomal suspensions (see Chapter 3), so that contamination by iron and high initial levels of lipid hydroperoxide are avoided, then this model can provide valuable data on electron flow from NADPH, probably via an obligatory iron-chelate, to initiate peroxidation.

(iii) *NADPH-dependent CCl_4-stimulated peroxidation.* This model (see 23) is important as it is a good example of metabolic activation of a toxic substance producing a reactive intermediate ($CCl_3OO^{\cdot}$) that can initiate peroxidation. The model is dependent on NADPH and the enzymes NADPH-cytochrome P_{450} reductase and cytochrome P_{450} (24). The latter enzyme can also participate in later initiating events by interaction with lipid hydroperoxide (25).

$$\text{NADPH-}P_{450}\text{ electron transport chain} \xrightarrow[]{+CCl_4} CCl_3^{\cdot} \xrightarrow[]{+O_2} CCl_3OO^{\cdot} \qquad \text{Equation 19}$$

$$CCl_3OO^{\cdot} + PUFA \rightarrow \text{lipid hydroperoxide (LOOH)} \qquad\qquad\qquad \text{Equation 20}$$

$$LOOH \xrightarrow{P_{450}} \text{new lipid free radicals, } LO^{\cdot},\ LOO^{\cdot},\ \text{etc} \qquad\qquad \text{Equation 21}$$

Because of its enzymic dependence this model is sensitive to changes in the temperature of incubation; most studies are done at 37°C. The peroxidation can be followed by estimating malonaldehyde, lipid hydroperoxide, appearance of diene conjugation, evolution of alkanes, and disappearance of PUFAs. Practical details are provided in Section 4.

(iv) *NADPH−ADP−iron stimulated peroxidation.* The catalytic effect of iron chelates on NADPH-dependent lipid peroxidation in liver microsomes was discovered by Hochstein and Ernster (26) and by Beloff-Chain *et al.* (27). Most studies use ADP as the chelating agent but other nucleotide phosphates and even pyrophosphate can also be used (28). The peroxidation that follows addition of ADP−iron in the presence of NADPH is very rapid and extensive; it can readily be followed by oxygen uptake (see Section 4) or by malonaldehyde production. Again, since it is dependent on enzymic activity, it is responsive to changes in temperature; most studies are done at 25°C or 28°C.

(v) *Ascorbate-iron dependent peroxidation.* This model (29) is similar to the one just described in terms of rapidity of peroxidation, and measurements of the reaction using O_2 uptake or the thiobarbituric acid reaction. However, unlike the model in Section 3.3.4, it is not enzyme catalysed. Ascorbate alone can also be used to stimulate microsomal lipid peroxidation; this system depends on the occurrence of iron complexes in the microsomal suspension, such as the iron complex of P_{450}, to initiate free radical chains.

(vi) *Cumene hydroperoxide-dependent peroxidation.* This model (see 30) was first described by Little and O'Brien (31) and is dependent on P_{450}.

(vii) *γ-Radiation-induced lipid peroxidation*. The use of ^{60}Co to give γ-irradiation of microsomal suspensions has some advantageous features for studying peroxidation that is initiated by OH˙. Firstly, the rate of initiation is largely independent of small concentrations of contaminating iron, and of initiating centres or species other than OH˙ that is produced at a rate that is dependent on the dose of radiation. Secondly, the model is independent of enzyme activity and is largely independent of temperature over a range such as $0-37°$C. Thirdly, the OH˙ radicals will attack all fatty acids in the membrane (although having some preference for PUFAs) unlike enzymic-catalysed processes that essentially deplete only $C_{20:4}$ and $C_{22:6}$.

3.3.4 *Plasma membrane*

Highly purified preparations of plasma membranes obtained from rat liver (see Chapter 3) do not significantly peroxidize when incubated with NADPH or NADH (32); such suspensions, however, do peroxidize readily with ascorbate-iron or with γ-radiation (32).

Phagocytosing leucocytes display a respiratory burst that results in the production of several reactive species; (for review see 33); this can be associated with lipid peroxidation.

3.4 **Isolated cells**

The isolated hepatocyte (see 34) is a convenient model for studying lipid peroxidation in a complex, organized biological environment. Compared with microsomal suspensions, for example, the intact cell provides additional anti-oxidant defences such as glutathione peroxidase, the glutathione reductases, glutathione itself (in the cytosol of liver cells its concentration is ~5 mM), superoxide dismutase, catalase, ascorbate, etc. In general, it is necessary to deplete these defensive systems of glutathione to obtain large stimulations of lipid peroxidation (see 35). Intact cells, of course, metabolize malonaldehyde (see Section 3.3.1); they also metabolize aldehydes and 4-hydroxyalkenals (36) to the corresponding acids and alcohols, and lipid hydroperoxides through the agency of glutathione peroxidase. Moreover, there is some indication (37) that diene conjugates are metabolized (or at least reduced) in liver. In consequence, the measurement of the rate of lipid peroxidation in isolated cells has some practical problems even though the demonstration that peroxidation is occurring is relatively easy. Methods that may be used to provide data on the kinetics of lipid peroxidation in the whole cell or in sub-cellular fractions of the peroxidized cell suspension are: alkane evolution, chemiluminescence, diene conjugation in microsomal lipid extracts, protein-bound carbonyls, loss of [^{14}C]arachidonate from pre-labelled microsomal phospholipid (see 38).

3.5 **Whole tissue and whole organ studies**

Measurement of lipid peroxidation that has been stimulated *in vivo* or in perfused organs (*in situ* or isolated) involves appreciating difficulties that arise when using material that is at a higher level of biological organization than are cell suspensions. Under conditions *in vivo* the tissue is an open system in that pro- and anti-oxidants can enter and leave. Moreover, all of the complications raised in Section 3.4 in relation to the metabolism/removal of peroxidation products also apply in these models.

With intact tissue that has been subjected to peroxidative attack it is best to process the tissue sample as quickly and efficiently as possible, in order to reduce artefactual peroxidation and additional metabolism of products under study during the sampling and work-up procedures. Freeze−clamping (see Chapter 3) followed by acid or solvent extraction is a recommended procedure; another suitable procedure for many purposes is to homogenize the fresh tissue sample immediately in acid containing anti-oxidant (see Chapter 3). These types of extraction, of course, give average values for the whole tissue sample that, in tissues such as liver, often contains many different cell types. Methods are now becoming available for cytochemical detection and measurement of lipid peroxidation in individual cells of stained *sections* of tissue (see 39); it is expected that major development of cytochemical techniques will occur in the near future.

For whole organ studies, either *in situ* or as isolated perfused organs, some non-invasive techniques have proved useful; for example, chemiluminescent studies on liver (40) and alkane production (41). With intact organ work it is also possible to follow the release of products (or consequences) of lipid peroxidation into the perfusing medium and, in the case of liver, into the bile. For example, stimulation of peroxidation in liver is accompanied by a rapid and large efflux of GSH and GSSG in bile (42,43).

3.6 Whole animal

The same general comments apply here as for Section 3.5. The only non-invasive methods available are alkane exhalation (see 44) and excretion of products such as malonaldehyde in the urine (45; but see 46). Invasive methods that have been used are biopsy analysis and blood analysis. The latter, naturally, has been much more widely used than the former. There is a considerable literature on changes in blood lipid hydro-peroxides in various diseases (see 47); and much interest has been generated by the reports (see 48) that liver disorders are accompanied by increased levels of a linoleic acid diene derivative (the octadeca-9,11-dienoic acid, 49) in plasma.

4. PRACTICAL ASPECTS

This section describes experimental protocols for several of the model systems described in Section 3. Firstly, details will be given for microsomal incubations.

4.1 Protocol for NADPH-dependent lipid peroxidation

The procedure is based on that given by Slater and Sawyer (23).

(i)   Prepare microsomal suspensions in ice-cold, 0.15 M KCl such that 1 ml of suspension contains microsomes equivalent to 1 g wet weight of original liver.

(ii)   Prepare a standard stock solution to contain: 83.5 mM KCl, 37 mM Tris buffer (pH 7.4), 5.5 mM glucose-6-phosphate (sodium salt), 0.25 mM $NADP^+$ (sodium salt), 106 mM acetamide, and 8 international units of glucose-6-phosphatase dehydrogenase, all contained in a volume of 32 ml. Make this stock solution freshly for each experiment. It serves as a buffered NADPH-generating system; once prepared, keep ice-cold until used.

(iii) Mix standard stock solution with microsomes in the proportions 22 ml:3 ml, and use immediately.

Lipid peroxidation

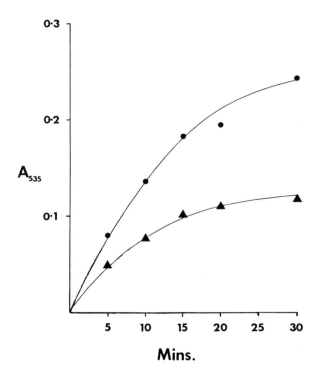

Figure 1. Lipid peroxidation in rat liver microsomal suspensions. The influence of increasing the incubation time on the colour produced in the thiobarbituric acid reaction, as measured by the optical absorption at 535 nm, is shown. Incubations were carried out at 37°C in the dark in the presence (●) or absence (▲) of CCl_4 added to the side-arms of Warburg flasks as a mixture (2 μl; 1:1) with liquid paraffin. The data shown are previously unpublished results of T.F.Slater and B.C.Sawyer. For other experimental details see Sections 4.1 and 4.2, and ref. 23.

(iv)   Place samples (2.5 ml) of the stock−microsomes mixture in tubes (∼15 ml capacity) fitted with ground glass sockets and stoppers; add 0.5 ml water (or solvent) or inhibitor solution under study.

(v)   Incubate the tubes in a water bath at 37°C for 0−60 min with gentle shaking and in the dark.

(vi)   At the end of the incubation period add 2 vol of 10% (w/v) trichloroacetic acid (TCA) and place the tubes in crushed ice.

(vii) After 10 min centrifuge the mixtures and use the supernatant solution for the thiobarbituric acid reaction as follows.

(viii) Mix the supernatant solution (2 ml) with 2 ml of 0.67% thiobarbituric acid and heat for 10 min in a boiling water bath.

(ix)   After cooling, measure the solutions spectrophotometrically at 535 nm, using a mixture of heated TCA−thiobarbituric acid as the blank.

(x)   Calculate the concentration of malonaldehyde in the incubated samples using the molar extinction coefficient of 1.49×10^5 M^{-1} cm^{-1} (23). Some typical results are shown in *Figure 1*.

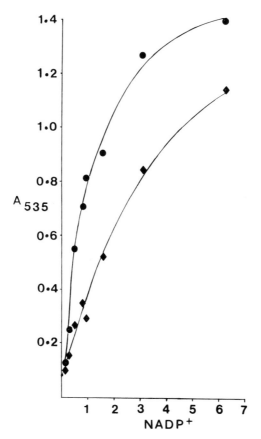

Figure 2. Lipid peroxidation in rat liver microsomal suspensions with (●) and without (◆) CCl_4. In these experiments (see Sections 4.1 and 4.2) lipid peroxidation was measured by the thiobarbituric acid reactions; the results are given as increases in the optical absorption at 535 nm. Incubations were for 30 min at 37°C, in the dark; the incubations were performed in Warburg flasks and the CCl_4 was placed in the side-arms as a mixture (2 μl; 1:1) with liquid paraffin. The results show an increase in the production of malonaldehyde-like material as the concentration (in mM) of $NADP^+$ is increased. The data shown are previously unpublished results of T.F.Slater and B.C.Sawyer.

4.2 Protocol of CCl_4-stimulated lipid peroxidation

The suggested protocol closely follows Section 4.1 above. The microsomes — stock mixture is prepared as already described above.

(i)   Incubate the mixture in 3.0 ml portions (see Section 4.1.iv) with and without addition of 10 μl of a CCl_4 solution in dimethyl sulphoxide (CCl_4:DMSO, 1:4, v/v) in stoppered tubes for 10—30 min at 37°C, with shaking and in the dark.

(ii)   Terminate the reaction with 10% TCA as in Section 4.1 and perform the thiobarbituric acid reaction on the acidic supernatant solution.

The protocol is as described by Slater and Sawyer (23); typical results are included in *Figure 1*.

Variants that have been used include:

(i) diffusing the CCl_4 into the microsomes−stock mixture, which is contained in the central compartment of a Warburg flask: the CCl_4 being placed in the side-arm;

(ii) using a saturated aqueous solution of CCl_4 in place of the CCl_4:DMSO mixture.

The concentration of $NADP^+$ used in the stock solution is a compromise between the cost of this nucleotide and the increased extent of the reaction observed with increasing levels of NADPH (see *Figure 2*).

The incubated mixture can also be used for measurement of:

(i) loss of PUFAs by gas-chromatographic methods;

(ii) diene conjugation measurement after lipid extraction;

(iii) lipid hydroperoxide measurements;

(iv) separation and measurement of aldehydic products, such as the 4-hydroxy-alkenals by h.p.l.c.

Details for these measurements are given later.

4.3 Protocol for NADPH−ADP−iron stimulated lipid peroxidation

This protocol (50) allows the measurement of peroxidation by oxygen uptake.

(i) Place the following in the oxygen electrode compartment (for example, a Gilson Instruments Oxygraph): 1.13 ml of 0.15 M KCl, 0.57 ml of 0.1 M Tris buffer (pH 7.4) and 0.1 ml of microsomal suspension (as described in Section 4.1).

(ii) Connect the electrode output to an appropriate recorder and set the recorder range such that 90% full range corresponds to total oxygen content of the mixture.

(iii) Start the reaction by the addition of NADPH (0.22 μmol in 15 μl; 6 mg of NADPH-Na$_2$ in 0.5 ml Tris buffer, 0.1 M pH 8) and by 30 μl of ADP−iron (38 mg ADP-Na in 1.0 ml Tris buffer, 0.1 M, pH 8.0 plus 0.67 ml of $FeSO_4 \cdot 7H_2O$, 38 mg in 100 ml of water). The total volume of the mixture is 1.845 ml.

(iv) Follow the reaction over a period of approximately 5 min; incubation is at 25°C, with magnetic stirring of the mixture in the electrode compartment. The small volumes of NADPH and ADP−iron are best added by using Hamilton-type microsyringes.

The buffer−microsomes mixture used has a dissolved oxygen content of approximately 240 nmol/ml; the chart range can be set to correspond to oxygen depletion by adding a small quantity of solid sodium dithionite to the electrode compartment filled with buffer. [Details on oxygen electrode and calibration can be found in Green and Hill (51). Intracellular O_2 concentrations can be calculated using an electron spin resonance spectroscopic method (see 52).] A typical experimental record is shown in *Figure 3*. By proportionally increasing the volumes of the mixture given above samples can also be used for measuring malonaldehyde production and PUFA consumption.

The protocol given above for NADPH−ADP−iron stimulated peroxidation can be modified to allow measurement of ascorbate-stimulated peroxidation as follows: instead of NADPH and ADP−iron use 0.1 ml of aqueous ascorbate (100 mg/10 ml water, neutralized to pH 7 with sodium hydroxide; prepare freshly). Variants on this are to

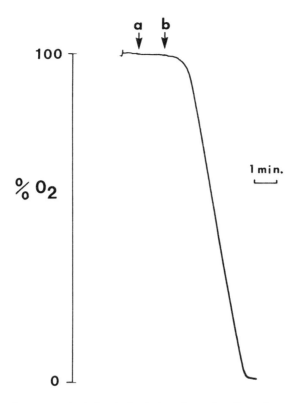

Figure 3. A trace of oxygen uptake during the incubation of normal rat liver microsomes. The incubation temperature was 25°C; the chart speed 0.2 mm/sec. The arrows indicate addition of **(a)** NADPH and **(b)** ADP−iron. For other experimental details see Section 4.3 and ref. 50.

use ascorbate−iron solutions (final concentrations 0.5 mM and 5 μM, respectively) or ascorbate−ADP−iron mixture (final concentrations 0.5 mM, 1.6 mM and 33 μM, respectively).

4.4 Protocol for peroxidation stimulated by cumene hydroperoxide

Incubate the following mixture for 15 min at 37°C, with shaking and in the dark: 1.1 ml of a Tris-KCl buffer mixture (Tris buffer, 0.1 M, pH 7.4:KCl, 0.15 M, 1:2 v/v), 0.1 ml microsomal suspension (as in Section 4.1), 0.15 ml cumene hydroperoxide solution (1 mM in water) and either 0.15 ml water (or solvent) or inhibitor under study in water (or solvent). Stop the reaction with 3 ml of 10% TCA and perform the thiobarbituric acid reaction as in Section 4.1.

4.5 Protocol for γ-irradiation

Place a mixture of 4 ml microsomes (see Section 4.1), previously diluted to 1 mg protein/ml 0.15 M KCl, in 20 ml phosphate buffer (0.1 M, pH 7.4) under a ^{60}Co source, at room temperature. The radiation dose is 0−500 Gray over a period of 30 or 60 min. The mixture can be analysed at the end of the irradiation period for thiobarbituric acid-

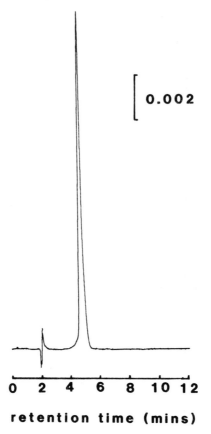

Figure 4. High-performance liquid chromatographic separation of malonaldehyde (10 μM standard) performed essentially as described by Esterbauer and Slater (54). Conditions: Merck Lichrosorb NH_2 column (25 cm × 4.0 mm); mobile phase of 0.03 M pH 7.4 Tris buffer/acetonitrile (9:1, v/v) at 1.0 ml/min; u.v. detection at 270 nm.

positive material, for lipid hydroperoxide, and for diene conjugates. For more experimental data see (53).

4.6 Malonaldehyde estimation

The protocols described above have been based in general on the final stage of the procedure being the thiobarbituric acid reaction. The latter reaction is not very specific for malonaldehyde, however, especially if the thiobarbituric acid reaction is performed with the complete acidified microsomal (or homogenate) suspension rather than the acidified supernatant. In the protocols given in Sections 4.1 −4.5 the thiobarbituric acid reaction has been carefully cross-checked with a direct h.p.l.c. estimation of malonaldehyde (54 − 56) and excellent agreement found. With some pure PUFAs, however, the correspondence is not good (57); thus, the thiobarbituric acid reaction should be carefully evaluated against a direct method for malonaldehyde before assuming that the coloured product observed is mainly a reflection of malonaldehyde (58). Full

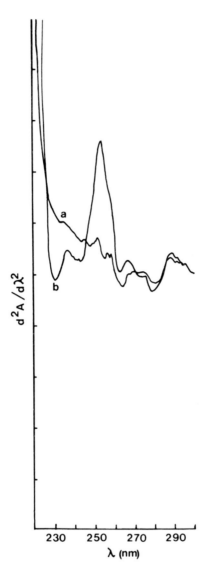

Figure 5. Second-derivative u.v. spectra of liver microsomal lipid extracts from (**a**) control rat and (**b**) rat dosed with CCl$_4$ (1.25 ml/kg; 3 h after dosing). The liver microsomes were extracted and the spectra recorded as described by Corongiu *et al.* (61). Note that absorption peak in the conventional sense appears as a minimum in the second-derivative spectrum. Note also that this method detects two such minima in the peroxidized sample at 233 nm and at 242 nm. These may represent two different classes of hydroperoxides (61).

experimental details of the h.p.l.c. method for malonaldehyde are given in reference (55). An illustration of the direct h.p.l.c. method is given in *Figure 4*.

4.7 Diene conjugation measurement

The standard method for diene conjugation measurement is based on lipid extraction, followed by difference spectrophotometry in the range 200−260 nm; full experimental details are given by Recknagel and Glende (59). This method suffers from a severe practical disadvantage, however, since the conjugation band is superimposed as a relatively small shoulder on a large background absorption. As a consequence it is often difficult to be sure of the precise wavelength of maximum absorption, and of the quantitative aspect of the absorption. An improved technique (60) uses second derivative spectrophotometry; this gives much better separation of the diene absorptions from background (*Figure 5*) and even allows identification of individual classes of diene absorption that are probably related to stereoisomerism of lipid hydroperoxides (61).

4.8 Lipid hydroperoxide measurement

These compounds can be measured in lipid extracts by classical titrimetric techniques, or by spectrophotometry of the iodide ion formed by reaction of the hydroperoxide with iodate (for review see 62). A simple, routine procedure (e.g. for plasma, 63) is not very sensitive but modifications (64) have greatly increased sensitivity and stoichiometry although, unfortunately, the experimental procedures thereby become exacting and time-consuming.

A very sensitive method for lipid hydroperoxides, based on the effects of low concentrations of these substances on purified cyclo-oxygenase (65) is a method that is suited to measurements on tissue extracts (see Chapter 12).

If lipid hydroperoxides are present in relatively high concentration then they can be separated, and later identified by h.p.l.c. (see 8,66).

4.9 Procedures for measuring alkane production

These are all based on collecting samples of head-space gas above an incubation mixture and subsequently analysing by gas chromatography. The experimental design of equipment, and practical problems are well described by Muller and Sies (41). It should be noted that pentane is metabolized by the liver cytochrome P_{450} system so that measurement is a balance of production versus metabolism.

4.10 Measurements of polyunsaturated fatty acids

Standard gas chromatographic methods are mostly used for these analyses (see 67) after prior extraction, hydrolysis and derivatization (68).

4.11 Measurements of 4-hydroxy-alkenals

This is a time-consuming method that is not suitable for routine measurements. The procedure (56) is based on derivatization, t.l.c. and, finally, separation by h.p.l.c.

5. CONCLUDING REMARKS

The protocols given above for liver microsomes, and details on several methods of analysis, can be readily modified for use with the various models described in Section 3 for studying lipid peroxidation in a wide range of biological materials.

6. REFERENCES

1. Smith,L.L. (1981) *Cholesterol Autoxidation.* Plenum Press, New York.
2. Porter,N.A., Weber,B.A., Weenen,H. and Khan,J.A. (1980) *J. Am. Chem. Soc.,* **102**, 5597.
3. Porter,N.A., Lehman,L.S., Weber,B.A. and Smith,K.J. (1981) *J. Am. Chem. Soc.,* **103**, 6447.
4. Slater,T.F. (1984) In *Methods in Enzymology.* Packer,L. (ed.), Academic Press, New York, Vol. 105, p. 183.
5. Packer,L., ed. (1984) *Methods in Enzymology.* Academic Press, New York, Vol. 105.
6. Forni,L.G., Packer,J.E., Slater,T.F. and Willson,R.L. (1983) *Chem.-Biol. Interactions,* **45**, 171.
7. Hasegawa,K. and Patterson,L.K. (1978) *Photochem. Photobiol.,* **28**, 817.
8. Chan,H.W.S. and Levett,G. (1977) *Lipids,* **12**, 99.
9. Willson,R.L. (1978) In *Biochemical Mechanisms of Liver Injury.* Slater,T.F. (ed.), Academic Press, London, p. 123.
10. Niki,E., Saito,T., Kawakami,A. and Kamiya,Y. (1984) *J. Biol. Chem.,* **259**, 4177.
11. Packer,J.E., Slater,T.F. and Willson,R.L. (1978) *Life Sci.,* **23**, 2617.
12. Wu,G-S., Stein,R.A. and Mead,J.F. (1982) *Lipids,* **17**, 403.
13. O'Connell,M.J., Ward,R.J., Baum,H. and Peters,T.J. (1985) *Biochem. J.,* **229**, 135.
14. Doba,T., Burton,G.W. and Ingold,K.U. (1985) *Biochim. Biophys. Acta,* **835**, 298.
15. Ekstrom,G. and Ingelman-Sundberg,M. (1984) *Biochem. Pharmacol.,* **33**, 2521.
16. Hunter,F.E., Gebicki,J.M., Hoffsten,P.E., Weinstein,J. and Scott,J. (1963) *J. Biol. Chem.,* **238**, 828.
17. Vladimirov,Y.A., Olenev,V.I., Suslova,T.B. and Cheremisina,Z.P. (1980) *Adv. Lipid Res.,* **17**, 173.
18. Siu,G.M. and Draper,H.H. (1982) *Lipids,* **17**, 349.
19. Bachur,N.R., Gee,M.V. and Friedman,R.D. (1982) *Cancer Res.,* **42**, 1078.
20. Mimnaugh,E.G., Kennedy,K.A., Trush,M.A. and Sinha,B.K. (1985) *Cancer Res.,* **45**, 3296.
21. Rushmore,T.H., Lim,Y.P., Farber,E. and Ghoshal,A.K. (1984) *Cancer Lett.,* **24**, 251.
22. Perera,M.I.R., Demetris,A.J., Katyal,S.L. and Shinozuka,H. (1985) *Cancer Res.,* **45**, 2533.
23. Slater,T.F. and Sawyer,B.C. (1971) *Biochem. J.,* **123**, 805.
24. Slater,T.F. (1982) In *Free Radicals, Lipid Peroxidation and Cancer.* McBrien,D.C.H. and Slater,T.F. (eds), Academic Press, London, p. 243.
25. Svingen,B.A., Buege,J.A., O'Neal,F.O. and Aust,S.D. (1979) *J. Biol. Chem.,* **254**, 5892.
26. Hochstein,P. and Ernster,L. (1963) *Biochem. Biophys. Res. Commun.,* **12**, 388.
27. Beloff-Chain,A., Catanzaro,R. and Serlupi-Crescenzi,G. (1963) *Nature,* **198**, 351.
28. Hochstein,P., Nordenbrand,K. and Ernster,L. (1964) *Biochem. Biophys. Res. Commun.,* **14**, 323.
29. Barber,A.A. (1963) *Radiat. Res. Suppl.,* **3**, 33.
30. Kulkarni,A.P. and Hodgson,E. (1981) *Int. J. Biochem.,* **13**, 811.
31. Little,C. and O'Brien,P.J. (1969) *Can. J. Biochem.,* **47**, 493.
32. Le Page,R.N., Cheeseman,K.H. and Slater,T.F. (1987) *Cell. Biochem. Function,* in press.
33. Baehner,R.L., Boxer,L.A. and Ingraham,L.M. (1982) In *Free Radicals in Biology.* Pryor,W.A. (ed.), Academic Press, New York, Vol. 5, p.91
34. Harris,R.A. and Cornell,N.W. eds (1983) *Isolation, Characterization and Use of Hepatocytes.* Elsevier, Amsterdam.
35. Smith,C.V., Hughes,H., Lauterburg,B.H. and Mitchell,J.R. (1983) In *Functions of Glutathione: Biochemical, Physiological, Toxicological and Clinical Aspects.* Larsson,A., Holmgren,A., Orrenius,S. and Mannervik,B. (eds), Raven Press, New York, p. 125.
36. Esterbauer,H., Zollner,H. and Lang,J. (1985) *Biochem. J.,* **228**, 363.
37. Slater,T.F. (1972) *Free Radical Mechanisms in Tissue Injury.* Pion, London.
38. Benedetti,A., Esterbauer,H., Ferrali,M., Fulceri,R. and Comporti,M. (1982) *Biochim. Biophys. Acta,* **711**, 345.
39. Benedetti,A., Malvaldi,G., Fulceri,R. and Comporti,M. (1984) *Cancer Res.,* **44**, 5712.
40. Cadenas,E. and Sies,H. (1984) In *Methods in Enzymology.* Packer,L. (ed.), Academic Press, New York, Vol. 105, p. 221.
41. Muller,A. and Sies,H. (1984) In *Methods in Enzymology.* Packer,L. (ed.), Academic Press, New York, Vol. 105, p. 311.
42. Akerboom,T.P.M., Bilzer,M. and Sies,H. (1982) *J. Biol. Chem.,* **257**, 4248.
43. Krieter,P.A., Ziegler,D.M., Hill,K.E. and Burk,R.F. (1985) *Biochem. Pharmacol.,* **34**, 955.
44. Dillard,C.J. and Tappel,A.L. (1979) *Lipids,* **14**, 989.
45. Draper,H.H., Polensek,L., Hadley,M. and McGirr,L.G. (1984) *Lipids,* **19**, 836.

46. Marnett,L.J., Buck,J., Tuttle,M.A., Basu,A.K. and Bull,A.W. (1985) *Prostaglandins*, **30**, 241.
47. Yagi,K., (ed.) (1982) *Lipid Peroxides in Biology and Medicine*. Academic Press, New York.
48. Fink,R., Margot,D.H., Cawood,P., Iverson,S.A., Clemens,M.R., Patsalos,P., Norden,A.G. and Dormandy,T.L. (1985) *Lancet,* (**ii**), 291.
49. Iversen,S.A., Cawood,P., Madigan,M.J., Lawson,A.M. and Dormandy,T.L. (1984) *FEBS Lett.,* **171**, 320.
50. Slater,T.F. (1968) *Biochem. J.,* **106**, 155.
51. Green,M.J. and Hill,H.A.O. (1984) In *Methods in Enzymology*. Packer,L. (ed.), Academic Press, New York, Vol. 105, p. 3.
52. Swartz,H.M. and Swartz,S.M. (1983) In *Methods of Biochemical Analysis*. Glick,D. (ed.), John Wiley, New York, Vol. 29, p. 207.
53. Garner,A., Jamal,Z. and Slater,T.F. (1986) *Int. J. Radiat. Biol.,* **50**, 323.
54. Esterbauer,H. and Slater,T.F. (1981) *IRCS Med. Sci.,* **9**, 749.
55. Esterbauer,H., Lang,J., Zadravec,S. and Slater,T.F. (1984) In *Methods in Enzymology*. Packer,L. (ed.), Academic Press, New York, Vol. 105, p. 319.
56. Poli,G., Dianzani,M.U., Cheeseman,K.H., Slater,T.F., Lang,J. and Esterbauer,H. (1985) *Biochem. J.,* **227**, 629.
57. Esterbauer,H. (1985) In *Free Radicals in Liver Injury*. Poli,G., Cheeseman,K.H., Dianzani,M.U. and Slater,T.F. (eds), IRL Press, Oxford and Washington, D.C., p. 29.
58. Slater,T.F. (1984) *Biochem. J.,* **222**, 1.
59. Recknagel,P.O. and Glende,E.A. (1984) In *Methods in Enzymology*. Packer,L. (ed.), Academic Press, New York, Vol. 105, p. 331.
60. Corongiu,F.P. and Milia,A. (1983) *Chem.-Biol. Interactions,* **44**, 289.
61. Corongiu,F.P., Poli,G., Dianzani,M.U., Cheeseman,K.H. and Slater,T.F. (1986) *Chem.-Biol. Interactions,* **59**, 147.
62. Johnson,R.M. and Siddiqi,I.W. (1970) *The Determination of Organic Peroxides*. Pergamon Press, Oxford.
63. Yagi,K. (1984) In *Methods in Enzymology*. Packer,L. (ed.), Academic Press, New York, Vol. 105, p. 328.
64. Hicks,M. and Gebicki,J.M. (1979) *Anal. Biochem.,* **99**, 249.
65. Warso,M.A. and Lands,W.E.M. (1984) *Clin. Physiol. Biochem.,* **2**, 70.
66. Hamilton,J.G. and Karol,R.J. (1982) *Prog. Lipid Res.,* **21**, 155.
67. Gurr,M.I. and James,R.T. (1980) *Lipid Biochemistry*. 3rd Edition, Chapman and Hall, London.
68. McDonald-Gibson,R.G. and Young,M. (1974) *Clin. Chim. Acta,* **53**, 117.

CHAPTER 15

Quantitative measurement of arachidonic acid in tissues or fluids

ROBERT G.McDONALD-GIBSON

1. INTRODUCTION

Arachidonic acid ($C_{20:4\ n\text{-}6}$) is the precursor of by far the largest number of cyclo-oxygenase and lipoxygenase products that experimental scientists are interested in. Knowledge of the endogenous arachidonic acid concentration, especially non-esterified, is important in biosynthetic capacity and especially enzyme kinetic studies as well as studies involving incorporation of [^{14}C]arachidonic acid into cyclo-oxygenase and lipoxygenase products (Chapter 5). Although the present chapter deals particularly with arachidonic acid measurement, the methods described can be used to quantify other polyunsaturated fatty acid eicosanoid precursors. The most appropriate method for quantitative measurement of arachidonic acid is gas−liquid chromatography (g.l.c.) utilizing a suitable quantitative internal standard. This approach, with suitable adaptation, can be used to measure non-esterified (free), total (non-esterified + esterified) arachidonic acid or the arachidonic acid concentration of individual lipid esters. Quantitative measurement of long chain fatty acids by comparison with an internal standard using this type of procedure is similar in principle to the methods described by McDonald-Gibson and Young (1).

2. GENERAL THEORY

A suitable internal standard, either pentadecanoic acid ($C_{15:0}$) or heptadecanoic acid ($C_{17:0}$) is added to the lipid extraction medium at an early stage of the extraction procedure. After methylation or *trans*-methylation of fatty acids in the extract the mixture of volatile long chain fatty acid methyl esters is separated by g.l.c. and the arachidonic acid peak area compared quantitatively with the internal standard peak of known concentration. It is assumed that recovery of internal standard from the procedure will be the same as for endogenous arachidonic acid.

(i)   For total arachidonic acid measurement the whole lipid extract can be methylated or *trans*-methylated.

(ii)   For non-esterified arachidonic acid measurement the total non-esterified fatty acids as a group are separated from other lipids by thin-layer chromatography (t.l.c.) prior to methylation.

(iii)   For measurement of arachidonic acid in individual lipids such as triglycerides, phospholipids or cholesterol esters these major lipid classes are also separated by t.l.c. prior to saponification and *trans*-methylation.

3. INTERNAL STANDARDS

Either $C_{17:0}$ or $C_{15:0}$ fatty acid internal standards can be used. $C_{17:0}$ is the standard of choice since it has a retention time closer to arachidonic acid, but $C_{15:0}$ can be used if g.l.c. resolution of palmitoleic acid ($C_{16:1}$) from $C_{17:0}$ is a problem. This is more likely with packed column g.l.c. than with capillary column techniques.

For total and non-esterified arachidonic acid measurement non-esterified heptadecanoic acid should be used. For measuring the arachidonic acid content of triglycerides, phospholipids or cholesterol esters then triheptadecanoin, diheptadecanoyl phosphatidyl choline or cholesterol heptadecanoate are recommended (Sigma Chemical Co.).

When calculating the weight of heptadecanoic acid present in the standard note that this will be dependent on the percentage contribution of the $C_{17:0}$ to the total molecular weight of the lipid in question. To calculate the weight of $C_{17:0}$ standard multiply the weight of the parent compound by the following factors:

non-esterified heptadecanoic acid × 1.0
triheptadecanoin × 0.95
diheptadecanoyl phosphatidyl choline × 0.69
cholesterol hepatadecanoate × 0.41

The precise amount of $C_{17:0}$ standard to add to the extraction mixture will depend very much on the type and amount of tissue or fluid being investigated and will vary according to circumstances. The optimum amount must be determined by trial and error but something in the range $10-100$ μg should provide a good starting point.

4. TOTAL LIPID EXTRACTION

For non-esterified arachidonic acid measurements many of the general eicosanoid extraction procedures described elsewhere in this book are probably suitable. The $C_{17:0}$ internal standard, dissolved in a small volume of suitable solvent, should be added at an early stage in the extraction procedure.

For total arachidonic acid measurement and arachidonic acid content of specific lipids, the following chloroform−methanol procedure should be used. It is also suitable for non-esterified arachidonic acid measurement. This method is based on the classical Folch lipid extraction method (2) but has been simplified to use on a small scale as a rapid one-step procedure.

(i)   To 1 ml of aqueous solution (tissue homogenate, incubate, plasma, blood etc.) add 2 ml of methanol and mix well in a 10 ml glass-stoppered tube for 2 min, preferably using a mechanical vortex mixer.

(ii)   Add an appropriate amount of the relevant $C_{17:0}$ standard or standards (e.g. $10-100$ μg, see Section 3) dissolved in 0.1 ml of chloroform.

(iii)   Add 3.9 ml of chloroform.

(iv)   Add 0.2 ml of 4.2% KCl solution.

(v)   Mix well in the glass stoppered tube for 4 min using a mechanical vortex mixer.

(vi)   Remove the glass stopper and centrifuge the tube at low speed (a few hundred *g*) in a bench centrifuge to separate aqueous and organic solvent phases.

(vii) The lower, chloroform, phase contains extracted lipids. Protein-like material should separate out at the interface.

(viii) Remove the lower, chloroform, layer carefully by Pasteur pipette, transferring it to a 10 ml screw-cap culture tube for esterification (total arachidonic acid measurement) or a 10 ml glass-stoppered conical centrifuge tube for concentration and t.l.c. if non-esterified arachidonic acid or individual lipids are to be studied.

Note: if circumstances require it alternative volumes of aqueous sample solution can be used but the volumes of chloroform, methanol and KCl must also be scaled up or down so that the final ratios of all components remain as described.

5. THIN-LAYER CHROMATOGRAPHIC SEPARATION OF LIPID CLASSES

This is only carried out if it is intended to study the non-esterified arachidonic acid content or the arachidonic acid content of individual lipid esters. It is not necessary for measuring total arachidonic acid.

(i)   Concentrate the lipid extract in chloroform down to dryness by evaporation under a stream of nitrogen with, if necessary, application of gentle heat. Excessive heat must be avoided.

(ii)   Re-dissolve the lipid residue in about 0.1 ml of chloroform for application to the t.l.c. plate.

(iii) Prepare a pre-coated silica gel t.l.c. plate (e.g. Merck Kieselgel 60) by first spraying it with a 0.1% solution of rhodamine B in ethanol followed by activation in an oven at 100°C for 1 h.

(iv)   Apply the lipid extract to the 'origin' of the t.l.c. plate as a streak about 1.5−2.00 cm long close to the centre and about 1.5 cm above the bottom of the plate. Apply only a small amount of lipid extract at a time using a micro-syringe, allowing each application to dry before applying the next. Gradually build up the band of sample until all has been applied.

(v)   Either side of the sample apply as discrete spots standards of appropriate lipids, for example non-esterified arachidonic acid, a triglyceride, a phospholipid or a cholesterol ester. 2 μl of a 25 mg/ml stock solution of standards is adequate.

(vi)   Place the t.l.c plate in a glass t.l.c. tank containing 100 ml of the following solvent mixture: n-hexane:diethyl ether:glacial acetic acid (80:20:2 by vol). Put the solvent into the tank immediately before use. Do not pre-equilibrate the tank or line it with filter paper, this tends to impair resolution.

(vii) Put the lid on the tank and allow the t.l.c. plate to develop until the solvent is within 2 cm of the top of the plate.

(viii) Remove the plate from the tank. Allow solvent to evaporate and view the plate under u.v. light. Using a pencil, outline the position of standards and lipids separated from the extract by reference to the co-chromatographed standards.

(ix)   Using a small metal spatula or scalpel blade carefully scrape off the silica gel corresponding to the area of lipid required for arachidonic acid measurement, this is the non-esterified fatty acid, phospholipid, triglyceride or cholesterol ester band.

(x)   Transfer the silica gel scrapings carefully to a 10 ml culture tube for methylation.

6. PREPARATION OF METHYL ESTERS FOR GAS CHROMATOGRAPHY

Various methods are available for preparation of methyl esters of long chain fatty acids including the use of diazomethane, sodium methoxide and boron trifluoride − methanol. The method described here utilizes the boron trifluoride − methanol reagent and is based on that described by Morrison and Smith (3). The technique will methylate non-esterified fatty acids and *trans*-esterify already esterified fatty acids. As an insurance policy, especially when working with arachidonic acid lipid esters, prior saponification is carried out using methanolic sodium hydroxide. Under some conditions the saponification step may be omitted but with certain lipids this means longer incubation times with BF_3 − methanol and may not be desirable.

6.1 Equipment

(i)   10 ml screw-cap culture tubes (Pyrex).
(ii)   Caps for culture tubes should have PTFE-faced soft silicone rubber liners.
(iii)   Tubes should be acid-washed and both tubes and caps or liners should finally be washed with methanol to remove all traces of lipid.
(iv)   10 ml conical centrifuge tubes with ground glass stoppers.

6.2 Reagents

(i)   Boron trifluoride (14% in methanol, Sigma Chemical Co.).
(ii)   Methanolic NaOH (0.5 M). Dissolve NaOH in minimum volume of water and make up to volume with methanol.
(iii)   Petroleum ether (40−60°C).

6.3 Method

(i)   Place the sample in a screw-cap culture tube. Either:

    (a)   Total lipid extract from Section 4 (viii). Remove solvent by evaporation under a stream of nitrogen with gentle heat if necessary, or
    (b)   Lipid esters (e.g. phospholipids, triglycerides, cholesterol esters) or non-esterified fatty acid areas from t.l.c. plate. Scrape off the appropriate area of silica gel [Section 5(ix)] and transfer it to a screw-cap culture tube.

(ii)   Add 0.8 ml of 0.5 M methanolic NaOH.
(iii)   Screw the cap on firmly.
(iv)   Heat the tube in a boiling water bath (100°C) in a fume cupboard for 5 min.
(v)   Remove the tube from the water bath and allow to cool in cold running water for 2−3 min.
(vi)   Open the tube and add 1 ml of 14% BF_3 − methanol reagent.
(vii)   Replace the screw cap *firmly* to ensure a good gas-tight seal. This is important otherwise volatile fatty acid esters may be lost.
(viii) Mix well.

(ix)   Place the tube in a boiling water bath (100°C) for 2 min.
(x)   Remove the tube from the water bath and allow it to cool in cold running tap water for 2−3 min.
(xi)   Open the tube and add 0.5 ml of water and 2 ml of petroleum ether.
(xii) Replace the cap and *mix well* using a mechanical vortex mixer.
(xiii) Centrifuge the tube gently (a few hundred r.p.m.) at room temperature to separate the phases.
(xiv) Using a Pasteur pipette transfer the upper, petroleum ether, layer into a 10 ml glass-stoppered conical centrifuge tube. Remove the solvent by evaporation under nitrogen.
(xv)   Re-dissolve the remaining fatty acid methyl ester residue in 50−100 μl of petroleum ether for gas chromatography.

7. GAS−LIQUID CHROMATOGRAPHY

Both capillary and packed column techniques are available using a variety of stationary phases. The most useful stationary phases for separation of a wide range of long chain fatty acids by chain length and degree of unsaturation are the very polar phases. For packed column work these include simple polyesters such as diethylene glycol succinate (DEGS, 15%) or cyanosilicones such as SP-2330 (10%) which have the advantage of higher temperature limits and longer column life. For wall-coated capillary columns polar cyanosilicones such as SP-2330, SP-2340, CP-Sil 88 or OV-275 can be used.

As g.l.c. instrumentation will differ from one laboratory to another, mention will not be made of any particular model or make of equipment. Only general operating procedures and principles will be described. Reference should be made to the operating instruction manuals of the instrument in question.

7.1 General equipment

(i)   A suitable gas chromatograph equipped for packed column or capillary column operation and with flame ionization detectors.
(ii)   Necessary operating gases: helium or nitrogen carrier gas, hydrogen and air for the flame ionization detector (FID).
(iii) An electronic integrator for measuring peak areas and data processing. If an integrator is not available then the relevant peak areas can be measured manually or by cutting out the chart paper and weighing.

7.2 Packed column separations

7.2.1 *Operating conditions*

(i) *Column(s)*. Two glass columns are required; 2 m long × 2 mm internal diameter. Dual column operation is recommended to eliminate excessive base line drift due to column bleed during temperature-programmed operation. Refer to the instrument manual for details. The column should be packed with 10% SP-2330 on Supelcoport support material (Supelco).

(ii) *Detectors*. Dual FID. For hydrogen and air flow rates and operating pressures refer to instrument manual.

(iii) *Carrier gas*. Oxygen-free nitrogen. Flow-rate approximately 50 ml/min.

(iv) *Injection temperature*. 225°C.

(v) *Oven temperature programme*. Initial temperature 180°C for 2 min, temperature gradient 7.5°C/min, final temperature 240°C for 8 min.

7.2.2 Procedure

Inject a maximum of 1 μl of fatty acid methyl ester mixture (containing $C_{17:0}$ internal standard) on to the selected column and chromatograph using the conditions and temperature programme described in Section 7.2.1. Obtain the chart recorder trace and integrator print-out to include the $C_{17:0}$ internal standard peak and the arachidonic acid peak being measured. Although not 100% foolproof, peak identification is normally achieved for these purposes by comparing peak retention times with known fatty acid methyl ester standards.

7.3 Capillary column separations

7.3.1 Operating conditions

(i) *Column*. A 50 m long coiled fused silica column of inside diameter 0.22 mm, wall coated with CP-Sil 88 (Chrompack) film thickness 0.2 μm.

(ii) *Detector*. FID. For hydrogen and air flow-rates and operating pressures refer to instrument manual. Detector temperature 260°C.

(iii) *Carrier gas*. Helium. Inlet pressure approximately 1.9 bar. Linear gas velocity 21 cm/sec.

(iv) *Injector*. Split-splitless injector using a split ration of 50:1. Splitter vent 20 ml/min. Injection temperature 225°C.

(v) *Oven temperature programme*. Initial temperature 180°C for 5 min, followed by a temperature gradient of 5°C/min to 205°C, 2.5 min at 205°C, followed by a further temperature gradient of 5°C/min to a final temperature of 230°C for 9 min.

7.3.2 Procedure

The same procedure as for packed column separations (Section 7.2.2) should be used.

7.4 Calculations

$$\text{Weight of arachidonic acid/ml homogenate} = \frac{aAA}{aC_{17:0}} \times wC_{17:0} \times RF$$

where aAA = area of arachidonic acid peak; $aC_{17:0}$ = area of heptadecanoic acid internal standard peak; $wC_{17:0}$ = weight of heptadecanoic acid internal standard added/ml homogenate; RF = detector response factor: this must be determined for the g.c. instrument and detector system being used. It takes into account that on a weight for weight basis detector responses to arachidonic acid and internal standard may not be identical. The detector response factor should be determined by injecting equal weights of arachidonic acid and internal standard methyl esters on to the column and measuring the detector response in terms of peak areas. The ratio of peak areas will give the response factor to use.

In addition to providing a means for quantitative measurement of arachidonic acid, the methods described can also be adapted to measure the absolute amounts of other fatty acids separated by the gas chromatographic procedure. The same methodology will, of course, also give the percentage composition of the fatty acid mixture.

8. REFERENCES

1.   McDonald-Gibson,R.G. and Young,M. (1974) *Clin. Chim. Acta,* **53**, 117.
2.   Folch,J., Lees,M. and Sloane-Stanley,G.H. (1957) *J. Biol. Chem.,* **226**, 497.
3.   Morrison,W.R. and Smith,L.M. (1964) *J. Lipid Res.,* **5**, 600.

CHAPTER 16

Methods in prostanoid receptor classification

ROBERT A.COLEMAN

1. INTRODUCTION

The number of different naturally-occurring prostanoids, their widespread production throughout the bodies of animals and man and their possibly unparalleled range of biological actions give promise of a host of potentially useful therapeutic applications of agents interfering with or mimicking specific prostanoid actions. A major drawback with the prostanoids themselves as potential drugs is one of selectivity of action; prostaglandins of the D, E, F and I types have all been evaluated as therapeutic agents, but all are limited by their side-effects, particularly vasodilatation, flushing, nausea, uterine cramps and diarrhoea. The question of how to increase the pharmacological selectivity of any range of drugs which mimic naturally-occurring hormones or autacoids may be addressed in two ways. While both methods may require the synthesis of large numbers of structural analogues, one method is empirical and the other systematic. The empirical method requires a wide range of tests designed to identify both desired activities and potential side-effects, and as the nature and number of all of the possible side-effects cannot be known with any certainty, the number of tests to detect them must be somewhat uncertain. The systematic method requires the identification of receptors for the hormone/autacoid, and this having been done, the desired profile of a potential drug may be described in terms of its actions at the various receptor types. It may also be predicted which side-effects it is impossible to dissociate pharmacologically from the therapeutically desired effects due to their mediation through a common receptor type.

While both methods undoubtedly require a considerable degree of luck in the identification of potentially useful and acceptable drugs, we believe that using the systematic approach is far more likely to succeed. It is for this reason that we have characterized and classified prostanoid receptors using the techniques outlined by Furchgott (1972), namely the comparison of rank orders of agonist potency, and comparison of the affinities of receptor-blocking drugs. This approach has been successfully used in the classification of histamine receptors into H_1 and H_2 types (1,2) and of adrenoceptors into α- and β-types (3) and of their subdivision into β_1- and β_2- (4) and α_1- and α_2- (5) subtypes. In the case of prostanoid receptors, this approach has led us to the conclusion that there exist five basic types of prostanoid receptor, one for each of the naturally-occurring prostanoid (cyclo-oxygenase product) types: PGD_2, PGE_2, $PGF_{2\alpha}$, PGI_2 and TXA_2. Furthermore, there appear to be subdivisions within these classes, thus for example different subtypes of PGE_2-sensitive receptors clearly exist.

The following text describes the methods that may be used to classify prostanoid receptors, and to characterize the profiles of drugs acting at those receptors. All of the methods described, unless otherwise stated, are those which are or have been routinely used in our laboratories.

2. THE CLASSIFICATION AND NOMENCLATURE

It is not within the scope of this chapter to present and discuss the evidence for the prostanoid receptor classification; this has been dealt with at length elsewhere (6−9). However, a working outline of the classification and its nomenclature and details as to its use are presented below. Some essential details are summarized in *Table 1*.

The nomenclature devised for the prostanoid receptors is both logical and systematic. All prostanoid receptors are P-receptors, and to avoid confusion with the P-(purine) receptors described by Burnstock (10), in each case the P is preceded by a letter defining which of the standard prostanoid types is the most potent and hence probably the natural ligand; thus those receptors most sensitive to PGD_2 become DP-receptors, PGE_2, EP-receptors, $PGF_{2\alpha}$, FP-receptors, PGI_2, IP-receptors and TXA_2, TP-receptors. Where subdivision of a particular receptor type occurs, the subtypes are identified by use of a subscript, e.g. EP_1 and EP_2. The use of these subscript numbers does *not* imply that these receptors are specific for PGE_1 and PGE_2, respectively; we have obtained no evidence that specific receptors for 1-series prostanoids exist.

An important point which emerges from *Table 1* is that there is considerable cross-reactivity between each of the standard prostanoids and the various receptors. Thus the observation that for example $PGF_{2\alpha}$ contracts a given smooth muscle preparation is not evidence in itself that the preparation contains FP-receptors. Before this may be concluded, a number of other criteria must be fulfilled. The most important criterion is that $PGF_{2\alpha}$ should be the most potent natural prostanoid. However, if this is not so, and $PGF_{2\alpha}$ although potent in absolute terms (e.g. EC_{50}, $10-100$ nM), is no more potent than one or more of the other natural prostanoids, or even if the rank order of agonist potency does not correspond with that for FP-receptors in *Table 1*, this is not necessarily evidence against the presence of FP-receptors. It more likely results from the co-existence of prostanoid receptor types in that preparation. This co-existence of different prostanoid receptors (heterogeneous populations) is very common, and that is why many preparations classically used in studies on prostanoid action, such as rat

Table 1. The nomenclature and some characteristics of prostanoid receptors.

Receptor	Most potent agonist	Rank order of agonist potency[a]
DP	PGD_2	$D_2 > E_2, F_{2\alpha}, I_2, TXA_2$[b]
EP	PGE_2	$E_2 > I_2 \geq F_{2\alpha} > D_2$
FP	$PGF_{2\alpha}$	$F_{2\alpha} > D_2 > E_2 > I_2$
IP	PGI_2	$I_2 \gg D_2, E_2, F_{2\alpha}, TXA_2$[b]
TP	TXA_2	$TXA_2 \gg D_2 > F_{2\alpha}, I_2 > E_2$

[a]Absolute potency of TXA_2 uncertain due to its extreme instability.
[b]Absolute rank order of weaker agonists uncertain due to lack of preparations containing homogeneous DP- and IP-receptors.

fundic strip and gerbil colon, are of limited use in receptor studies. Indeed one of the greatest problems in prostanoid receptor studies is finding preparations which contain homogeneous receptor populations.

3. PHARMACOLOGICALLY ACTIVE AGENTS IN PROSTANOID RECEPTOR CLASSIFICATION

3.1 Use of the standard agonists

In initial studies the most important agonists to use are the naturally-occurring prostanoids, PGD_2, PGE_2, $PGF_{2\alpha}$, PGI_2 and TXA_2. All except TXA_2 are commercially available. Due to its extreme instability, TXA_2 must be generated as required (see below), but it is most common instead to use the stable TXA_2-mimetic, $11\alpha,9\alpha$-epoxymethano PGH_2 (U-46619) (11), which is available commercially. We have found no evidence for the existence of receptors specific for PGA_2, PGB_2 or PGC_2, nor that any of them are naturally-occurring. Similarly there is no convincing evidence for the existence of receptors specific for the prostaglandin endoperoxides, PGG_2 or PGH_2, as these are believed to act largely as intermediates in the biosynthesis of the other prostanoids. If PGG_2 and/or PGH_2 do act directly, they do so at receptors indistinguishable from TXA_2-sensitive receptors (see 6,12). There follow details on the solubility, storage and use of the naturally-occurring prostanoids, PGD_2, E_2, $F_{2\alpha}$ and I_2 as well as U-46619.

As the commercially available prostanoids are rather expensive, some thought must be given to making the most efficient use of them. For this reason I will mention where it is possible to repeatedly freeze−thaw stock solutions, and where it is not. These details are summarized in *Table 2*.

3.1.1 *Preparation of authentic TXA₂*

Although there is substantial evidence that U-46619 behaves as a potent, selective mimic of TXA_2, for some applications it is more appropriate to use authentic TXA_2. Due to its extreme instability, TXA_2 is not available commercially, but it may be prepared as and when required. There are two main methods of obtaining TXA_2.

(i)   The biosynthetic method by conversion of PGH_2 to TXA_2 with platelet-derived thromboxane synthetase. A description of this method is beyond the scope of this chapter, and appears elsewhere.

Table 2. Solubility and stability of the standard prostanoids.

Prostanoid	Solubility[a] in solvent named	Freeze−thaw	Stability	
			at 0°C	at −20°C
PGD_2	1% $NaHCO_3$ ≥ 10 mM	No	≥ 8 h	Months
PGE_2	1% $NaHCO_3$ ≥ 10 mM	Yes	≥ 8 h	Months
$PGF_{2\alpha}$	1% $NaHCO_3$ ≥ 10 mM	Yes	≥ 8 h	Months
PGI_2	Tris buffer (pH 9) ≥ 10 mM	No	≥ 8 h	Uncertain
U-46619	1% $NaHCO_3$ ≥ 10 mM	Yes	≥ 8 h	Months

[a]Dilutions of PGD_2, PGE_2, $PGF_{2\alpha}$ and U-46619 may be prepared in saline or physiological salt solution, and are all stable if kept on ice over the course of the day. Dilutions of PGI_2 may be prepared in Tris buffer (pH 8) immediately before use.

(ii) Generation from guinea-pig chopped lung of rabbit aorta contracting substance (identified as predominantly TXA_2) by mechanical agitation.

While also not strictly within the scope of this chapter, we have found that the isolated chopped lung preparation of the guinea-pig in association with the superfusion cascade technique is a simple, inexpensive and reliable method of generating and evaluating the biological actions of authentic TXA_2.

(i)   To prepare the chopped lung, kill a guinea-pig by a blow to the head followed by exsanguination, open up the thoracic cavity to reveal the lungs, and the lower neck to reveal the lower end of the trachea.

(ii)   With a pair of sharp scissors, cut through the trachea then, holding the trachea with a pair of forceps distal to the cut, lift the trachea away from the neck and carefully cut beneath the trachea and then the lungs pulling them away from the animal all of the time until they have been removed, with the heart, from the body cavity.

(iii)   Rinse the trachea, lungs and heart in a beaker of physiological salt solution and then place them in a Petri dish. Remove the heart and then cut the lung lobes away from the accessory tissue, trachea, bronchi and pulmonary vasculature. Place the lung lobes in a beaker of physiological salt solution.

(iv)   Next, taking one lobe at a time, and with a pair of sharp scissors, cut up the lung into pieces about 2 mm cube.

(v)   Place all of the pieces into a small nylon mesh bag which is held by means of a snug-fitting plastic collar in a 10 ml heated (37°C) organ bath (see *Figure 1*). The nylon mesh may conveniently be obtained from tights/stockings, and the plastic collar from the body of a parallel-sided centrifuge tube or similar plastic container.

(vi)   Drip heated (37°C) Krebs' solution over the lung at a rate of 5 ml/min and allow the effluent to superfuse the required assay tissues.

(vii)   To generate the TXA_2, stir the lung in an even, vigorous manner with a plastic rod (we have used the plunger from a 1 ml disposable syringe).

The quantity of TXA_2 released from the chopped lung is related to the degree of stirring; thus the more vigorous or longer the agitation, the more TXA_2 is generated. We have therefore found it simple to produce graded release of TXA_2 by stirring the lung at a constant rate for increasing periods of time (e.g. $1-30$ sec). Thus 'agitation/effect' curves may be obtained on the assay tissues in either a sequential or a cumulative fashion. If an interval of $20-30$ min is allowed between successive 'agitation/effect' curves they are usually highly reproducible for as many as six consecutive curves.

To demonstrate that the active principle generated by this procedure is indeed TXA_2, a specific TX synthase inhibitor should be added to the Krebs' solution superfusing the chopped lung. Such an agent will prevent the conversion of the prostaglandin endoperoxides, PGG_2 and PGH_2, into TXA_2 and this will be seen as an inhibition of activity on TX-sensitive (TP-) receptor-containing preparations, and a potentiation on preparations containing other types of prostanoid receptor where presumably unchanged endoperoxide acts through conversion to other, stable prostanoids. It is, however, important to remember that TX synthase inhibitors are unlikely to obliterate activity on TP-receptor-containing tissues, as PGH_2 itself is known to be a fairly potent TP-

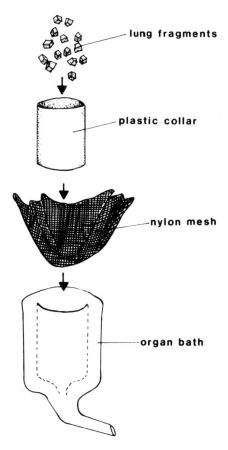

Figure 1. The basic equipment required for the generation of 'rabbit aorta contracting substance' (RCS) from guinea-pig lung.

receptor agonist. Examples of useful TX synthase inhibitors are imidazole and n-butyl-imidazole (which are commercially available), and dazoxiben and dazmagrel (which may only be obtained by gift from Pfizer UK Ltd.).

3.2 Synthetic agonists

While the natural 2-series prostanoids are invaluable tools in the classification and characterization of prostanoid receptors, the information that they provide on their own is limited. There are however a small number of synthetic prostanoid agonists which we have found equally valuable in receptor characterization, and which provide substantial complementary information to that obtained with the natural agonists. In addition, some of these agonists have provided evidence for the division of one class of receptor, the EP-receptor, into two subtypes, EP_1- and EP_2-. Some particularly useful synthetic agonists are summarized in *Table 3*, and their structures are shown in *Figure 2*. Details of these agonists are outlined below.

271

Table 3. Some useful synthetic prostanoid agonists, the receptor types for which they are selective and their potencies at those receptors.

Agonist	Receptor selectivity	Approximate equipotent concentration $\dfrac{EC_{50}\ agonist}{EC_{50}\ standard}$
BW245C	DP	0.03 (PGD$_2$ = 1)
16,16-dimethyl PGE$_2$	EP$_1$	0.1 (PGE$_2$ = 1)
Sulprostone	EP$_1$	1.0 (PGE$_2$ = 1)
Fluprostenol	FP	1.0 (PGF$_{2\alpha}$ = 1)
Cloprostenol	FP	0.4 (PGF$_{2\alpha}$ = 1)
Iloprost	IP/EP$_1$	1.0 (PGI$_2$ = 1)/1.0 (PGE$_2$ = 1)
U-46619	TP	> 1.0 (TXA$_2$ = 1)[a]

[a]Absolute potency of TXA$_2$ unknown due to extreme instability.

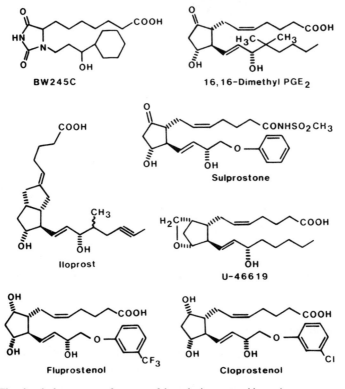

Figure 2. The chemical structures of some useful synthetic prostanoid agonists.

3.2.1 *BW245C*

BW245C (13) is a highly selective DP-receptor agonist (9). It appears to have little or no agonist activity at EP-, FP-, IP- or TP-receptors. It is about 30-times more potent than PGD$_2$ at DP-receptors and is more selective than PGD$_2$, having no agonist activity at FP- or TP-receptors. It is therefore of particular value in the identification of DP-receptors where they exist within a heterogeneous (mixed) receptor population.

BW245C is soluble in 1% $NaHCO_3$ to a concentration of at least 1 mM. It is stable in solution at $-20°C$ for long periods (>12 months). It also seems to withstand a degree of freeze−thawing. BW245C is not commercially available at present, and may only be obtained by gift from the Wellcome Foundation.

3.2.2 16,16-dimethyl PGE₂

16,16-dimethyl PGE_2 is of limited use in receptor classification, its chief application being for prostanoid studies *in vivo*, where unlike its parent, PGE_2, it resists inactivation in the lung. In one respect, it is less selective than PGE_2, having considerably higher potency at TP-receptors. However, it does have one useful feature, and that is its selectivity of action within EP-receptors, being at least 10 times more potent on EP_1-receptors than on EP_2-receptors. 16,16-dimethyl PGE_2 may therefore be regarded as a moderately selective EP_1-receptor agonist compared wth PGE_2 (9).

16,16-dimethyl PGE_2 is soluble in 1% $NaHCO_3$ to concentrations of at least 1 mM. It is stable in solution at $-20°C$ for long periods (>12 months). It also stands repeated freeze−thawing. It is now available from a number of commercial sources.

3.2.3 Sulprostone

Sulprostone (14), a stable acyl sulphonamide analogue of PGE_2, is a very valuable compound, and is a highly selective EP-agonist, being a more selective EP-agonist than PGE_2. Thus although sulprostone is slightly less potent than PGE_2 (~ 3-fold) on EP_1-receptors, it is essentially inactive at EP_2-, DP-, FP-, IP- and TP-receptors. Sulprostone may therefore be regarded as a potent, selective EP_1-receptor agonist (9).

Sulprostone is not soluble in $NaHCO_3$, but to prepare a stock 1 mM emulsion, first dissolve the compound in sufficient ethanol to yield a final 3% v/v concentration, add Tween 80 to yield a final 0.01% v/v concentration and make up to volume with 0.9% w/v saline. On addition of saline, the preparation takes on a milky appearance, but in this form sulprostone is stable at $-20°C$ for long periods (>12 months), and will withstand repeated freeze−thawing. Sulprostone is not available commercially, but only as a gift from Schering AG.

3.2.4 Fluprostenol (ICI81008)

Fluprostenol (15), a stable analogue of $PGF_{2\alpha}$ ranks with BW254C and sulprostone as one of the most selective compounds that we have examined. While it is a potent FP-agonist, being equipotent with $PGF_{2\alpha}$, it is far more selective than its parent compound, having essentially no demonstrable agonist activity at any of the other four prostanoid receptor types (DP, EP, IP or TP) (9). Because it is much more selective than $PGF_{2\alpha}$, it is useful in identifying FP-receptors in mixed receptor populations. While fluprostenol has been commercially available in a 0.104 mM solution as the veterinary product Equimate (ICI), it has now unfortunately been taken off the market in the UK.

3.2.5 *Cloprostenol (ICI80996)*

Cloprostenol (15), a close analogue of fluprostenol, has essentially the same pharmacological profile except that it is slightly more potent (2- to 3-fold) as an FP-agonist. However, unlike fluprostenol, cloprostenol has similar potency to $PGF_{2\alpha}$ on EP- and TP-receptors. Therefore, while cloprostenol is a potent FP-agonist, it is less selective than fluprostenol. Cloprostenol may be obtained commercially in a 0.56 mM solution as the veterinary product Estrumate (ICI), in which form it is stable at room temperature for 3 years.

3.2.6 *Iloprost*

Iloprost (16), a 16-methyl carbacyclin analogue, is a potent, chemically stable IP-agonist. It is as potent as PGI_2 at IP-receptors, but also has high potency at EP_1-receptors, for example in guinea-pig fundus it is approximately equipotent with PGE_2 and is in fact about 20-times more potent than PGI_2. It has one pharmacological advantage over PGI_2, and that is its apparent inactivity at TP-receptors. Although PGI_2 is a weak TP-agonist, iloprost is considerably weaker still. Iloprost is soluble in 1% $NaHCO_3$ in concentrations greater than 1 mM. It is stable at $-20°C$ and will stand some degree of freeze−thawing. Iloprost is not available commercially at present and may only be obtained by gift from Schering AG.

3.2.7 *U-46619*

See Section 3.1.

Table 4. Some prostanoid receptor blocking drugs.

Receptor	Antagonist	Range of reported pA_2 values
DP	AH6809	6.5
	N-0164	−
	DPP	−
EP_1	SC-19220	5.2−5.6
	AH6809	6.4−7.0
	N-0164	−
	PPP	−
	DPP	−
EP_2	None	
FP	None	
IP	None	
TP	AH19437	5.9−6.8
	AH23848	7.8−9.5
	Pinane thromboxane	−
	EP045	6.1−7.5
	EP092	7.3−8.0
	AH6809	5.8
	SQ28053	7.9−8.5
	ICI 159,995	6.2−6.8
	BM13177	5.4−6.3
	13-Azaprostanoic acid	5.3

3.3 **Antagonists**

While agonists can provide much useful information regarding receptor classification, definitive evidence can really only be provided with antagonists as these are the only ones for which pharmacological activity is a reflection of receptor affinity. Unfortunately, there exist few, if any, antagonists at most types of prostanoid receptor, the only exception to this being TP-receptors for which there exist a wide range of antagonists of very different structural types. *Table 4* lists the prostanoid receptor types and drugs which we and others have found to block them. The chemical structure of these antagonists are shown in *Figure 3*. Details of these antagonists are outlined below.

3.3.1 *SC-19220*

SC-19220 (17) was one of the earliest prostanoid antagonists identified. Although it is rather weak, it is specific in its prostanoid antagonism, and in addition is a selective EP_1-receptor blocking drug, having no antagonist activity at EP_2-receptors. It was the selectivity of antagonism of EP-receptors by SC-19220 that first indicated the necessity

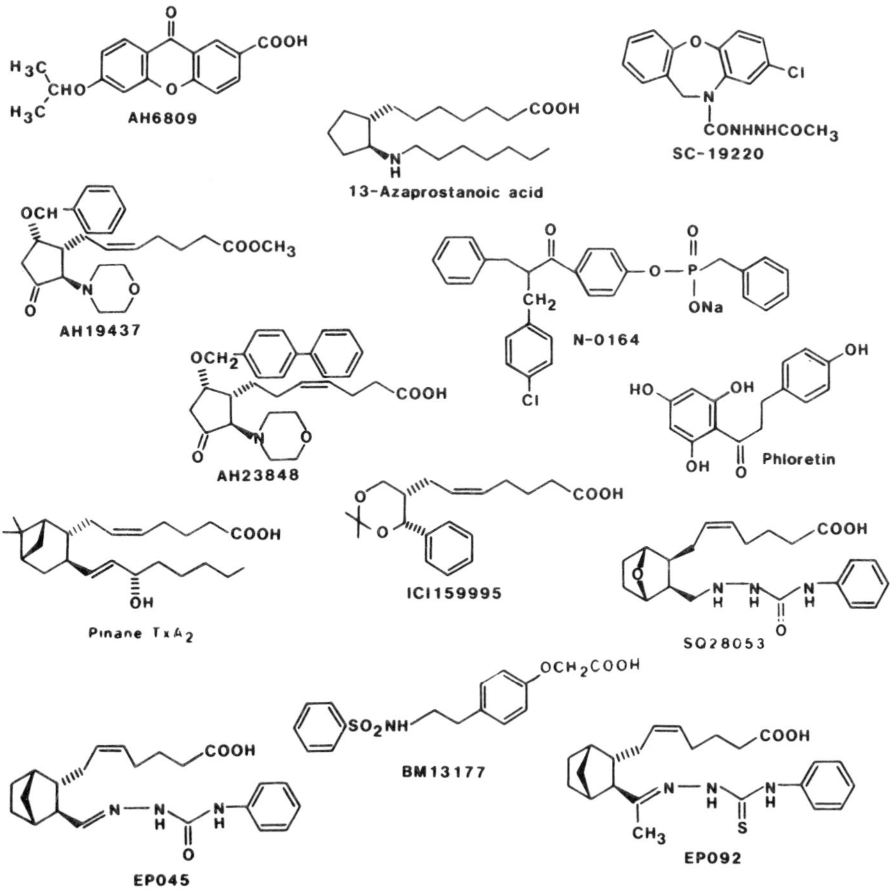

Figure 3. The chemical structure of some prostanoid antagonists.

275

for subdivision of this receptor type (6). SC-19220 is insoluble in aqueous media at the concentrations of stock solution required (0.3–3.0 mM), and we have found that while it is soluble in organic solvents, the most satisfactory preparation of SC-19220 is a suspension. This is prepared by the addition of sufficient ethanol to yield a final concentration of 3% v/v, to this is added Tween 80 to give a final concentration of 0.01% v/v. Saline is then added to give the final desired concentration of SC-19220 — the preparation is clearly milky. Suspensions of SC-19220 should be prepared immediately before use as on leaving the preparation to stand, the SC-19220 tends to flocculate and sediment out, and while this does not appear to influence its potency, the concentrations of successive samples from the stock solution are progressively less reliable. Even ultrasonic agitation will not reconvert the preparation to a fine suspension.

SC-19220 has a reasonably fast onset of action, and a 30 min pre-treatment period is sufficient for maximal antagonism. SC-19220 is not suitable for use *in vivo* particularly by the intravenous route due to its low potency, poor solubility and some albumen binding ($\sim 80\%$). SC-19220 is supplied as a white powder, and in this form it appears to be stable for prolonged periods at room temperature (>2 years). For reasons of the physical instability of the suspension, we have not tried to store such preparations.

SC-19220 is not available commercially, and may only be obtained by gift from Searle Research and Development Company.

3.3.2 *AH6809*

AH6809 (9), like SC-19220, is a selective EP_1-receptor blocking drug, having little or no antagonist activity at EP_2-receptors. However, unlike SC-19220 it has a degree of antagonist activity at some other prostanoid receptors. At concentrations slightly higher than those blocking EP_1-receptors, AH6809 blocks DP-receptors, and again at higher concentrations still it also blocks some TP-receptors (e.g. rat aorta, dog saphenous vein, dog coronary artery, dog splenic capsule), but not others (e.g. guinea-pig lung, human platelets, rabbit aorta) suggesting the existence of some subdivision within TP-receptors. While AH6809 is specific in its prostanoid antagonist activity at lower concentrations (up to 10 μM), at higher concentrations it can have spasmolytic activity unrelated to its prostanoid receptor blocking activity, and at these concentrations it can inhibit the enzyme phosphodiesterase.

AH6809 has a reasonably rapid onset of action, and a 30 min pre-treatment time is sufficient for maximal antagonism. AH6809 is soluble in aqueous media as the sodium salt, thus it may be dissolved in concentrations of at least 3 mM in 1% $NaHCO_3$. Solutions of AH6809 appear to be stable at 0°C over the course of the day, but there may be loss of activity if the solutions are kept at 0°C overnight. Therefore, AH6809 solutions are always made up fresh on the day of the experiment.

AH6809 is not suitable for use *in vivo* due to its substantial albumen binding ($\sim 98\%$). It is not available commercially, and may only be obtained by gift from Glaxo Group Research Ltd.

3.3.3 *AH19437 and AH23848*

These two analogues have similar profiles of action, both being selective TP-receptor blocking drugs (9,18). The main difference between the two being that AH23848 is

30–100 times more potent than AH19437. As AH19437 is not very potent, its specificity and selectivity of action cannot be rigorously tested due to limitations in solubility; but for AH23848, concentrations of over 1000 times its pA_2 at TP-receptors have no antagonist activity versus non-prostanoid agonists (e.g. 5-HT and KCl) on vascular smooth muscle, and versus adenosine diphosphate on platelets. Similarly, these high concentrations of AH23848 have no antagonist activity at DP-, EP_1-, EP_2-, FP- or IP-receptors.

AH23848 has a reasonably rapid onset of action, and a 45 min pre-treatment time appears to be sufficient for equilibration. AH23848 is a white powder, which is soluble in 1% $NaHCO_3$ in saline in concentrations greater than 1 mM. While solutions of AH23848 appear to be stable in solution at 0°C over the course of the day, it is not advised to keep solutions for longer periods. Therefore, solutions of AH23848 are made up fresh on the day of the experiment and are kept on ice.

One interesting feature of AH19437 and AH23848 as well as a number of other TP-receptor blocking drugs (see below) is that they appear, under some circumstances, to possess some partial agonist activity. This activity is most easily observed *in vivo* where on intravenous administration a transient (1–2 min duration) broncho- and vaso-constriction is observed. After oral administration this agonist activity is not observed. Prior exposure of an animal to a TP-receptor blocking drug including AH19437 or AH23848 prevents the transient agonist activity. Interestingly, it is not easy to demonstrate this partial agonist activity *in vitro*, and we have found that prior exposure of vascular or bronchial smooth muscle preparations to a TP-agonist such as U-46619 will prevent AH23848 demonstrating its inherent agonist activity. In order to observe this, naive preparations (i.e. not previously exposed to a TP-receptor agonist) must be used, and in such cases a transient agonist response may be observed on antagonist administration. This transient partial agonist activity has never been observed on blood platelets.

AH19437 and AH23848 are both active *in vivo* at relatively low doses, and are therefore suitable for prostanoid receptor studies in whole animals. AH19437 is no longer available, but AH23848 may be obtained by gift from Glaxo Group Research Ltd.

3.3.4 *N-0164, DPP and PPP*

N-0164, DPP and PPP (9,20,21) have similar profiles of action in so far as we have examined them. While they all clearly possess prostaglandin antagonist activity, none appear to be competitive in that they all cause a flattening of prostaglandin concentration effect curves. All three compounds appear to block EP_1- and TP-receptors, and N-0164 and DPP also block DP-receptors, although in this latter action they are weak and their specificity unreliable.

3.3.5 *13-Azaprostanoic acid*

Although 13-azaprostanoic acid (13-APA)(19) is a specific TP-receptor blocking drug, its lack of potency limits its general usefulness. It has one interesting feature, and that is its apparent platelet selectivity, being at least five times more potent in blocking TP-receptors in human platelets than those in rat aorta.

13-APA is not very soluble in aqueous media, and to make up a 10 mM stock solution it is necessary to dissolve the compound in sufficient ethanol to yield a final 12% concentration and to make up to volume with saline. It is then necessary to use solutions immediately after they are prepared as within minutes of addition of saline, 13-APA will come out of solution. Solutions of 13-APA are therefore never stored. Optimal tissue contact times for 13-APA have not been determined, but 10 min on platelets and 60 min on vascular smooth muscle appear to be sufficient.

13-APA is not commercially available.

3.3.6 *Other TP antagonists*

A number of other TP-antagonists have been reported (see *Table 4*). While we have no experience of their use, there is considerable literature evidence that they do exhibit selective TP-receptor blocking activity, and should therefore be as useful as AH19437 and AH23848 in studies on prostanoid receptors (see 9).

4. DETERMINATION OF POTENCY OF PHARMACOLOGICALLY ACTIVE AGENTS

4.1 **Determination of agonist potency**

4.1.1 *Smooth muscle*

In order to compare prostanoid agonist potencies on different preparations, it is necessary to select a standard agonist against which all others are compared. While comparisons would be most easily made if the same prostanoid agonist served as standard on all preparations, this is not possible as no one prostanoid is highly active at all prostanoid receptors. Therefore, as it is important that a potent agonist is chosen as standard for each prostanoid receptor type, the standard selected is what may be regarded as the natural agonist for that receptor type, that is the most potent natural agonist (except in the case of TXA_2, where U-46619 is used).

Smooth muscle may contract or relax in response to prostanoids, and as smooth muscle is, in the absence of any outside influence, in a relaxed state, the contractile actions may be simply studied on normal 'resting' smooth muscle preparations. However, in order to study relaxant actions, the smooth muscle must be in a contracted state. Such a contracted state is usually obtained by addition of a spasmogen to the physiological solution bathing the preparation or, alternatively, it may be achieved by stimulation of excitatory nerve fibres within the tissue by exposing it to repeated trains of electrical pulses. Spasmogen-induced contractions may be maintained by the continued presence of that spasmogen in the bathing fluid or, if the tissue will not support such a maintained contracture, repeated responses to spasmogen may be obtained with washout and recovery between doses. Similarly, contractile responses to electrical stimulation are usually obtained at regular intervals. *Figure 4* shows these various methods of achieving contraction, as well as the responses obtained with a spasmolytic agent.

Relative potencies of agonists compared with the standard may be determined as follows:

(i)   First, construct a cumulative concentration – effect curve to the standard agonist (see *Figure 5*). This should be achieved by addition to the tissue bathing fluid of the threshold effective concentration of the agonist (x nM) and waiting for

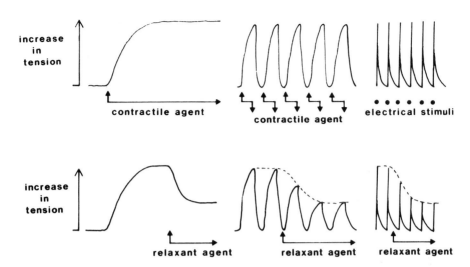

Figure 4. Methods of studying the effects of relaxant agonists. (a) Induction of elevated tone (left hand panel), or reproducible contractile responses to repeated administration of agonist (middle panel) or trains of electrical pulses (right hand panel). (b) Inhibition of these responses by administration of a relaxant agent.

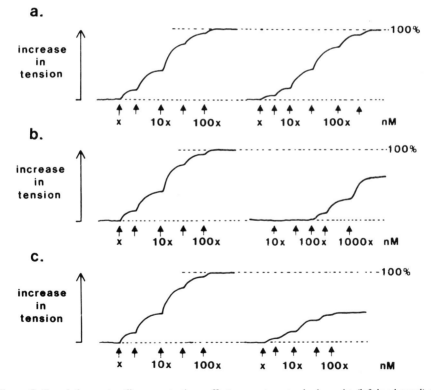

Figure 5. Cumulative contractile concentration−effect curves to a standard agonist (left hand panel) and a test agonist (right hand panel). (a) Test agonist a full agonist with respect to the standard. (b) Test agonist weak, such that a full concentration−effect curve cannot be constructed. (c) Test agonist a partial agonist with respect to the standard.

the preparation to respond. If a response is obtained, wait until it has equilibrated, then add the next concentration, which should be either $+2x$ nM or $+9x$ nM, depending on whether '3'-fold dose increment (i.e. 1, 3, 10, 30, etc.) or a 10-fold dose increment (i.e. 1, 10, 100, 1000, etc.) is being used. Once more wait until the response obtained has equilibrated, then add the next concentration, that is $+7x$ nM or $+90x$ nM (see above). Continue this procedure until further addition of drug causes no further increase in response, then wash the drug from the bath by two or three changes of bathing fluid, repeat this changing of the bathing fluid at approximately 15 min intervals.

(ii)   If, after addition of the first concentration of drug to the bathing fluid, the tissue does not respond within $2-3$ min, for most tissues it is almost certainly not going to, so administer the next concentration in the dosing sequence, and proceed as above. Some tissues (e.g. some vascular preparations) may take longer than 3 min to start to respond to drug administration, and these will be identified experimentally.

(iii)   On completion of the full concentration−effect curve, and after a suitable washout period of at least 30 min, and preferably $45-60$ min, construct a second concentration−effect curve to the standard agonist in the same way as above, but using information gained during the construction of the first as to suitable starting concentration and dose increments.

(iv)   Repeat such concentration−effect curves to the standard agonist using the same washout period and number of washes each time until the curves are reproducible such that there is no more than a 2-fold change in EC_{50} (see below).

(v)   Now construct a concentration−effect curve to the test agonist using the same dose increments as for the standard. The starting concentration for the test agonist may be determined by reference to previous experiments, or by assuming a similar potency to the standard; if this is inappropriate, it will be obvious in the first experiment, and a suitably higher or lower starting concentration may be used in subsequent experiments.

(vi)   If little or no tissue response has been obtained after the highest practicable concentration of test compound has been added to the bathing solution, in the absence of any extenuating circumstances, it is safe to say that the test compound has little or no agonist activity at the receptor present in that tissue.

(vii)   Now test it for possible antagonist activity by constructing a further concentration−effect curve to the standard agonist in the continued presence of the test compound (see *Figure 6*); a reduction in potency of the standard in this final curve indicates some sort of antagonist activity of the test compound (see next section).

All of the concentration−effect curves from these studies should be plotted on log-linear graph paper. Contractile responses may be expressed in terms of either absolute changes in tissue tension (isometric method, see Section 5.2.1) or length (isotonic method, see Section 5.2.1) or as percentage increase, where 100% is defined as the maximum response obtainable with the standard agonist on that preparation (see *Figure 5*).

Relaxant responses should be expressed in terms of percentage decrease in tension

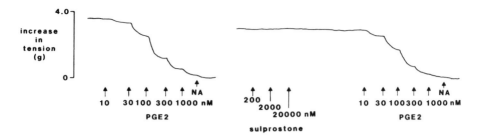

Figure 6. Construction of cumulative concentration–effect curves to a standard agonist in the absence (left hand panel) and in the presence (right hand panel) of a high concentration of a test compound which itself has no agonist activity in this preparation. In this example, the standard agonist is PGE$_2$, the test compound is sulprostone (see Section 3.2.3), the tissue is cat tracheal strip (see Section 5.2.2) and the response is smooth muscle relaxation.

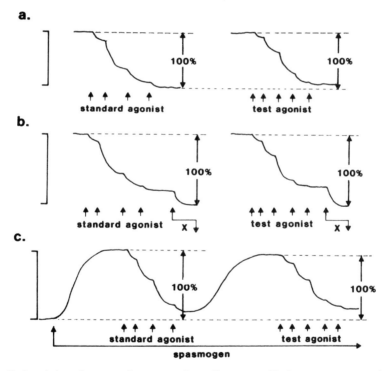

Figure 7. Cumulative relaxant agonist concentration–effect curves. Maximum responses may be defined as: **(a)** the greatest response obtained in the final control concentration–effect curve (left hand panel), **(b)** the response obtained to a high concentration of a standard spasmolytic drug (X) added at the end of each concentration–effect curve, or **(c)** the degree of each contraction induced by the spasmogenic stimulus.

or length, where 100% is defined as that decrease from the spasmogen-induced tone to the pre-spasmogen level, or the maximum response obtainable with the standard agonist on that preparation, or the response obtained to a maximally effective concentration of a non-prostanoid relaxant agent added at the end of each prostanoid concentration–effect curve (see *Figure 7*). The absolute potencies of the agonists studied should be expressed as EC_{50}, where EC_{50} is defined as that concentration of agonist causing a response equal to 50% of the maximum obtainable to the standard agonist.

The potency of the test compound relative to that of the standard is expressed as equipotent concentration (standard agonist $= 1$), and to determine this value, divide the EC_{50} value for the test compound by that for the standard, that is:

$$\text{equipotent concentration} = \frac{EC_{50} \text{ (test agonist)}}{EC_{50} \text{ (standard agonist)}}$$

A value greater than 1.0 means that the test compound is weaker than the standard, a value of less than 1.0 means that it is more potent. It is important to stress that values of equipotent concentration can only be determined if the concentration–effect curves to standard and test agonist are parallel. Attempts to generate data in this way from curves which are clearly not parallel can only result in misleading information. Reasons for non-parallel concentration–effect curves are most commonly:

(i)   the standard and test agonists are not acting at the same receptor type;
(ii)   one (or both) of the agonists has a low efficacy and so tends to act as a partial agonist; or
(iii) the preparation contains receptors mediating opposing effects and the standard and test agonists have different potencies at them. This is particularly common in the case of prostanoid receptors.

4.1.2 *Blood platelets*

Agonist activity is assessed on blood platelets in essentially the same manner as in smooth muscle except that only one concentration of one agonist can be studied on each aliquot of blood or platelet-rich plasma (PRP). Therefore in order to compare a range of concentrations of a given prostanoid against a similar range of concentrations of the standard, a blood or PRP sample must be divided into a sufficient number of aliquots, and concentration–effect curves are neither truly 'cumulative' nor 'sequential' (see Section 5.2.1), but are 'composite'.

Anti-aggregatory agonist activity is demonstrated by the ability of the agonist to inhibit the aggregatory response to a standard agonist (e.g. adenosine diphosphate, $0.1 - 10 \ \mu M$). This anti-aggregatory activity is quantified by determining the concentration of agonist required to cause a pre-determined decrease in the aggregatory potency of ADP (e.g. 10-fold). The method used is the same as that for the determination of pA_2 for an antagonist (see Sections 4.2.1 and 4.2.2). The use of whole blood rather than PRP suffers from the serious disadvantage that blood contains high concentrations of serum proteins which may well bind and thus effectively inactivate agonist drugs. At the very least this would seriously limit the quantitative relevance of results obtained in studies where whole blood is used.

4.2 **Antagonists**

4.2.1 *Smooth muscle*

While an indication of antagonist activity may be obtained by comparing responses to a single concentration of agonist, first in the absence and then in the presence of a potential antagonist agent, such information has no quantitative value. Thus the expression of potency of an antagonist as a percentage inhibition of a submaximal response to an agonist is meaningless as this will vary with the size of the agonist response, or rather where it lies on the agonist concentration – effect curve. Antagonist potency should be expressed in terms of degree of shift of agonist concentration – effect curves. The most useful antagonists are competitive receptor blocking drugs, as for these compounds a measure of affinity for the receptor may be determined (see 22). This measure is termed the pA_2, which is defined as the negative molar concentration of antagonist which will cause a 2-fold reduction in potency of an agonist. In order to determine the pA_2 for an antagonist, the effects of a range of concentrations of antagonist on agonist concentration – effect curves should be determined, and the data obtained used to calculate the pA_2 as outlined below. Before this is undertaken however it is important to establish the specificity of prostanoid antagonism. To achieve this, concentrations of antagonist sufficient to produce a substantial rightward shift ($>$ 10-fold) of the prostanoid agonist concentration – effect curve on the tissue in question should be shown to be without effect against similar curves to agonists acting at sites other than prostanoid receptors.

To determine pA_2 for an antagonist, at least three different concentrations of antagonist should be used, these being, preferably, in 10-fold increments. However, due to low potency and limitations of solubility or specificity of the antagonist, this is not always possible. The procedure is as follows:

(i)   Construct and repeat cumulative concentration – effect curves (see Section 5.2.1) to the standard agonist until constant (as outlined in the previous section).

(ii)   Once reproducible curves have been obtained, immediately after washout add a suitable concentration of antagonist, and replace it after each further washout such that the tissue has the maximum possible exposure to it between agonist curves, then construct a further agonist concentration – effect curve.

Ideally, this procedure should be repeated using the same concentration of antagonist, to make sure that any antagonist effect has had sufficient time to come to equilibrium. Thus, if four tissues are used simultaneously, four different concentrations of antagonist may be evaluated simultaneously. Alternatively, one tissue can serve as an untreated control to which no antagonist is administered and with which spontaneous alterations in agonist potency with time can be determined, while on the other three preparations different concentrations of antagonist can be tested. With some tissues it is possible to test different concentrations of antagonist in sequence on each preparation. Such preparations must have a reasonably rapid response to the agonist, and the antagonist equilibration time must be relatively short. Obviously, in such cases antagonist concentrations should be progressively increased and not decreased. And finally, if a series of different concentrations of antagonist are to be evaluated on the same preparation, it is particularly important to run in parallel a control preparation treated with agonist but not antagonist to determine spontaneous change in agonist potency with time. Where parallel control preparations are used, there are two views on what to do with the data obtained from them:

(i)   the preparation should be used solely as an indicator; thus, if spontaneous change in agonist potency exceeds a pre-determined amount (e.g. 2- or 3-fold) then the whole experiment is abandoned;

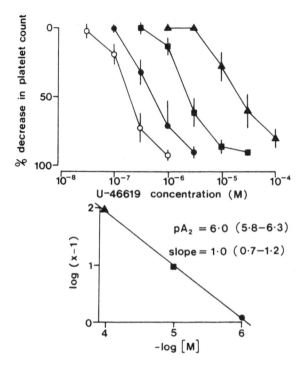

Figure 8. Determination of antagonist potency of AH19437 (see Section 3.3.3) against U-46619 on human platelets — the construction of a Schild plot. Upper panel, mean concentration−effect curves to U-46619 in the absence (○) and presence of AH19437, 1 μM (●), 10 μM (■) and 100 μM (▲). Lower panel, Schild plot, where x = agonist concentration ratio $\frac{(EC_{50} + antagonist)}{EC_{50}\ control}$ and [M] is the concentration of antagonist (AH19437).

(ii)   the changes in agonist potency occurring after addition of antagonist should be 'corrected' by a factor corresponding to the spontaneous change in potency on the control preparations.

It is a matter of personal choice as to which course to follow.

Degree of antagonism by any given concentration of antagonist is expressed as concentration ratio (CR), which is calculated by dividing the EC_{50} for the agonist in the presence of the antagonist by that in its absence (i.e. the EC_{50} from the final control concentration−effect curve). Thus:

$$CR = \frac{EC_{50} + antagonist}{EC_{50} - antagonist}$$

This can only be done however if the two curves are parallel. If they are not, then quantification of antagonist potency cannot be simply achieved.

The values of CR are used to determine pA_2 by plotting, on linear graph paper, log (CR−1) on the ordinate against −log antagonist molar concentration (−log [M]) on the abscissa (see *Figure 8*). The regression may be fitted by eye or preferably by means of regression analysis. The point at which the resulting regression crosses the abscissa [i.e. where $\log (CR-1)=0$] corresponds to the pA_2 value. The slope of the regression describes the relationship between antagonist concentration and degree of antagonism, thus if the antagonism is competitive in nature, the slope should be 1.0. If the slope is significantly different from 1.0, then this is evidence that the antagonism is not of a simple competitive nature and means usually either

(i)   that the antagonist is not a receptor blocking drug but interferes at some other stage intermediate between receptor activation and tissue response; or

(ii)   in that tissue the agonist acts through more than one receptor type, at which the antagonist has different potencies.

If the latter is the case, the use of agonists with high degrees of selectivity for the various receptors present (if such agonists are available) will help clarify the situation.

4.2.2 *Blood platelets*

Again antagonist activity is assessed on blood platelets in essentially the same manner as on smooth muscle, except that agonist concentration—effect curves in the absence and presence of antagonist must be constructed in a composite fashion (see Section 4.1.2). Thus, in order to evaluate the effect of a single concentration of an antagonist against a given agonist concentration—effect curve, sufficient aliquots of blood or PRP must be prepared to allow one for each concentration of agonist in the absence of antagonist, and one for each concentration of agonist in the presence of the antagonist. If a pA_2 value is to be determined, it will be necessary to evaluate a minimum of three concentrations of antagonist. Due to the time taken in the estimation of aggregation in the large number of aliquots arising from such an experiment, a time control has to be run; this is important as platelets have a limited life-span and will deteriorate much more rapidly than isolated smooth muscle. Thus the experiment should be designed as follows:

(i)   Construct a concentration—effect curve to the agonist in the absence of antagonist.

(ii)   Construct, in random sequence, concentration—effect curves to the agonist in the presence of the various concentrations of antagonist.

(iii)   Construct a further concentration—effect curve to the agonist in the absence of antagonist.

(iv)   Mean the two agonist curves in the absence of antagonist, and compare the curves obtained in the presence of agonist with this mean control curve.

Antagonist studies carried out in whole blood suffer the same disadvantage as previously mentioned for agonist studies (see Section 4.1.2), namely the presence of serum proteins.

5. USEFUL PREPARATIONS IN PROSTANOID RECEPTOR CLASSIFICATION

5.1 **Criteria**

Preparations of potential use in prostanoid receptor classification should ideally fulfil the following two criteria.

(i)   They should demonstrate an uncomplicated response to prostanoids. For example, smooth muscle should contract *or* relax in response to one or more of the standard prostanoids, but should not do both.

(ii)   They should demonstrate a well-defined rank order of agonist potency, with one standard agonist substantially (at least an order of magnitude) more potent than any of the others. A less well-defined rank order is usually indicative of the preparation bearing a heterogeneous receptor population.

These criteria are ideal, and often compromises have to be made. Thus, in some instances, it may be necessary to employ preparations which show a complicated response to prostanoids because uncomplicated ones bearing the desired receptor type have not as yet been identified. If this is the case, the preparations chosen are usually those which show the biggest difference in prostanoid potency in eliciting the two effects. The second criterion presupposes that our receptor classification is correct, and that if two or more of the standard prostanoids are highly potent agonists, this constitutes evidence for a heterogeneous prostanoid receptor population. While this may not always be so, to date we have found no exceptions, but for definitive proof we require the development of potent, selective blocking drugs for all of the postulated receptor types. Despite the complications resulting from using preparations with mixed receptor populations, there are instances where such preparations can be of use, and some of these will be discussed below.

Most of the preparations that we have found useful in our prostanoid receptor studies are either preparations of smooth muscle or blood platelets from a range of species including man. In the case of smooth muscle preparations, responses are either contraction or relaxation, whereas in the case of blood platelets the responses are either aggregation or inhibition of aggregation (anti-aggregation).

5.2 Smooth muscle

Some particularly useful smooth muscle preparations containing essentially homogeneous prostanoid receptor populations are listed in *Table 5*.

Table 5. Some smooth muscle preparations containing homogeneous prostanoid receptor populations.

Preparation	Response	Receptor type	Most potent prostanoid	Effective concentration range (nM)	EC_{50} (nM)	Maximum response (g)
Guinea-pig fundus	↑	EP_1	PGE_2	1−1000	8	1−4
Guinea-pig ileum[a]	↑	EP_1	PGE_2	3−3000	33	1−2
Dog fundus	↑	EP_1	PGE_2	3−10 000	47	3−6
Cat trachea	↓	EP				
		2_2	PGE_2	1−10 000	20	3−5
Guinea-pig ileum[b]	↓	EP_2	PGE_2	10−10 000	102	3−4
Dog iris	↑	FP	$PGF_{2\alpha}$	1−1000	11	0.1 −0.2
Cat iris	↑	FP	$PGF_{2\alpha}$	10−10 000	38	0.15−0.3
Guinea-pig lung	↑	TP	U-46619	3−30 000	143	0.15−0.3
Rat aorta	↑	TP	U-46619	1−3000	6	0.5 −1.0
Rabbit aorta	↑	TP	U-46619	3−3000	24	1.5 −3.0

[a]Longitudinal muscle preparation.
[b]Circular muscle preparation.
↑ Contraction.
↓ Relaxation.

Some smooth muscle preparations containing heterogeneous receptor populations are listed together with the receptors they contain in *Table 6*.

5.2.1 *General conditions of use*

(i)   Tissues may be removed from freshly killed or anaesthetized animals.

(ii) Animals may be killed either by a blow to the head followed by exsanguination or by an overdose of sodium pentobarbitone (Expiral).

(iii) Tissues may be used immediately after removal from the body, or may be stored in oxygenated, physiological salt solution at 4°C overnight. Some tissues may be stored even longer under these conditions.

(iv) Tissues may be removed from freshly killed experimental animals at the end of an experiment. This avoids the necessity of killing animals solely for the purpose of obtaining tissues for isolated tissue work. This is particularly appropriate with larger animals such as cats and dogs. It is important however to find out and to note the drugs with which that animal has been treated in the course of its primary experiment. Clearly, drug treatment can make the tissue unsuitable for further use, such as for prostanoid work; it seems unwise to use tissues from an animal which has previously been dosed with prostanoids or their antagonists. Tissues taken from these experimental animals may either be used directly or be stored in physiological salt solution at 4°C until required.

(v)   Tissue preparations should have cotton threads attached at either end. These should

Table 6. Some smooth muscle preparations containing heterogeneous prostanoid receptor populations.

Preparation	Response	Receptor type	Most potent prostanoid	Effective concentration range (nM)	EC_{50} (nM)	Maximum response (g)
Guinea-pig trachea	↑	EP_1	PGE_2	1 – 100	11	0.5 – 1.5
	↑	TP	U-46619	3 – 1000	11	1 – 3
	↓	EP_2	PGE_2	10 – 30 000	530	0.5 – 1.5
Pig fundus	↑	EP_1	PGE_2	3 – 3000	145	2 – 5
	↑	TP	U-46619	10 – 30 000	1290	1 – 4
Dog lung	↑	FP	$PGF_{2\alpha}$	10 – 100 000	3150	0.2 – 0.4
	↑	TP	U-46619	10 – 10 000	180	0.2 – 0.4
Cat lung	↑	FP	$PGF_{2\alpha}$	10 – 100 000	5330	0.2 – 0.5
	↑	TP	U-46619	3 – 10 000	46	0.2 – 0.5
Rat fundus	↑	EP_1	PGE_2	3 – 10 000	48	3 – 7
	↑	FP	$PGF_{2\alpha}$	3 – 30 000	164	3 – 7
	↑	TP	U-46619	3 – 30 000	148	3 – 7
Dog saphenous vein	↑	TP	U-46619	0.3 – 1000	2	2 – 6
	↓	DP	PGD_2	30 – 30 000	2600	1 – 2
	↓	EP_2	PGE_2	0.1 – 10 000	50	0.7 – 1.5
Dog splenic capsule	↑	TP	U-46619	10 – 10 000	208	0.3 – 0.5
	↓	?[a]	–	–	–	–

[a]Although dog splenic capsule contains inhibitory receptors, these have not as yet been characterized.
↑ Contraction.
↓ Relaxation.

be either tied or sewn to the tissue, whichever is most appropriate. One thread should be tied in a small loop by which the preparation can be anchored in an organ bath, the other should be left long for attachment to the arm of a strain gauge mounted above the bath.

(vi)   Strain gauges are most commonly isometric (allowing changes in tension but not length) or possibly isotonic (allowing changes in length but not tension).

(vii) Each preparation should be anchored in an organ bath by means of a hook (preferably glass). Organ baths should be heated (usually to $37°C$) and should contain physiological salt solutions oxygenated with 5% CO_2 in O_2.

(viii) A generally useful physiological salt solution is Krebs' solution which has the following composition (in g/l): NaCl, 6.9; KCl, 0.35; KH_2PO_4, 0.16; $MgSO_4$. $7H_2O$, 0.15; glucose, 2.0; $NaHCO_3$, 2.1 and $CaCl_2.6H_2O$, 0.28.

(ix)   In some experiments a high potassium (66 mM, dipolarizing) Krebs' solution is used. In these cases, NaCl, 3.4 g/l and KCl, 4.8 g/l are used. All other constituents are as above.

(x)   In all studies involving prostanoids on smooth muscle, it is important that endogenous prostanoid synthesis should be prevented. Failure to do so can result in problems in analysing the results obtained. Addition of indomethacin (2.8 μM) to the bathing fluid effectively eliminates any endogenous prostanoid production.

(xi)   A resting tension should be applied to the preparation when mounted in the organ bath. The same degree of tension should be maintained throughout an experiment even if this means constant re-setting. The degree of tension may either be predetermined and constant for any given tissue, or an optimal tension determined for each individual preparation. To determine optimum tension, tension/response curves are constructed at the outset of each experiment by repeating a single dose of spasmogen (e.g. K^+) on preparations exposed to increasing levels of tension. By this means, the level of tension may be determined in the presence of which the spasmogen elicits the greatest tissue response.

(xii) Agonist concentration–effect curves may be constructed in either a sequential or a cumulative fashion. The sequential method involves the administration of a range of concentrations of agonist with washout and tissue recovery between each administration and the next. The cumulative method involves the testing of the full range of concentrations of agonist with no washout or recovery between, thus a full tissue response may be built up in a stepwise fashion (see Section 4.1.1). Only at the completion of the full tissue response is there washout and tissue recovery, after which another curve to the same or a different agonist is constructed in the same manner. The advantage of the sequential method is that any effect of one concentration on another will be minimal. However the disadvantage is that unlike the cumulative method it can be extremely time-consuming. For this reason, we have always used the cumulative method and have found it to be reliable in most, if not all, preparations.

5.2.2 *Particular isolated smooth muscle preparations*

Bearing in mind the general conditions for the use of smooth muscle preparations summarized above, there follow detailed descriptions of the preparation of the tissues listed in *Tables 5* and *6*.

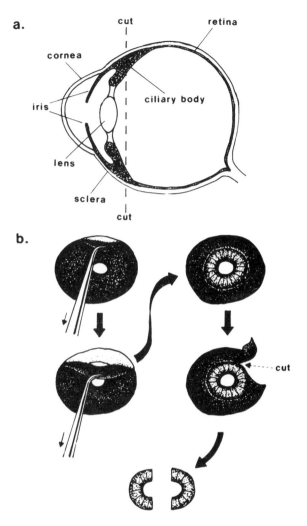

Figure 9. Preparation of the isolated iris sphincter muscle. **(a)** Section of eye showing line of cut. **(b)** Separation of iris and ciliary body from sclera, then of ciliary body from iris, and finally section of iris to form two preparations.

(i) *Dog and cat iris sphincter muscle.* Eyes may be removed from freshly killed dogs or cats; the use of barbiturate anaesthetics to kill the animals has no obvious detrimental effect on the iris preparations from them.

Iris preparations may be used fresh, or if they are not required until the following day, intact eyes may be stored in physiological salt solution at 4°C overnight; preparations are not viable if stored in this way for longer than 24 h, nor are iris preparations removed from the eye viable on storage for even this length of time.

(1)   When the preparation is required, using sharp scissors, cut through the sclera just behind the cornea to separate the anterior part from the body of the eye (see *Figure 9*).

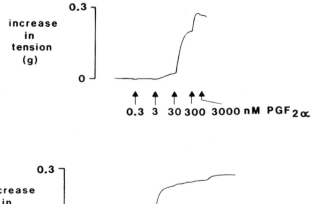

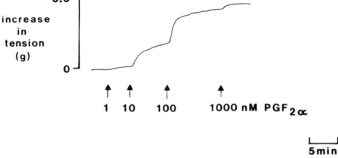

Figure 10. Typical concentration−effect curves to PGF$_{2\alpha}$ on **(a)** dog iris sphincter muscle, and **(b)** cat iris sphincter muscle. Note the more sustained nature of the contractile responses of cat iris than of dog iris.

(2) Within this anterior part lies the lens supported by its suspensory ligaments; remove this carefully but firmly by pushing it away with some blunt instrument, curved forceps are a convenient shape. Viewed from behind with the lens removed, the lining of the anterior part of the eye, the uveal tunic appears as a black ring, the centre of which is the pupil.

(3) Using curved forceps, carefully peel the lining layer away from the body of the anterior part of the eye, the cornea and surrounding ring of sclera. Remember this is a very fragile preparation and should be treated with the greatest care.

(4) Turn over the black ring of uveal tunic removed from the eye; it is clearly seen to consist of coloured iris surrounded by a black area which is ciliary body. Using sharp scissors cut away the ciliary body leaving a ring of iris (see *Figure 9*).

(5) While the iris consists of both radial and sphincter muscles, the latter is more robust and reliable for physiological use. Two sphincter muscle preparations can be obtained from each iris simply by cutting across the iris to leave two half rings.

(6) Tie the threads to each end of each half iris, and mount the iris in an organ bath. Iris preparations from both cat and dog will only contract in response to prostanoids, and these contractions must be measured isometrically; attempts at using isotonic recording methods have always been unsuccessful in our hands.

(7) Bathe the preparations in oxygenated physiological salt solution at 37°C.

(8) Use a resting tension of 0.5 g, dog iris preparations particularly will not sustain resting tensions of 1 g or greater. Preparations of cat iris are somewhat more

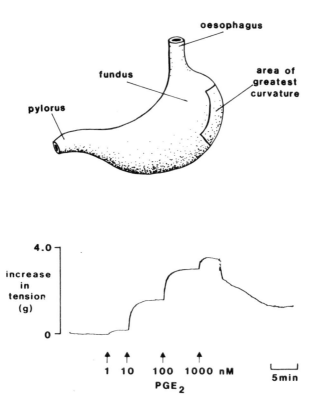

Figure 11. The fundic strip preparation and its response to PGE$_2$. (a) Typical stomach showing area of greatest curvature from which fundic strips are cut. (b) Typical concentration–effect curve to PGE$_2$ on guinea-pig fundic strip preparation.

robust than those of dog iris and they respond to prostanoids with greater, better maintained maximal contractions.

(9)   Construct concentration–effect curves in either a sequential or a cumulative dosing fashion. Typical cumulative concentration–effect curves to PGF$_{2\alpha}$ on iris sphincter preparations from both dog and cat are illustrated in *Figure 10*.

(ii) *Fundic strip preparations of guinea-pig, dog, rat and pig.* Longitudinal fundic strip preparations from the stomachs of many species are responsive to a range of prostanoids, the predominant response to which is contraction. Whole stomachs or sections of stomach fundus may be taken from animals killed either by a blow to the head followed by exsanguination (guinea-pigs, rats and young piglets 1–2 days old). Dogs and larger pigs may be killed by an overdose of barbiturate anaesthetic. Whole stomachs and sections of fundus from which all gastric contents have been washed may be stored overnight or even over two nights in physiological fluid at 4°C without detriment. The preparation of fundic strips is essentially the same for all species, and may be achieved as follows:

(1)   Cut strips of approximately 10 mm × 3 mm from the fundus along the axis of

291

the stomach from the part of greatest curvature (see *Figure 11*); by this means longitudinal muscle fibres will be obtained.

(2)   Having cut the strips, remove the gastric mucosal layer by holding one end of a strip with a pair of forceps, and using another pair to carefully pull the mucosal (inner) layer away.

(3)   When all of the mucosa has been removed, tie the cotton threads to each end of the strip and mount the preparation in an organ bath containing oxygenated physiological salt solution maintained at 37°C.

(4)   Contractions of the preparation may be measured isometrically. Impose a resting tension of 1 g on the preparation and re-set it regularly as the tissue tends to stretch and the tension falls.

Agonist concentration−effect curves can be constructed in a cumulative fashion on fundic strip preparations from all four species. A typical cumulative concentration−effect curve to PGE_2 on a fundic strip preparation from the guinea-pig is illustrated in *Figure 9*.

(iii) *Guinea-pig isolated ileum.* Like the guinea-pig isolated fundic strip preparation, the isolated longitudinal preparation of guinea-pig ileum responds to prostanoids with contraction.

(1)   Kill a guinea-pig by means of a blow to the head and exsanguination.

(2)   Open the abdominal cavity of the guinea-pig, and remove the section of ileum between approximately 15 and 25 cm from the stomach.

(3)   Cut 1 cm lengths from this section of ileum.

(4)   Sew the cotton threads to each end of each section of ileum.

(5)   Mount the resulting preparations in organ baths containing oxygenated physiological salt solution maintained at 32°C.

Contractions of the preparation may be measured either isometrically or isotonically. The use of an isotonic recording method can serve to reduce the degree of spontaneous myogenic activity should this become limiting. Where isometric recording is used, a resting tension of 1 g is used, and where isotonic recording is used, a 1 g weight is applied to the tissue. Agonist concentration−effect curves can be constructed in a cumulative fashion. A typical cumulative concentration−effect curve to PGE_2 is illustrated in *Figure 12*.

(iv) *Guinea-pig ileum circular muscle.* Circular muscle preparations of guinea-pig ileum are obtained essentially as those of longitudinal muscle except that the ileum is cut into rings of approximately 3 mm width. Cut open the rings to form strips, and at the end of each sew a cotton tie. Preparations should be mounted in organ baths containing Krebs' solution in the same way as the longitudinal preparations, except that they may be maintained at 37°C. Also, on either side of each preparation should be placed a platinum or stainless steel rod electrode.

Electrical stimulation of these preparations every 2 min with 4 sec trains of pulses of frequency 7.5 Hz, pulse width 1 msec and supramaximal voltage causes neuronally-mediated, transient contractile responses of approximately 3−4 g magnitude. Prostanoids inhibit such electrically-induced spike responses, and PGE_2 is the most potent natural

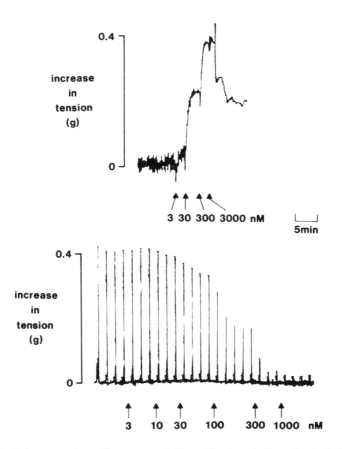

Figure 12. Typical concentration–effect curves to PGE_2 on **(a)** guinea-pig ileum (longitudinal muscle) and **(b)** electrically-stimulated guinea-pig ileum (circular muscle). Note the very much more rapid response of the longitudinal preparation to PGE_2.

agonist. Unlike longitudinal muscle preparations, circular muscle preparations of guinea-pig ileum are not contracted by prostanoids. A typical cumulative concentration–effect curve to PGE_2 is illustrated in *Figure 12*.

(v) *Isolated vascular strip preparations.* A number of vascular smooth muscle preparations are useful in terms of their responsiveness to prostanoids, including rat and rabbit aortic strips and dog saphenous vein. Aorta preparations should be removed from dead animals, while saphenous vein preparations may be removed from either dead or anaesthetized animals. Rats and rabbits are usually killed by a blow to the head followed by exsanguination. Dogs are usually anaesthetized with barbitone solution, and are killed by an overdose of sodium pentobarbitone. The smooth muscle in nearly all blood vessels is oriented circularly, around the vessel. Thus this must be taken into account when preparing isolated vascular strips. We use two different methods which are: spiral strip preparations, and isolated ring preparation. The removal of the tissue from the animal is the same in both cases and is as follows.

(1)   Firstly expose the vessel by opening up the thorax and/or abdomen (for aorta)

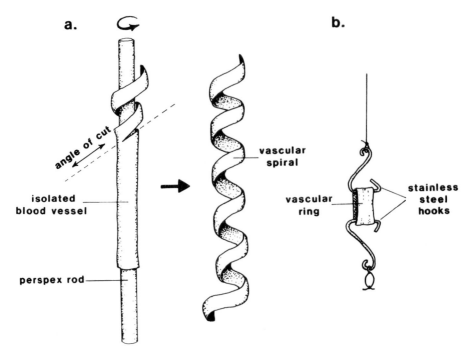

Figure 13. Vascular smooth muscle preparation. (a) Cutting a vascular spiral. (b) A vascular ring mounted on stainless steel hooks.

or by carefully cutting open the skin on the outer side of a hind limb from heel to knee (for saphenous vein).

(2)   In the case of removal of saphenous veins from anaesthetized dogs, tie off all side branches of the vein, and also tie the vein itself both proximally and distally to the section to be removed.

(3)   Using sharp scissors snip a small hole in the wall of the distal end of the section of vein to be removed, and via this hole introduce a Perspex rod into the lumen of the vessel and push it carefully up its length. The rod should be of sufficient diameter to fit fairly comfortably into the vascular lumen.

(4)   Next, dissect the vessel free from the surrounding tissue and away from the animal.

(5)   With the vessel on the Perspex rod, remove all connective tissue, to leave the tissue as clean as possible. At this stage, the tissue may be prepared either as a spiral or as isolated rings.

(6)   To cut a spiral, place one end of the Perspex rod protruding from the blood vessel into a lump of plasticene on the bench, and while rotating the rod slowly with one hand, cut the vessel with a scalpel blade at an angle of 45°, starting at the top and working down, or at the bottom and working up. This will result in the vessel being cut in a spiral fashion, leaving a long ribbon of tissue (see *Figure 13*).

(7)   Cut the ribbon into 1 cm lengths, and tie the cotton threads onto each end.

(8)   To prepare isolated rings, simply cut the vessel transversely into 3 mm lengths.

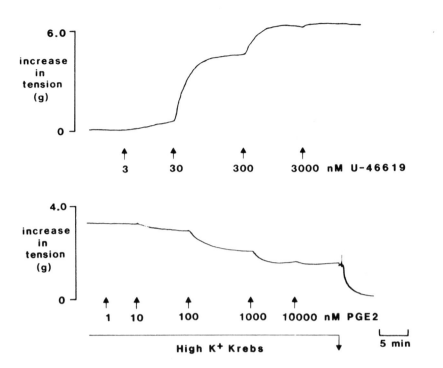

Figure 14. Dog saphenous vein preparation (spiral strip). **(a)** Contractile concentration–effect curve to U-46619. **(b)** Relaxant concentration–effect curve to PGE$_2$.

Through the lumen of each length, pass two stainless steel hooks (made of wire, gauge 25 swg, see *Figure 13*). The cotton threads should be tied to the hooks.

(9)   Mount preparations, whether spiral or ring, in organ baths containing oxygenated physiological solution maintained at 37°C.

(10) Apply resting tension of 1 g to dog saphenous vein and rabbit aorta, and of 0.5 g to rat aorta.

Both aortic preparations and dog saphenous vein are capable of responding to spasmo-gens with increases in tension of several grams. Aortas from both rat and rabbit respond to prostanoids with contractions only, while dog saphenous vein will either contract or relax, depending on the conditions of the study, and the particular prostanoid used. Prostanoid-induced contractile responses of all three vascular preparations are mediated by TP-receptors. It is important to note that many workers who have used rabbit aorta have made two observations: firstly, a proportion of preparations, while quite responsive to non-prostanoid agonists (e.g. noradrenaline and serotonin), do not respond at all to prostanoids, presumably due to a lack of functional TP-receptors, the reason for which is unknown. Secondly, the TP-receptors in rabbit aorta, and probably in the rabbit generally, appear different from those in vascular preparations from other species, par-ticularly with regard to the low potency of some types of TP-receptor blocking drugs.

In addition to receptors mediating contraction, dog saphenous vein also contains recep-tors mediating relaxation, these being predominantly E$_2$-receptors. To evaluate the

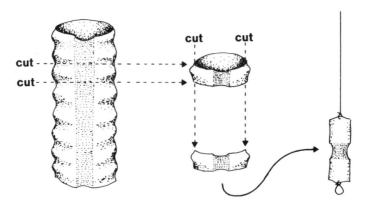

Figure 15. Preparation of the cat isolated tracheal strip.

relaxant actions of prostanoids on dog saphenous vein, the preparation should be contracted by the use of high-K^+ Krebs' solution (see Section 5.2.1). The use of high K^+ Krebs' solution results in a well-maintained contraction of the vascular smooth muscle on which cumulative relaxant concentration−effect curves can be constructed. Prostanoid-induced relaxant responses of dog saphenous vein are mediated by EP- and DP-receptors, thus PGE_2 and PGD_2 are the most potent agonists. Typical contractile and relaxant cumulative concentration−effect curves are illustrated in *Figure 14*.

(vi) *Cat trachea strip.* Lengths of trachea may be removed from either anaesthetized or dead cats, the use of barbiturate anaesthetics does not adversely affect tracheal preparations. Cat tracheal preparations may be used fresh, but appear to 'behave' better if stored over one or, better still, two nights at $4°C$; storage seems to reduce the incidence of spontaneous myogenic activity which can limit the usefulness of some preparations. Tracheas may be excised from directly below the larynx down to the tracheal bifurcation. The structure of the trachea is a series of cartilaginous rings, incomplete on the dorsal side (see *Figure 15*). The incomplete part of each ring consists of a smooth muscle connection.

(1)   To prepare cat tracheal smooth muscle, cut the trachea into individual rings, then cut away the ventral, cartilaginous portion of each ring to leave two small plates of cartilage joined by smooth muscle as shown in *Figure 15*.
(2)   Sew the cotton threads, one through each of the cartilaginous plates.
(3)   Mount this preparation in an organ bath containing oxygenated physiological salt solution maintained at $37°C$.
(4)   Apply a resting tension of 1 g to the tissue.

   Cat tracheal smooth muscle only relaxes in response to prostanoids, the receptors involved being of the EP $_2$-type, therefore preparations must be contracted by some other agent to allow relaxant responses to be measured. Both acetylcholine and carbachol contract cat trachea, carbachol being the most potent. Concentrations of approximately 50 μM acetylcholine or 0.5 μM carbachol normally produce just submaximal, well-maintained contractile response usually of between 3 and 5 g in magnitude. In the

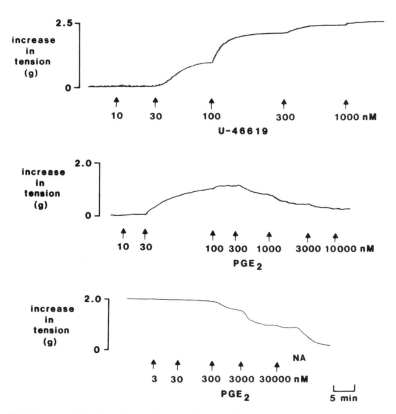

Figure 16. Guinea-pig isolated tracheal strip. Typical contractile concentration−effect curves to **(a)** U-46619 and **(b)** PGE$_2$ (note its bell-shaped nature), and relaxant concentration−effect curve to **(c)** PGE$_2$.

presence of spasmogen, prostanoids cause concentration-related relaxations, with PGE$_2$ being the most potent agonist. A typical cumulative concentration−effect curve to PGE$_2$ is illustrated in *Figure 6*.

(vii) *Guinea-pig tracheal strip.* Guinea-pig tracheal smooth muscle, unlike the same preparation from the cat, is capable of both contracting and relaxing in response to prostanoids.

The method by which the tissue is prepared is essentially the same as the cat tracheal strip preparation, except that, being substantially smaller, guinea-pig trachea is cut into sections each containing three or four cartilaginous rings, and instead of cutting away the bulk of the cartilage, it is merely cut through on the ventral side, that is opposite the smooth muscle leaving half of the cartilage attached to each end of the smooth muscle band for attachment of the cotton threads. The further preparation of guinea-pig trachea is exactly the same as that of cat trachea.

Guinea-pig trachea contains both TP- and EP$_1$-receptors mediating contraction, the most potent agonists being U-46619 and PGE$_2$. While U-46619 causes concentration-related contractile responses, PGE$_2$ gives a bell-shaped concentration−effect curve, causing contraction at lower concentrations, but relaxations at higher ones. The relaxant

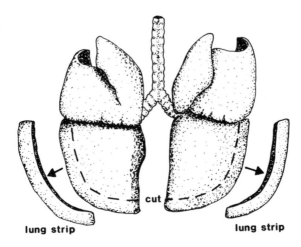

Figure 17. Guinea-pig isolated lung strip. Preparation of lung parenchymal strips from the lower lobes. Similar strips may also be prepared from the upper lobes.

responses are mediated by EP_2-receptors. In order to more effectively study PGE_2-induced inhibitory responses, guinea-pig tracheal strips can be pre-contracted by acetylcholine. Acetylcholine causes well-maintained, submaximal contraction of guinea-pig trachea, and this contraction may be partly reversed in a concentration-related fashion by PGE_2. Typical concentration−effect curves to the contractile effects of PGE_2 and U-46619, and to the relaxant effects of PGE_2, are illustrated in *Figure 16*.

(viii) Guinea-pig isolated lung strip. Guinea-pig lung strip preparations contract in response to prostanoids.

(1) Kill guinea-pigs by a blow to the head and exsanguination.

(2) Open the thoracic cavity via the ventral wall by cutting up through the rib cage and then the clavicles into the throat exposing lungs, bronchi and lower trachea.

(3) Remove the trachea and lungs as described in Section 3.1.1.

(4) Place the lungs, trachea and heart, if still attached, into physiological salt solution to rinse away any blood, then place in a Petri dish containing a small quantity of physiological salt solution and, if necessary, cut away the heart.

(5) To prepare lung strips, cut strips of about 3 mm width from the margins of the larger lung lobes (see *Figure 17*).

(6) Cut these strips into 10 mm lengths and tie the cotton threads to each end. Great care must be taken in tying the threads to the lung strip preparations as they are delicate and the threads will cut through them if they are tied too tightly. However, failure to tie a thread tightly enough will result in the preparation pulling itself from its tie during the course of the experiment.

(7) Mount the preparations in organ baths containing oxygenated physiological salt solution maintained at $37°C$. Apply a resting tension of 0.5 g to the tissue.

Guinea-pig lung strips respond to prostanoids predominantly with a contraction which is mediated by TP-receptors. However, some preparations will exhibit small relaxations

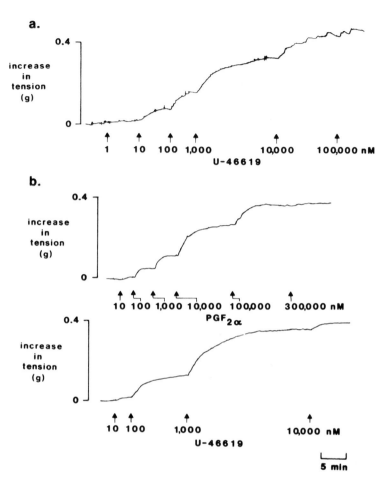

Figure 18. Typical contractile concentration−effect curves to U-46619 on **(a)** guinea-pig lung strip, and to PGF$_{2\alpha}$ and U-46619 on **(b)** dog lung strips.

to PGE$_2$ and particularly PGE$_1$, responses believed to be mediated by EP$_2$-receptors. Concentration−effect curves to the contractile actions of prostanoids can be constructed in a cumulative fashion. A typical concentration−effect curve to U-46619 is illustrated in *Figure 18*.

(ix) Cat and dog isolated lung strips. Lung strip preparations may be obtained from both dog and cat. In the case of these species, dead animals usually killed by an overdose of anaesthetic may be used. Whole lungs need not be removed, rather single lung lobes, and these may be stored overnight in physiological salt solution at 4°C without detriment. Lung strips should then be prepared exactly as for the guinea-pig, and should be mounted in organ baths containing oxygenated physiological salt solution maintained at 37°C. Apply a resting tension of 1 g to the preparations. Prostanoids will only cause contractions on dog and cat lung strips, these being mediated by both TP- and FP-

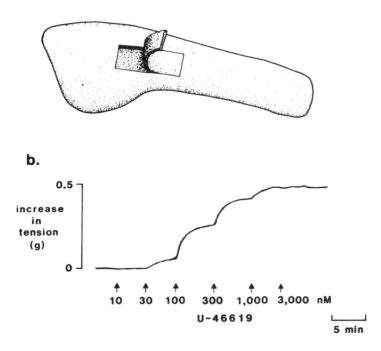

Figure 19. Dog splenic strip. (a) The preparation of a splenic strip. (b) The response of an isolated splenic strip preparation to cumulative administration of U-46619.

receptors; U-46619 and $PGF_{2\alpha}$ are approximately equipotent. Typical concentration–effect curves to $PGF_{2\alpha}$ and U-46619 on cat lung strip preparations are illustrated in *Figure 18.*

(x) Dog splenic capsule. Splenic capsular strips may be cut from spleens of dogs killed by an overdose of barbiturate anaesthetic. The strips may be cut from spleens removed from the dog or *in situ.*

(1)   Cut strips of capsular smooth muscle approximately 25 mm wide and 50 mm long from one face of the spleen, along its length, as illustrated in *Figure 19.* The capsule closely and firmly adheres to the underlying splenic tissue and may not be simply pulled away from it. It must, therefore, be cut away from the body of the spleen.

(2)   The resulting strip of splenic capsule will have a substantial amount of the underlying splenic tissue still attached to it. To remove this, place the strip, capsule downwards, on a cork board or on a gauze swab and, using curved forceps, working along the length of the strip, press down upon the splenic tissue to crush it.

(3)   When the tissue has been crushed in this way along the whole length of the strip, use the curved forceps to stroke the damaged splenic tissue away. One such treatment will *not* remove all of the splenic tissue, so the procedure should be repeated as often as is necessary to completely clear the capsular strip of all adherent tissue. It is important to remember to keep the tissue moist with the physiological salt

Table 7. Some platelet preparations containing heterogeneous prostanoid receptor populations.

Species	Response	Receptor	EC_{50} for most potent prostanoid (nM)	
Man	Aggregation	TP	160	(U-46619)
	Anti-aggregation	IP	0.65	(PGI$_2$)
		DP	29	(PGD$_2$)
Guinea-pig	Aggregation	TP	24	(U-46619)
	Anti-aggregation	IP	< 10	(PGI$_2$)
		DP	75	(PGD$_2$)
Rat	Aggregation	TP	9300	(U-46619)
	Anti-aggregation	IP	7	(PGI$_2$)
Rabbit	Aggregation	TP	930	(U-46619)
	Anti-aggregation	IP	0.7	(PGI$_2$)

solution throughout this procedure. It is also important to take the greatest care with the removal of the splenic tissue, or the capsular strip will be damaged.

(4)   When the capsular strip has been prepared, cut it into sections of about 3 mm wide and 12 mm long, and tie threads to either end of each resulting strip.

(5)   Mount the preparations in organ baths containing oxygenated Krebs' solution maintained at 37°C.

(6)   Apply a resting tension of 1 g to the tissue.

Dog splenic capsular smooth muscle responds to prostanoids predominantly with a contraction which is mediated by TP-receptors, and concentration−effect curves to the contractile actions of prostanoids can be constructed in a cumulative fashion. A typical concentration−effect curve to U-46619 is illustrated in *Figure 19*. This preparation is particularly useful when studying the biological actions of authentic TXA$_2$ as it has a very rapid response time, an important consideration when using an agonist with such a short half-life.

When in a pre-contracted state, dog splenic capsular smooth muscle will respond to some prostanoids (e.g. PGE$_1$) with relaxation. The nature of the receptors mediating this relaxation has however not yet been investigated.

5.3 **Blood platelets**

Platelet preparations from a number of species have proved useful in prostanoid receptor classification. Details of species and receptor differences are listed in *Table 7*. It is clear that all of the preparations contain heterogeneous prostanoid receptor populations.

5.3.1 *General conditions of use*

(i)   Blood may be drawn from conscious or anaesthetized animals or people.

(ii)   The blood or PRP should be used as soon after removal as possible (see Chapter 3).

(iii)   Platelet activity may be studied either by the turbidometric method using PRP or by direct platelet counting in whole blood or PRP (see Chapter 9).

(iv)   While agonist concentration−effect curves may be obtained for both the aggre-
         gatory and anti-aggregatory activities of prostanoids on blood/PRP samples, they
         are of necessity composite as only a single concentration of agonist may be
         evaluated on any one aliquot. Concentration−effect curves on any single blood
         or PRP sample therefore have to be built up from the effects of single concen-
         trations on single aliquots of the sample.

(v)   Similarly, to study the effect of any particular concentration of antagonist on
         an agonist concentration−effect curve, agonist concentration−effect curves
         should be constructed as in (iv), but both in control aliquots and in aliquots to
         which have been added known concentrations of antagonist.

(vi)   In all studies on platelets, as on smooth muscle, it is important to inhibit end-
         ogenous prostanoid synthesis. In order to achieve this, aspirin (2 mM) should
         be added to all blood/PRP samples.

(vii)   All blood should be prevented from coagulating by immediate addition of the
         anti-coagulant trisodium citrate (12.9 mM — human and guinea-pig blood, and
         8.5 mM — rabbit blood) or heparin (10 U/ml rat blood) to all blood samples
         immediately on removal from the donor.

5.3.2 *Methods of study of platelet preparations.*

(i) *Turbidometric method.* As this method is dealt with at length elsewhere in this publication it will not be described in this chapter.

(ii) *Platelet counting method.* This method has one advantage over the previous method,
and that is that whole blood may be used. There is no need, therefore, to expose the
platelets to the traumatic procedures involved in the preparation of PRP. This, however,
is probably its only clear advantage and it does have one serious drawback, and that
is the expense of the particle counter, and for this reason the method is unlikely ever
to be of any general practical use to many of those interested in the classification of
platelet prostanoid receptors. Thus this method will not be described in detail here,
but it has previously been thoroughly detailed elsewhere (see 23).

6. CONCLUDING REMARKS

The purpose of this chapter has been to provide sufficient information for potential
students of prostanoid receptors to embark upon their task. However, the information
provided is by no means comprehensive. Thus, for example, there are no doubt many
useful agonists and antagonists as well as isolated tissues which I have not included,
either because I am unaware of them or because I have not used them myself. There
is of course no reason why a worker in the area should not use any tools at his disposal,
but he must be aware of their possible limitations. Also, while I have presented a working
classification of prostanoid receptors, I do not mean to suggest that it is complete or
even necessarily wholly correct, just that it is the culmination of a considerable amount
of study in the area and is consistent with the evidence obtained to date. There is no
doubt considerable room for extension and even, if necessary, modification.

Finally, I have restricted this chapter to the pharmacological approach to receptor
classification, that is a comparison of rank orders of agonist and antagonist potency.

There is also however the increasingly popular and sometimes fruitful alternative approach of ligand binding. The reasons that I have not covered this in the present chapter are firstly, my limited experience of its use and secondly its questionable relevance to pharmacological receptors. While the first is no reason for avoiding the technique, it is important that, where possible, results obtained from such studies are supported by functional (i.e. pharmacological) data, as a cell may contain many ligand-specific binding sites unrelated to pharmacological receptors.

In conclusion, I hope that this chapter will provide the means by which to elucidate the profiles of action of prostanoid agonists and antagonists, to identify the prostanoid receptor types present in particular isolated tissues and also to attempt to extend and if necessary modify the proposed prostanoid receptor classification.

7. ACKNOWLEDGEMENTS

I would like to thank Bob Sheldrick for his substantial contribution to the development of many of the techniques described, Phil Lumley for permission to include data relating to blood platelets and Beverley Shambrook and Sandra Roe for typing the manuscript.

8. REFERENCES

1. Ash,A.S.F. and Schild,H.O. (1966) *Br. J. Pharmacol.*, **27**, 427.
2. Black,J.W., Duncan,W.A.M., Durant,G.J., Ganellin,C.R. and Parsons,M.E. (1972) *Nature*, **236**, 385.
3. Ahlquist,R.P. (1948) *Am. J. Physiol.*, **153**, 586.
4. Lands,A.M., Arnold,A., McAuliff,J.P., Luduena,F.P. and Brown,T.G. (1967) *Nature*, **214**, 597.
5. Dubocovich,M.L. and Langer,S.Z. (1974) *J. Physiol.*, **237**, 505.
6. Kennedy,I., Coleman,R.A., Humphrey,P.P.A., Levy,G.P. and Lumley,P. (1982) *Prostaglandins*, **24**, 667.
7. Kennedy,I., Coleman,R.A., Humphrey,P.P.A. and Lumley,P. (1983) In *Advances in Prostaglandin, Thromboxane and Leukotriene Research*. Samuelsson,B., Paoletti,R. and Ramwell,P.W. (eds), Raven Press, New York, Vol. 11, p. 327.
8. Coleman,R.A., Humphrey,P.P.A., Kennedy,I. and Lumley,P. (1984) *Trends Pharmacol. Sci.*, **5**, 303.
9. Coleman,R.A., Humphrey,P.P.A. and Kennedy,I. (1985) In *Trends in Autonomic Pharmacology*. Kalsner,S. (ed.), Taylor and Francis, London and Philadelphia, Vol. 3, p. 35.
10. Burnstock,G. (1978) In *Cell Membrane Receptors for Drugs and Hormones: A Multi-Disciplinary Approach*. Straub,R.W. and Bolis,L. (eds), Raven Press, New York, p. 107.
11. Coleman,R.A., Humphrey,P.P.A., Kennedy,I., Levy,G.P. and Lumley,P. (1981) *Br. J. Pharmacol.*, **73**, 773.
12. Mais,D.E., Kochel,P.J., Saussy,D.L. and Halushka,P.V. (1985) *Mol. Pharmacol.*, **28**, 163.
13. Caldwell,A.G., Harris,C.J., Stepney,R. and Whittaker,N. (1980) *J. Chem. Soc.* [Perkin I], 495.
14. Hess,H.-J., Schaaf,T.K., Bindra,J.S., Johnson,M.R. and Constantine,J.W. (1979) In *International Sulprostone Symposium*. Friebel,K., Schneider,A. and Wurfel,H. (eds), Schering, Berlin and Bergkamen, p. 29.
15. Dukes,M., Russell,W. and Walpole,A.L. (1974) *Nature*, **250**, 330.
16. Schrör,K., Darius,H., Marzky,R. and Ohlendorf,R. (1981) *Naunyn-Schmiedeberg's Arch. Pharmacol.*, **316**, 252.
17. Sanner,J.H. (1969) *Arch. Int. Pharmacodyn. Ther.*, **180**, 46.
18. Brittain,R.T., Boutal,L., Carter,M.C., Coleman,R.A., Collington,E.W., Geisow,H.P., Hallett,P., Hornby,E.J., Humphrey,P.P.A., Jack,D., Kennedy,I., Lumley,P., McCabe,P.J., Skidmore,I.F., Thomas,M. and Wallis,C.J. (1985) *Circulation*, **72**, 1208.
19. LeBreton,G.C., Venton,D.L., Enke,S.E. and Halushka,P.V. (1979) *Proc. Natl. Acad. Sci. USA*, **76**, 4097.
20. Eakins,K.E., Rajadhyaksha,V. and Schroer,R. (1976) *Br. J. Pharmacol.*, **58**, 333.
21. Bennett,A. (1974) *Prog. Drug Res.*, **8**, 83.
22. Arunlakshana,O. and Schild,H.O. (1959) *Br. J. Pharmacol. Chemother.*, **14**, 48.
23. Lumley,P. and Humphrey,P.P.A. (1981) *J. Pharmacol. Methods*, **6**, 153.

CHAPTER 17

Paf-acether (platelet-activating factor)

JACQUES BENVENISTE

1. INTRODUCTION

A substance capable of aggregating rabbit platelets was obtained in 1972 upon challenge with a specific antigen of leucocytes obtained from sensitized rabbits. It was named platelet-activating factor (PAF) (1). Later, its formation and release in appropriately challenged cells or organs has led to its acceptance as a pivotal molecule in a variety of pathophysiological conditions. More recently its molecular structure has been elucidated: 1-O-alkyl-2-acetyl-*sn*-glycero-3-phosphocholine (2,3) and total synthesis has been achieved (4) (*Figure 1*). Thus, the trivial name paf-acether was coined, emphasizing the main structural features of the molecule.

2. SYNTHESIS OF PAF-ACETHER

The procedures for obtaining paf-acether from cell types and organs that form the mediator are more or less derived from the original work (1). The prerequisites for a good yield of the mediator are the removal of platelets that, when in excess, are capable of removing the molecule from the cell suspension, and addition of bovine serum albumin (BSA) (lipid-free) as a carrier for the phosphoether lipid. It was realized recently that part of the formed mediator was not released in the extracellular medium. Hence the use of ethanol extraction (that was shown in our laboratory to be as efficient as the classical Bligh and Dyer method for lipid extraction) to obtain the cell-bound paf-acether.

2.1 The formation and release of paf-acether

The formation and release of paf-acether from human leucocytes are illustrated in *Table 1* using data from ref. 5.

2.1.1 *Preparation of cells*

Blood polymorphonuclear neutrophils are prepared as follows.

(i)   Collect 10 ml of venous blood as a mixture with 5 mM EDTA (final concentration) and dilute with 1 volume of 0.15 M NaCl and layer on 10 ml of Ficoll-Paque.

(ii)   After centrifugation (375 g, 40 min, 20°C), collect the bottom layer and dilute with two volumes of 2.5% gelatin in 0.15 M NaCl.

(iii)   After sedimentation for 30 min, remove the upper layer (devoid of erythrocytes), centrifuge (350 g, 15 min, 20°C), and wash twice in Hepes-buffered solution

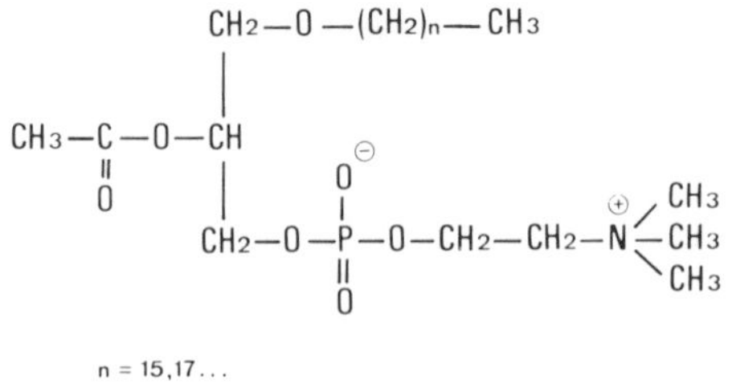

$$CH_2-O-(CH_2)_n-CH_3$$

$$CH_3-C-O-CH$$

Figure 1. Paf-acether: chemical structure

$n = 15,17\ldots$

Figure 1. Paf-acether: chemical structure

Table 1. Formation and release of paf-acether.

	p mol paf-acether
Lymphocytes	1.0 ± 0.4 (0)[a]
Monocytes	17.8 ± 1.3 (47)
Neutrophils	100.3 ± 8.3 (49)

[a]Mean $\pm$ 1 SD of five experiments (percentage of paf-acether released in supernatants.

(4.2 mM) containing (mM): 2.6 KCl, 137 NaCl, 5.6 glucose, and 0.25% BSA, pH 7.4.

(iv)   Finally, resuspend the cells in washing buffer supplemented with 1.3 mM $CaCl_2$ and 1 mM $MgCl_2$.

Human mononuclear cells can be obtained from heparinized venous blood by centrifugation on Ficoll–Triosil gradient.

(i)   Separate cells collected from the interface into adherent (monocytes) and non-adherent (lymphocytes) cells by plating 1×10^7 cells in Hank's balanced salt solution (HBSS) containing 10% fetal calf serum for 1 h at 37°C on 7 cm diameter plastic Petri dishes (Falcon Plastics, Becton Dickinson and Co., Oxnard, CA).

(ii)   Recover the non-adherent cells by washing the plates twice with cold HBSS and then centrifuge (200 g, 10 min, 4°C); the cell pellet is resuspended in HBSS.

(iii) Plate the non-adherent cells again for 1 h, recover them as described above, and finally resuspend in Hepes buffer as already described.

(iv)   Scrape the adherent cells from the plates in cold HBSS by using a rubber policeman, sediment by centrifugation (200 g, 10 min, 4°C), and resuspend in Hepes buffer.

2.1.2 Formation and release of paf-acether

Suspend lymphocytes, monocytes or neutrophils (1×10^6) in 1 ml of Hepes buffer; add ionophore A-23187 (2 μg/ml) and incubate at 37°C for 1 h.

The release of paf-acether is assessed as follows: stop the reaction by adding EDTA (2 mM final concentration); sediment the cells by centrifugation (275 g, 10 min, 4°C), and store the supernatants at −20°C until assay. For cell-associated paf-acether, the reaction is stopped by adding 4 ml of absolute ethanol to the 1 ml suspension. After 1 h centrifuge the samples (1500 g, 20 min, 20°C) and store the ethanolic supernatants at −20°C until assay.

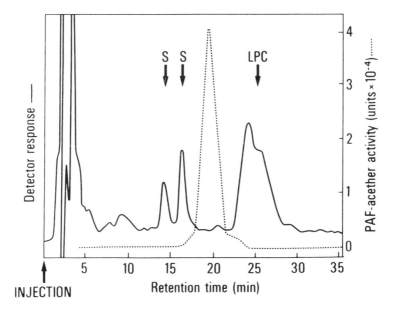

Figure 2. The h.p.l.c. illustrated was performed with a Varian-Aerograph liquid chromatograph, model 8500 (maximum operating pressure of 600 bars) (Varian USA) equipped with a differential refractometer model R 401 (Waters Associates SA, USA) and a recorder Omniscribe TM (Houston Instruments, USA). Micropak Si-5 columns, 25 cm × 6.356 mm (2 mm i.d.) or 25 cm × 12.7 mm (8 mm i.d.) were used. Samples were applied to the columns with a high pressure septum-less injector. Maximum injection volume was 35 μl. Several experiments were first carried out with a mixture of phosphatidylcholine (PC), sphingomyelin (S), and lysophosphatidylcholine (LPC) in order to establish the conditions required for obtaining a complete separation of these three phospholipids within short retention times. On 2 mm i.d. columns, efficient separations were achieved when dichloromethane/methanol/water (60:50:5, by vol) system was used at a flow-rate of 200 ml/h (100 bars). Under the latter conditions, PC exhibited a retention time of 9 min; S was eluted in two fractions (corresponding to two different populations with respect to the fatty acid composition), with retention times of 14 and 17 min, respectively; LPC started to be eluted at 22 min.

2.2 Assay and characterization of paf-acether

Precise criteria must be met before biological activity can be accepted as evidence of paf-acether (6). The substance in question should aggregate washed rabbit platelets (pretreated for 15 min with the cyclo-oxygenase inhibitor aspirin lysine salt 0.1 mM), in Tyrode's buffer containing an ADP-scavenger system (creatine phosphate 0.7 mM and creatine phosphokinase 3.9 IU/ml). The assay is performed in an aggregometer (Icare, Marseille, France), and the results are expressed in pmol paf-acether, calculated using a calibration curve established with synthetic paf-acether. In addition, the compound must migrate with synthetic paf-acether in thin layer chromatography as well as coeluting with it using high-performance liquid chromatography (*Figure 2*).

Moreover, the substance must be inactivated by phospholipases A_2 (PLA$_2$), C and D, and must exhibit a resistance to *Rhizopus arrhizus* lipase (7) (*Table 2*). Finally, the substance to be characterized should induce tachyphylaxis when cross-examined against synthetic paf-acether in washed rabbit platelets and its effect on platelets should be suppressed by the specific paf-acether antagonists (see below). Structural analysis such as mass spectrometry would, of course, provide the most persuasive evidence for the

Table 2. Action of lipases on paf-acether activity.

Lipases (concentrations/ml)		Medium	Activity (units/ml)
Lipase	(*R. arrhizus*)[a] 0.1 mg	Borate, 0.1 M pH 6.5 CaCl$_2$ 10 mM Deoxycholate, 1 mg/ml BSA, 0.4 mg/ml	148
A2	(Porcine pancreas[a] or *Crotalus*) 0.1 mg	TBS, pH 8 CaCl$_2$ 10 mM	0[c]
A2	(*Naja naja*), purified[b] 0.05 unit	TBS, pH 8 CaCl$_2$ 10 mM	0[c]
A2	(*Crotalus*), purified[b] 0.5 unit	TBS, pH 8 CaCl$_2$ 10 mM	0[c]
C	(*Bacillus cereus*)[a] 0.001 mg	TBS, pH 8 CaCl$_2$ 10 mM	0[c]
D	(cabbage)[a] 0.01 mg	Acetate buffer, 0.1 M pH 5.6 CaCl$_2$ 50 mM	0[c]
C	(*Staphylococcus aureus*)[b] Sphingomyelinase, purified 4 units	TBS, pH 8 CaCl$_2$ 10 mM MgCl$_2$ 0.25 mM	136

Experimental conditions were 15 min incubation at 37°C except for lipase from *R. arrhizus* which was incubated for 18 h at 30°C with constant agitation and phospholipase D, incubated 1 h at 20°C. These experiments were repeated five times with identical results. Paf-acether activity is expressed in units, as defined in refs 3 and 6. Starting solution of paf-acether contained 140 units/ml.
[a]From Boehringer-Mannheim.
[b]Gift from Dr Zwaal, Utrecht, The Netherlands.
[c]Same experiments done in the presence of 0.01 M EDTA: paf-acether activity was identical to that of starting solution. (From ref. 7).

presence of paf-acether, but the amount of material formed is usually too low to permit the routine use of such a procedure (8).

3. SOURCES AND METABOLISM OF PAF-ACETHER

The presence of this compound has now been reported for a wide variety of cell types including rodent peritoneal macrophages (9), alveolar macrophages (10) and polymorphonuclear cells (11). While paf-acether was first isolated from rabbit basophils (1), its detection in human basophils is still somewhat controversial. Rabbit and human platelets have also been shown to produce paf-acether. More recently, two cell types quite relevant to lung, vascular and allergic diseases were shown to synthesize and release large amounts of paf-acether: endothelial cells and eosinophils (13,14).

A series of enzymatic steps appears to be involved in the formation of paf-acether upon stimulation of various cells, namely peritoneal and alveolar macrophages, neutrophils and platelets (reviewed in 15). Through the activity of several substrates and enzymes, including acyl-CoA and acyltransferase, the substrate for phospholipase A$_2$ (PLA$_2$) is eventually formed, namely 1-alkyl-2-acyl-*sn*-glycero-3-phosphocholine, an analog of phosphatidylcholine. The PLA$_2$ is then capable of hydrolysing this pro-

Table 3. Acetyltransferase activity in human leucocytes.

Ionophore	Acetyltransferase activity (nmol paf-acether/10 min/mg protein)		
µg/ml	Lymphocytes	Monocytes	Neutrophils
0	0.5 ±0.1	4.0 ± 2.3	17.8 ± 5.3
2	0.9 ± 0.3	8.8 ± 1.3	37.5 ±4.0

duct to form 1-alkyl-2-lyso-glycero-phosphocholine (lyso paf-acether) which in turn serves as a substrate for acetyltransferase and for the formation of paf-acether. The inactivation of paf-acether depends on acetylhydrolase and acyltransferase activities. Although the overall rate of biosynthesis of both intracellular and extracellular paf-acether depends on the balance between the various anabolic and catabolic enzymes, the main topic of interest up to now has been the determination of the acetyltransferase activity (16); values for this activity in human leucocytes are shown in *Table 3*.

The acetyltransferase activity in control cells (*Table 3*) or in cells treated for 10 min at 37°C with ionophore (2 µg/ml) was measured as described in (16). The cells (1×10^7 cells in 1 ml 0.15 M NaCl) were sonicated (three pulses of 5 sec, Bronson Sonic Power Co., Danbury, CT) in an ice bath and were centrifuged (500 g, 5 min, 4°C). NaCl solution (0.15 M) was added to the resulting cell lysate to obtain about 0.6 mg of protein/ml. Protein concentrations were determined by the method of Lowry. The cell lysate (50 µl) was added to the reaction mixture (0.5 ml, pH 7.0), which contained (mM) 4.2 Hepes, 137 NaCl, 2.6 KCl, 0.65 $CaCl_2$, 0.5 $MgCl_2$ and 0.25% BSA, and the following substrates: 200 µM [^{3}H]acetyl-CoA (0.3 µCi/100 nmol) and 40 µM lyso paf-acether. The reaction was carried out for 10 min at 37°C and was then stopped by adding 1 ml of methanol containing 1-[^{14}C]palmitoyl-2-acetyl-*sn*-glycero-3-phosphocholine (1500 d.p.m.) as an internal standard. Extraction procedures were performed as described previously (16).

4. EFFECTS OF PAF-ACETHER

Since the original observation that paf-acether potently activates washed rabbit platelets, its activity has been assessed on cells (neutrophils, eosinophils) and platelets from a wide variety of species (reviewed in 17,18).

A hypotensive effect of an intravenous injection of paf-acether in rabbits, guinea pigs, baboons and rats has been reported. In fact, paf-acether is the same or a similar molecule as the anti-hypertensive polar renomedullary lipid described 25 years ago (19). In dogs paf-acether induces an acute circulatory collapse (20). When injected in isolated heart Langendorff preparations, paf-acether causes both a negative inotropic effect and a reduction in coronary flow (21). When administered intradermally to the rat or human, paf-acether induces oedema independently of platelet and neutrophil activation (22).

The presence of a specific IgE response in alveolar macrophages from asthmatic patients, resulting in the release of a lysosomal enzyme as well as paf-acether has been described (23,24). This release was not observed in alveolar macrophages obtained from theophylline- or cortico-steroid-treated patients. Intravenous or aerosol administration of paf-acether to guinea-pigs induces an immediate increase of inspiratory pressure, reflecting bronchoconstriction (25). Recently, the acute bronchomotor effect of paf-acether has been demonstrated in primates, namely the baboon (26), and *Macaca mulatta* (27), and in comatose (cerebral death) patients (28). Significant cardiac modifications, such as a severe drop in left ventricle stroke work index also occurred in the latter study. More recently, paf-acether has been suspected of increasing bronchial reactivity in the guinea-pig and in man (29,30).

5. SPECIFIC INHIBITION OF PAF-ACETHER-INDUCED PLATELET ACTIVATION

Specific binding sites for paf-acether have been detected on platelets, leucocytes and in lung (reviewed in 31). The recent demonstration that the paf-acether analogue CV 3988, and the extract of a Chinese plant Kadsurenone, are specific inhibitors of paf-acether effects and possess anti-receptor properties, is of great interest (reviewed in 31). Many other analogues and inhibitors have been described. Analogues of paf-acether devoid of agonistic activity are: SaRI 62586, SaRI 62436, SRI 63-073, Ro 18-7953, Ro 18-8736, Ro 19-1400 and Ro 19-3704. Specific inhibitors with structure not related to paf-acether include: lignans called Kadsurenone and L-652,731, triazolobenzodiazepines, WEB 2086 from Boehringer-Ingelheim, terpenoids such as BN 52021, calcium channel blocking drugs (gallopamil-diltiazem) and 48740 RP.

Using human platelet-rich plasma and washed platelets, BN 52021 activity and specificity compared with those of Kadsurenone and CV 3988 (32). Washed platelets, which were prepared so as to render them specifically sensitive either to ADP, arachidonic acid or paf-acether (2.5 nM), were inhibited by BN 52021 in a concentration-dependent manner (IC_{50}:1.6 $\pm$ 0.3 μM). Aggregations triggered by ADP or by arachidonic acid were either not or only marginally inhibited by 220 μM BN 52021. Kadsurenone affected only the paf-acether aggregation (IC_{50}:0.8 $\pm$ 0.4 μM), CV 3988 inhibited paf-acether-, arachidonic acid- and ADP-induced aggregation with IC_{50} of 1.0 $\pm$ 0.1 μM, 2.2 $\pm$ 0.1 μM and 10.2 $\pm$ 2.3 μM, respectively. Nevertheless CV 3988 is a specific anti-paf-acether compound when tested in platelet-rich plasma. In the presence of plasma, CV 3988, Kadsurenone and BN 52021 inhibited paf-acether-induced aggregation with IC_{50} of 27.6 $\pm$ 9.3 μM, 19.6 $\pm$ 10.4 μM and 3.3 $\pm$ 1.8 μM, respectively. The concentration of paf-acether necessary for inducing 50% aggregation (EC_{50}) in platelet-rich plasma was increased 5- and 47-fold with 1 μM and 5 μM BN 52021, respectively, indicating a competitive type of inhibition. As such, these paf-acether antagonists represent useful tools to explore the pathophysiological role of paf-acether. Given the potential importance of this mediator in immunopathology, they might lead to the development of new anti-allergic and anti-inflammatory drugs.

6. REFERENCES

1. Benveniste,J., Henson,P.M. and Cochrane,C.G. (1972) *J. Exp. Med.*, **136**, 1356.
2. Benveniste,J., Tencé,M., Varenne,P., Bidault,J., Boullet,C. and Polonsky,J. (1979) *C.R. Acad. Sci. Paris*, **289D**, 1037.
3. Demopoulos,C.A., Pinckard,R.N. and Hanahan,D.J. (1979) *J. Biol. Chem.*, **254**, 9355.
4. Godfroid,J.J., Heymans,F., Michel,E., Redeuilh,C., Steiner,E. and Benveniste,J. (1980) *FEBS Lett.*, **116**, 161.
5. Jouvin-Marche,E., Ninio,E., Beaurain,G., Tencé,M., Niaudet,P. and Benveniste,J. (1984) *J. Immunol.*, **133**, 892.

6. Roubin,R., Tencé,M., Mencia-Huerta,J.M., Arnoux,B., Ninio,E. and Benveniste,J. (1983) *Lymphokines.* Pick,E. (ed.), Academic Press, New York, Vol. 8, p. 249.
7. Benveniste,J., Le Couedic,J.P., Polonsky,J. and Tencé,M. (1977) *Nature*, **269**, 170.
8. Hanahan,D.J., Demopoulos,C.A., Liehr,J. and Pinckard,R.N. (1980) *J. Biol. Chem.*, **255**, 5514.
9. Mencia-Huerta,J.M. and Benveniste,J. (1979) *Eur. J. Immunol.*, **9**, 409.
10. Arnoux,B., Duval,D. and Benveniste,J. (1980) *Eur. J. Clin. Invest.*, **10**, 437.
11. Lotner,G.Z., Lynch,J.M., Betz,S.J. and Henson,P.M. (1980) *J. Immunol.*, **124**, 676.
12. Chignard,M., Le Couedic,J.P., Tencé,M., Vargaftig,B.B. and Benveniste,J. (1979) *Nature*, **279**, 799.
13. Camussi,G., Aglietta,M., Malavasi,F., Tetta,C., Piacibello,W., Sanavio,F. and Bussolino,F. (1983) *J. Immunol.*, **131**, 2397.
14. Lee,T-c., Lenihan,D.J., Malone,B., Roddy,L.L. and Wasserman,S.I. (1984) *J. Biol. Chem.*, **259**, 5526.
15. Snyder,F. (1985) *Med. Res. Rev.*, **5**, 107.
16. Ninio,E., Mencia-Huerta,J.M. and Benveniste,J. (1983) *Biochim. Biophys. Acta*, **751**, 298.
17. Vargaftig,B.B., Chignard,M., Benveniste,J., Lefort,J. and Wal,F. (1981) *Ann. N.Y. Acad. Sci.*, **370**, 119.
18. Pinckard,R.N., McManus,L.M. and Hanahan,D.J. (1982) *Advances in Inflammation Research.* Weissmann,G. (ed.), Raven Press, New York, Vol. 4, p. 147.
19. Muirhead,E.E. and Stirman,J.A. (1958) *Am. J. Pathol.*, **34**, 561.
20. Bessin,P., Bonnet,J., Apffel,D., Soulard,C., Desgroux,L., Pelas,I. and Benveniste,J. (1983) *Eur. J. Pharmacol.*, **86**, 403.
21. Benveniste,J., Boullet,C., Brink,C. and Labat,C. (1983) *Br. J. Pharmacol.*, **80**, 81.
22. Björk,J. and Smedegard,G. (1983) *Eur. J. Pharmacol.*, **96**, 87.
23. Joseph,M., Tonnel,A.B., Torpier,G., Capron,A., Arnoux,B. and Benveniste,J. (1983) *J. Clin. Invest.*, **71**, 221.
24. Arnoux,B., Simoes-Caeiro,M.H., Landes,A., Mathieu,M., Duroux,P. and Benveniste,J. (1982) *Am. Rev. Resp. Dis.*, **125**, 70.
25. Vargaftig,B.B., Lefort,J., Chignard,M. and Benveniste,J. (1980) *Eur. J. Pharmacol.*, **65**, 185.
26. Denjean,A., Arnoux,B., Masse,R., Lockhart,A. and Benveniste,J. (1983) *J. Appl. Physiol.*, **55**, 799.
27. Patterson,R. and Harris,K.E. (1983) *J. Lab. Clin. Med.*, **102**, 933.
28. Gateau,O., Arnoux,B., Deriaz,H., Viars,P. and Benveniste,J. (1984) *Am. Rev. Resp. Dis.*, **129** (4 Suppl.), A3.
29. Morley,J., Sanjar,S. and Page,C.P. (1984) *Lancet*, **II**, 1142.
30. Cuss,M., Dixon,C.M.S. and Barnes,P.J. (1986) *Lancet*, **II**, 189.
31. Braquet,P. and Snyder,F. (1986) In *Platelet-Activating Factor.* Snyder,F. (ed.), Plenum, New York.
32. Nunez,D., Chignard,M., Korth,R., Le Covedic,J.P., Norel,X., Spinnewyn,B., Braquet,P. and Benveniste,J. (1986) *Eur. J. Pharmacol.*, **123**, 197.

Eicosanoids: structure, availability, storage and stability

SANTOSH NIGAM

Table 1.

Eicosanoid	Formula	Mol. wt	Available as/in	Storage	Stability	Commercially available from[a]
Arachidonic acid		272.2	10 mg/ml in ethanol (98%)	4°C	no data available	Cayman
PGA_1		336.6	crystalline solid light yellow (99%)	4°C	at least for 6 months	Upjohn Seragen Cayman
PGA_2		334.5	colourless oil (99%)	4°C	expected to be comparable with PGA_1	Upjohn Seragen Cayman
PGB_1		336.6	white crystalline powder (99%)	4°C	at least for 6 months	Upjohn Seragen Cayman
PGB_2		334.5	colourless oil at room temperature (99%)	4°C	no data available expected to be as PGB_1	Upjohn Seragen Cayman
PGD_2		337.6	white, crystalline power (>99%)	4°C	no data available	Upjohn Seragen Cayman
PGE_1		354.5	light yellow to white needles (99%)	4°C	for 2 years at 4°C	Upjohn Seragen Cayman
PGE_2		352.5	light yellow to white needles (99%)	4°C	for 2 years at 4°C	Upjohn Seragen Cayman
$PGF_{1\alpha}$		356.5	white, crystalline solid (99%)	4°C	no data available	Upjohn Seragen
$PGF_{2\alpha}$ -free acid		413.6	white, crystalline solid (99%)	4°C	no data available	Seragen Cayman Ultrafine
-trimethamine		475.6	crystalline solid (>99%)	4°C	1 year at room temperature	Upjohn Cayman NEN

313

Table 1 contd.

Eicosanoid	Formula	Mol.wt	Available as/in	Storage	Stability	Commercially available from[a]
11-PGF$_{2\alpha}$		413.6	white, crystalline solid (99%)	4°C	no data available	Cayman
PGG$_2$		427.6	50 μg/ml in hexane, ethylacetate, HOAc 1%	−78°C	no data available	Cayman
PGH$_2$		411.6	50 μg/ml in pentane, ethylacetate, HOAc 1%	−78°C	no data available	Cayman
PGI$_2$ sodium salt		367.8	white, crystalline powder (99%)	4°C	no data available	Cayman Upjohn Seragen
13,14-dihydro-15-keto-PGA$_2$		337.5	colourless, viscous oil (98%)	4°C	no data available	Cayman
13,14-dihydro-15-keto-PGD$_2$		338.5	colourless, viscous oil (99%)	−78°C	no data available	Cayman
6-keto-PGE$_1$		368.7	white crystalline powder (99%)	4°C	no data available	Upjohn Cayman
15-keto-PGE$_2$		351.6	white granular crystals (99%)	4°C	no data available	Cayman
13,14-dihydro-15-keto-PGE$_2$		352	light, yellow viscous oil (98%)	−78°C	no data available	Upjohn Seragen Cayman
11-deoxy-13,14-dihydro-15-keto-11β-16δ-cyclo-PGE$_2$ (mixture of isomers)		322	waxy solid to viscous yellow oil	4°C	no data available	Cayman
16,16-dimethyl PGE$_2$		372.5	(a) 2.2 mg/ml in triacetin (b) yellow solid (unstable to heat, oxygen and moisture)	−78°C	no data available	Upjohn Cayman
6-keto-PGF$_{1\alpha}$		370.5	white crystalline powder (>99%)	−10°C 20°C	no data available	Upjohn Seragen Cayman NEN
6,15-diketo-PGF$_{1\alpha}$		369.5	colourless viscous oil (99%)	4°C	no data available	Cayman
15-keto-PGF$_{2\alpha}$		412.6	light yellow viscous oil (99%)	4°C	no data available	Cayman

Table 1 contd.

Eicosanoid	Formula	Mol.wt	Available as/in	Storage	Stability	Commercially available from[a]
13,14-dihydro-15-keto-PGF$_{2\alpha}$		414.6	light yellow viscous oil (99%)	$-20°C$	no data available	Upjohn Cayman Seragen
9,11-dideoxy-9α, 11α-methano-epoxy-PGF$_{2\alpha}$		409.6	light yellow viscous oil (99%)	$4°C$	no data available	Upjohn Cayman
9,11-dideoxy 9α, 11α-epoxy-methano-PGF$_{2\alpha}$		409.6	light yellow viscous oil (99%)	$4°C$	no data available	Upjohn Cayman
LTA$_4$ (methylester)		334.2	solution in 98:2 hexane/triethylamine 1 mg/ml (97%)	$-78°C$	3 months at $-20°C$	Cayman Upjohn Ultrafine
LTB$_4$		336.2	absolute ethanol 5 μg/ml (98%)	$-78°C$	3 months at $-20°C$	Cayman Upjohn Ultrafine
20-hydroxy-LT-B$_4$		352.6	50 μg/ml ethanol	$-78°C$	3 months at $-20°C$	Cayman
20-carboxy-LTB$_4$		354.6	50 μg/ml ethanol	$-78°C$	3 months $-20°C$	Cayman
LTC$_4$		628.8	phosphate-buffered saline (97%)	$-78°C$	3 months at $-20°C$	Ultrafine Cayman Upjohn
LTD$_4$		496.7	phosphate-buffered saline (97%)	$-78°C$	3 months at $-20°C$	Cayman Upjohn Ultrafine
LTE$_4$		439	phosphate-buffered saline (99%)	$-78°C$	3 months at $-20°C$	Cayman Upjohn Ultrafine
LTF$_4$		613	phosphate-buffered saline (99%)	$-78°C$	3 months at $-20°C$	Cayman Ultrafine
N-acetyl-LTE$_4$		449	50 μg/ml ethanol	$-78°C$	3 months at $-20°C$	Cayman

Table 2.

HETEs	Formula	Mol.wt	Available as/in	Storage	Stability	Commercially available from[a]
5-HETE		320.4	5 mg/ml absolute ethanol (99%)	−20°C	for 3 months	Cayman NEN Seragen
12-HETE		320.4	5 mg/ml absolute ethanol (99%)	−20°C	for 3 months	Cayman NEN Seragen
15-HETE		320.4	5 mg/ml absolute ethanol (99%)	−20°C	for 3 months	Cayman NEN Seragen
5-HETE (methyl ester)		334.4	5 mg/ml absolute ethanol (99%)	−20°C	for 3 months	Cayman
12-HHT		324.4	5 mg/ml absolute ethanol (99%)	−20°C	for 3 months	Cayman
5,6-EET		283.4	0.1 mg/ml in 98:2 hexane/ triethylamine	−20°C	for 3 months	Cayman
8-HETE (hydroxy-5,9,11,14-eicosaenoic acid)		320.4	50 μg/ml ethanol	−20°C	for 3 months	Cayman
9-HETE (9-hydroxy-5,7,11,13 eicosatetraenoic acid)		319.4	50 μg/ml ethanol	−20°C	for 3 months at −20°C	Cayman
11-HETE (11-hydroxy-5,8,12,14 eicosatetraenoic acid)		319.4	50 μg/ml ethanol	−20°C	for 3 months at −20°C	Cayman
5-HETE (5-hydroperoxy-6,8,11,14, eicosatetraenoic acid)		335.4	50 μg/ml 987:12:1 hexane/ isopropanol/ acetic acid	−20°C	for 3 months at −20°C	Cayman
12-HPETE		304.3	50 μg/ml 987:12:1 hexane/ isopropanol/ acetic acid	−20°C	for 3 months at −20°C	Cayman
15-HPETE		302.3	50 μg/ml 980:24:1 hexane/ isopropanol/ acetic acid	−20°C	for 3 months at −20°C	Cayman
5,6-DHETE		335.4	50 μg/ml ethanol	−20°C	for 3 months at −20°C	Cayman
5,12-DHETE		335.4	50 μg/ml ethanol	−20°C	for 3 months at −20°C	Cayman
5,15-DHETE		335.4	50 μg/ml ethanol	−20°C	for 3 months at −20°C	Cayman

Table 2 contd.

HETEs	Formula	Mol. wt	Available as/in	Storage	Stability	Commercially available from[a]
8,15-DHETE		335.4	50 μg/ml ethanol	−78°C	for 2 months at −78°C	Cayman
EPA Eicosapentaenoic Acid		270.2	10 mg/ml in ethanol (98%)	−78°C	for 2 months at −78°C	Cayman
5,6 ETE		303.2	1 mg/ml in 98:2 hexane/ triethylamine	−20°C	for 3 months at −20°C	Cayman
14,15-EPETE		303.2	95−98% hexane 2% triethylamine	−78°C	for 3 months at −20°C	Cayman
14,15-DHETE		335.4	50 μg/ml ethanol	−20°C	for 3 months at −20°C	Cayman

Table 3.

Thromboxane	Formula	Mol. wt	Available as/in	Storage	Stability	Commercially available from[a]
TXB$_2$		370.5	white crystalline powder (99%)	the powder: −10°C to −20°C solution: 4°C or below	at least for 4 weeks	Cayman Upjohn Seragen
11-keto-TXB$_2$		369.5	colourless, viscous oil (99%)		at least for 4 weeks	Cayman
Pinane-TXA$_a$		333.5	0.275 mg/ml absolute ethanol (99%)	the powder: −10°C to −20°C solution: 4°C or below	at least for 4 weeks	Cayman
Carbocyclic-TXA$_2$		346.5	50 μg/ml ethanol	the powder: −10°C to −20°C solution: 4°C or below	at least for 4 weeks	Cayman

317

Table 4.

PAF	Formula	Mol.wt	Available as/in	Storage	Stability	Commercially available from[a]
C$_{16}$	CH$_2$–O–(CH$_2$)$_{15}$–CH$_3$ CH$_3$CO–C–H CH$_2$–O–P–O–(CH$_2$)$_2$–N–(CH$_3$)$_3$ O$^-$	523.7	white powder, soluble in ethanol (70%)	$-20°C$	powder: stable, the solution for 4 weeks	BACHEM
C$_{18}$	CH$_2$–O–(CH$_2$)$_{17}$–CH$_3$ CH$_3$CO–C–H CH$_2$–O–P–O–(CH$_2$)$_2$–N–(CH$_3$)$_3$ O$^-$	551.8	white powder, soluble in ethanol (70%)	$-20°C$	powder: stable, the solution for 4 weeks	BACHEM
Enantio-PAF (C$_{16}$)	CH$_2$–O–P–O–(CH$_2$)$_2$–N–(CH$_3$)$_3$ HO–C–H O$^-$ CH$_2$–O–(CH$_2$)$_{15}$–CH$_3$	523.7	white powder, soluble in ethanol (70%)	$-20°C$	powder: stable, the solution for 4 weeks	BACHEM
rac-PAF (C$_{16}$)	CH$_2$–O–(CH$_2$)$_{15}$–CH$_3$ H–C–OH CH$_2$–O–P–O–(CH$_2$)$_2$–N–(CH$_3$)$_3$ O$^-$	523.7	white powder, soluble in ethanol (70%)	$-20°C$	powder: stable, the solution for 4 weeks	BACHEM
Lyso-PAF (C$_{16}$)	CH$_2$–O–(CH$_2$)$_{15}$–CH$_3$ HO–C–H CH$_2$–O–P–O–(CH$_2$)$_2$–N–(CH$_3$)$_3$ O$^-$	481.7	white powder, soluble in ethanol (70%)	$-20°C$	powder: stable, the solution for 4 weeks	BACHEM
Lyso-PAF (C$_{18}$)	CH$_2$–O–(CH$_2$)$_{17}$–CH$_3$ HO–C–H CH$_2$–O–P–O–(CH$_2$)$_2$–N–(CH$_3$)$_3$ O$^-$	509.8	white powder, soluble in ethanol (70%)	$-20°C$	powder: stable, the solution for 4 weeks	BACHEM
Enantio-lyso-PAF (C$_{16}$)	CH$_2$–O–P–O–(CH$_2$)$_2$–N–(CH$_3$)$_3$ CH$_3$CO–C–H O$^-$ CH$_2$–O–(CH$_2$)$_{15}$–CH$_3$	481.7	white powder, soluble in ethanol (70%)	$-20°C$	powder: stable, the solution for 4 weeks	BACHEM
rac-Lyso-PAF (C$_{16}$)	CH$_2$–O–(CH$_2$)$_{15}$–CH$_3$ H–C–CH$_3$CO CH$_2$–O–P–O–(CH$_2$)$_2$–N–(CH$_3$)$_3$ O$^-$	481.7	white powder, soluble in ethanol (70%)	$-20°C$	powder: stable, the solution for 4 weeks	BACHEM
Dehydro-PAF (C$_{18}$)	CH$_2$–O–(CH$_2$)$_8$–CH=CH–(CH$_2$)$_7$–CH$_3$ CH$_3$CO–C–OH CH$_2$–O–P–O–(CH$_2$)$_2$–N–(CH$_3$)$_3$ O$^-$	521.6	white powder, soluble in ethanol (70%)	$-20°C$	powder: stable, the solution for 4 weeks	BACHEM

Table 5.

Antisera Sera	Commercially available from[a]
PGA$_1$	Seragen, Institut Pasteur
PGB$_1$	Seragen, Institut Pasteur
PGD$_2$	Seragen
PGE$_1$	Institut Pasteur
PGE$_2$	Seragen, Cayman, Institut Pasteur
PGF$_{1\alpha}$	Institut Pasteur
PGF$_{2\alpha}$	Seragen, Cayman, Institut Pasteur
13, 14-Dihydro-15-keto- PGE$_2$	Institut Pasteur

Table 5 contd.

Antisera Sera	Commercially available from[a]
6-keto-PGF$_{1\alpha}$	Seragen, Cayman
15-keto-PGF$_{2\alpha}$	Cayman
13, 14-dihydro-15-keto-PGF$_{2\alpha}$	Seragen, Cayman, Institut Pasteur
TXB$_2$	Seragen, Cayman, Institut Pasteur
5-HETE	Seragen
12-HETE	Seragen
15-HETE	Seragen

Table 6.

Radioimmunoassay kits	Commercially available from[a]
^{3}H-Kits	
PGD$_2$	Seragen
PGE$_1$	Seragen
PGE$_2$	
PGF$_{2\alpha}$	Seragen, Amersham, NEN
11-deoxy-13, 14-dehydro-15-keto-11β, 16δ-cyclo-PGE$_2$	Amersham
6-keto-PGF$_{1\alpha}$	Seragen, Amersham, NEN
13, 14-dihydro-15-keto-PGF$_{2\alpha}$	Seragen
TXB$_2$	Seragen, Amersham, NEN
LTB$_4$	Amersham
LTC$_4$	NEN
5-HETE	
12-HETE	Seragen
15-HETE	
^{125}I-Kits	
PGE$_2$	Seragen, NEN
PGF$_{2\alpha}$	Seragen
6-keto-PGF$_{1\alpha}$	Seragen, NEN
TXB$_2$	Seragen, NEN

Enzyme immunoassay kits

PGD$_2$	
PGF$_{2\alpha}$	Laboratoire des
6-keto-PGF$_{1\alpha}$	Stallergenes
TXB$_2$	

[a]Addresses
Upjohn Diagnostics, Kalamazoo, MI 49001, USA
Cayman Chemical, 2280 Peters Road, Ann Arbor, MI 48103, USA
Bachem Chemikalien, Hauptstr. 44, CH-4416 Bubendorf, Switzerland
Ultrafine Chemical, Chemistry Tower, University of Salford, Salford M5 4WT, UK
Seragen Inc., 54, Clayton Street, Boston, MA 02122, USA
Amersham International, White Lion Road, Amersham, Buckinghamshire HP7 9LL, UK
NEN Research Products, 6072 Dreieich, FRG
Institut Pasteur, 3 Bd. Raymond Poincaré, BP3-92430 Marnes la Coquette, France
Laboratoire des Stallergenes, 7, Alleé des Platanes, 24264 Fresnes Cedex, France

INDEX

Acetylsalicylate,
  cyclo-oxygenase inhibitor, 235
Aggregometry,
  basic principles, 151−155
  lipoxygenase products, 164
  platelet aggregation, 153
  species sensitivity, 159
  thromboxane A_2, 164
  whole blood, 155
Agonists,
  prostanoid receptor, 164
  standard, use in classifying receptors,
    269
  synthetic, 271−274
Antagonists,
  of paf-acether, 310
  prostanoid receptor, 163
  thromboxane receptor, 164
  use of receptor classification, 275
Arachidonic acid,
  availability, 310
  extraction of lipids containing, 266
  gas-liquid chromatography by capillary
    column, 267
  gas-liquid chromatography by packed
    column, 263
  methyl esters for gas chromatography,
    262
  quantitative measurement in tissues and
    fluids, 259
  stability, 310
  structure, 310
  substrate for cyclo-oxygenase, 224
  thin-layer chromatography of lipids
    containing, 260
  use of internal standard in measurement,
    260
Argentation h.p.l.c.,
  applications, 85
  mechanism, 83, 84
  separation of isotopically labelled from
    unlabelled eicosanoids, 85
Ascorbate,
  -iron dependent lipid peroxidation, 247
Autoradiography,
  of thin-layer chromatograms, 72
Availability,
  of eicosanoids and related compounds,
    313−318

Bioassay,
  of eicosanoids, 143−150
  of inhibitory prostanoids, 161

  of leukotrienes, 144, 146
  of prostaglandins, 145
  of thromboxanes, 146
  sensitivity, 145
  slow-reacting substances, 146
  tissues used, 144
Blood,
  enzyme immunoassay of eicosanoids,
    203, 207
  radioimmunoassay of eicosanoids, 191
  sampling and storage procedures, 29
  whole, aggregometry, 155
Bovine,
  coronary artery in eicosanoid bioassay,
    144
BW 755C,
  cyclo-oxygenase pathway inhibitor, 235
  lipoxygenase inhibitor, 235
Carbocyclin,
  stable prostacyclin mimetic, 159
Cat,
  iris in receptor classification, 286, 291
  lung in receptor classification, 286, 291
  trachea in receptor classification, 286,
    291
Chemical detection,
  in thin-layer chromatography, 60
Chick rectum,
  in eicosanoid bioassay, 144
Cyclo-oxygenase,
  absorbance spectrum, 218
  fatty acid substrates, 224
  haem requirement, 218
  hydroperoxide initiator, 200
  inhibitor interactions, 224
  measurement, 209
  oxygen electrode assay, 210
  pathway of arachidonic acid metabolism,
    4, 6
  properties, 217
  purification, 215
  radioisotope assay, 214
  size and sub-unit composition, 217
  spectrophotometric assay, 215
Cytochrome P-450,
  discrimination from lipoxygenase, 234
  NADPH-cytochrome P-450 reductase
    and lipid peroxidation, 246
Diene conjugation,
  measurement of lipid peroxidation, 255
13,14-Dihydro-15-keto-metabolites,
  availability, 314, 315
  enzyme immunoassay, 199

321